OXFORD MEDICAL PUBLICATIONS

GADDUM'S PHARMACOLOGY

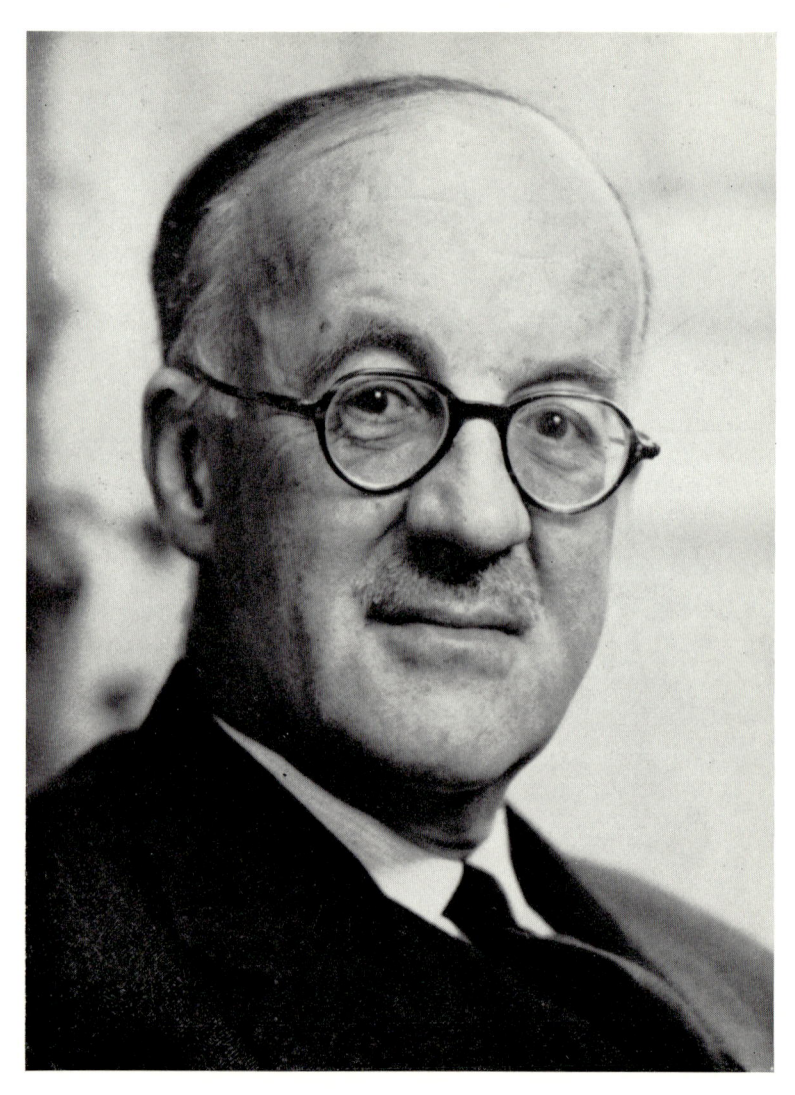

SIR JOHN GADDUM, F.R.S.

GADDUM'S PHARMACOLOGY

SEVENTH EDITION

REVISED BY

A. S. V. BURGEN, M.D., F.R.C.P., F.R.S.

Director, National Institute for Medical Research, Mill Hill
Formerly Sheild Professor of Pharmacology, University of Cambridge

AND

J. F. MITCHELL, M.A., B.Sc., Ph.D.

Professor of Pharmacology, University of Bristol

LONDON
OXFORD UNIVERSITY PRESS
NEW YORK   TORONTO
1972

Oxford University Press, Ely House, London W. 1

GLASGOW NEW YORK TORONTO MELBOURNE WELLINGTON
CAPE TOWN IBADAN NAIROBI DAR-ES-SALAAM LUSAKA ADDIS ABABA
DELHI BOMBAY CALCUTTA MADRAS KARACHI LAHORE DACCA
KUALA LUMPUR SINGAPORE HONG KONG TOKYO

ISBN 0 19 261113 5

© OXFORD UNIVERSITY PRESS 1959, 1968, 1972

FIRST EDITION 1940
SEVENTH EDITION 1972

All rights reserved. No part of this publication may be reproduced, stored in a retrieval system, or transmitted, in any form or by any means, electronic, mechanical, photocopying, recording, or otherwise, without the prior permission of Oxford University Press

For copyright reasons this book may not be issued on loan or otherwise except in its original soft cover

PRINTED IN GREAT BRITAIN
AT THE UNIVERSITY PRESS, OXFORD
BY VIVIAN RIDLER
PRINTER TO THE UNIVERSITY

CONTENTS

1. **GENERAL PHARMACOLOGY**   1
   Principles of drug action—antagonists—receptors—distribution and absorption of drugs—metabolism—excretion.

2. **CENTRAL NERVOUS SYSTEM DEPRESSANTS I**   15
   Experimental methods—general anaesthesia—theories of anaesthesia—signs of anaesthesia—premedication—volatile and gaseous anaesthetics—anaesthetic solutions.

3. **CENTRAL NERVOUS SYSTEM DEPRESSANTS II**   25
   Hypnotics and sedatives—anticonvulsants—tranquillizers—analgesics.

4. **CENTRAL NERVOUS SYSTEM STIMULANTS**   39
   Antidepressants—convulsants—analeptics—hallucinogens.

5. **LOCAL ANAESTHETICS**   49
   Mode of action—individual local anaesthetics.

6. **CHOLINERGIC SYSTEM**   54
   Methods of studying cholinergic system—nicotinic receptors—muscarinic receptors—mixed receptor sites—individual cholinergic drugs and their antagonists.

7. **ADRENERGIC SYSTEM**   78
   Catecholamine synthesis—storage and metabolism—release and block of release—sympathomimetic substances—α and β antagonists.

8. **SMOOTH MUSCLE**   92
   Histamine—antihistamines—serotonin—peptides—ergot—prostaglandins—slow reacting substance—xanthines.

9. **CIRCULATION**   101
   Circulatory homeostasis—sympathomimetics—hypotensives—anti-anginal drugs—cardiac glycosides—antiarrhythmics.

10. **BODY TEMPERATURE AND THE ANTIPYRETIC—ANALGESICS**   112
    Body temperature control.

11. **ALIMENTARY CANAL**   117
    Gastric secretion—antacids—vomiting—bile—purgatives—protectives—demulcents—astringents.

12. **VITAMINS**   125
    Water-soluble vitamins—fat-soluble vitamins.

13. BLOOD — 135
   Iron—cobalamins—folic acid—anticoagulants—heparin—coumarols.

14. HORMONES — 142
   The pituitary—the thyroid—the parathyroids—the pancreas—the adrenal steroids—the sex hormones.

15. RENAL PHARMACOLOGY — 168
   Diuretics—uricosurics—drugs altering urine pH.

16. CHEMOTHERAPY I: BACTERIA, FUNGI, VIRUSES — 177
   Historical—principles of chemotherapeutic action—resistance—chemotherapeutic spectra—individual antibacterial agents—antifungal and antiviral agents—antiseptics.

17. CHEMOTHERAPY II: PROTOZOA AND WORMS — 195
   Malaria—amoebic dysentery—leishmania—trypanosomes—helminthes.

18. CHEMOTHERAPY III: CANCER — 205
   General principles of cancer chemotherapy—drugs used in the chemotherapy of cancer.

19. QUANTITATIVE AND HUMAN PHARMACOLOGY — 211
   Bioassay—development of new drugs—drug toxicity.

ADDITIONAL GENERAL READING IN PHARMACOLOGY — 228

UNITS OF MEASUREMENT — 229

AQUEOUS SOLUTIONS — 230

INDEX OF CHEMICAL RINGS — 231

INDEX — 233

PREFACE TO THE SEVENTH EDITION

Our objectives in the sixth edition were to provide within a manageable compass a survey of modern pharmacology, suitable as an introductory text for students of medicine, pharmacy, and science. The enthusiasm with which it has been received suggests that on the whole we have hit the target. In the present edition the main change is an expansion of the section on chemotherapy, otherwise we have revised the text to accommodate new drugs and new ideas that have come to the fore since the last edition.

A. S. V. B.
J. F. M.

University Department of Pharmacology
Cambridge
August 1971

1

GENERAL PHARMACOLOGY

Drugs are chemical substances which, by interacting with biological systems, change their behaviour. In complex organisms the nervous system is so important that we will find that many drugs act on synaptic areas either in the central nervous system or in autonomic or somatic nerves, others act on peripheral structures directly affecting contraction of muscles, or secretion, yet others affect the growth and development or metabolism of tissues or invading organisms. The fact that drugs have different actions means that they have selectivity in the structures and systems with which they react; only rarely is this selectivity so high that it may be termed specific, much more often drugs have more than one action and we are then inclined to talk of a main action (i.e. that to be used pharmacologically or therapeutically) and side actions (those that are undesired in the particular application). This division is quite arbitrary and may just serve the needs of the moment. For instance, when morphine is used as an analgesic we may deprecate the constipation it causes by an action on the intestine, but this same intestinal action may be made use of therapeutically in diarrhoea. In the following section we will explore the quantitative nature of drug action and some of the factors responsible for selective action.

The basic phenomena of drug actions are most easily investigated on isolated systems of which one of the simplest is the intestine. If a short piece of small intestine is placed in a warm oxygenated salt solution whose compositiod is similar to that of blood plasma it will survive and respond to suitable drugs for long periods. Magnus was the first to use such a preparation for studying the action of drugs on the longitudinal muscle of the gut [Fig. 1.1].

In vivo this muscle layer contracts when acetylcholine is released from the terminals of the cholinergic nerves originating in the myenteric plexus and we may produce a similar response by adding acetylcholine to the bath in which the intestine is immersed. The longitudinal muscle contracts within a few seconds and if the bath fluid is replaced by fresh medium the muscle equally rapidly relaxes back to its original length. If the concentration of acetylcholine is reduced the response will usually be smaller and by systematically studying the effect of dose of the drug we can build up a dose–response curve from which we can see that very small doses produce no response, larger doses a graded increase in response until finally a maximum is produced and further increase in dose produces no greater effect. This is the usual behaviour of drugs—the intensity of the response is proportional to the amount of drug used.

Acetylcholine is the natural excitant agent for this muscle but we must not assume that this chemical structure is uniquely effective; we can explore whether this is so by making chemical alterations in the molecule and seeing if activity is retained. The simplest and most satisfactory way of investigating this is by a homologous series. To do this we prepare a series of compounds based on the original drug in which a particular chemical group is modified by the addition or removal of carbon atoms. We may do this in the present case by preparing esters of choline with the series of aliphatic acids—formic, acetic, propionic, butyric, valeric [Fig. 1.3]. In Figure 1.2 it is seen that propionylcholine also causes contraction of the longitudinal muscle of the ileum and can produce the same maximum response as acetylcholine but to produce

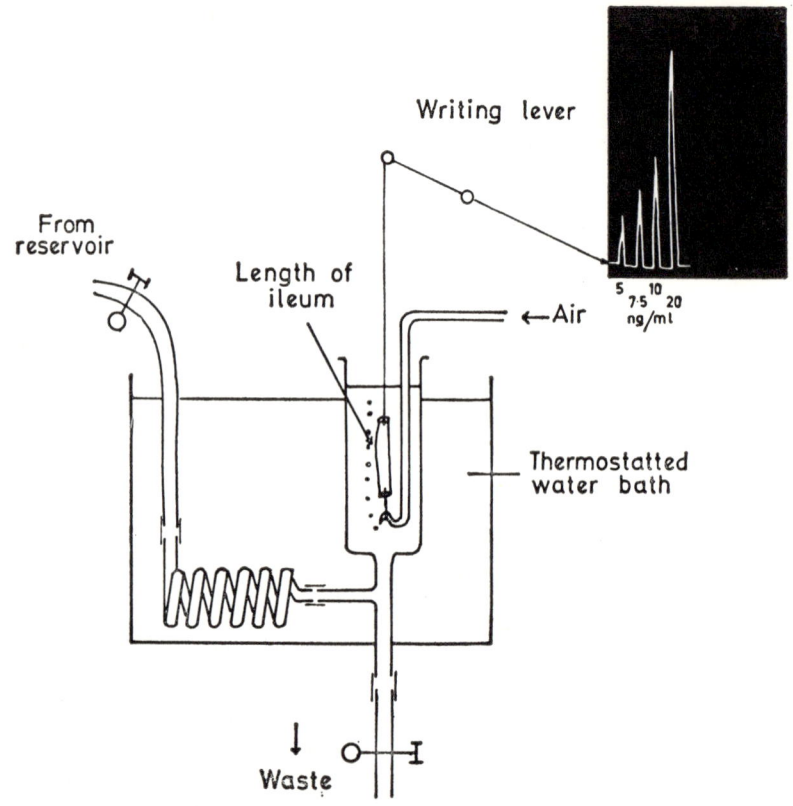

FIG. 1.1. Arrangements for recording the contractions of the longitudinal muscle of the small intestine. The water bath is usually kept at about 35° C.

any particular extent of contraction about twenty times the amount of propionylcholine is needed compared with that of acetylcholine. Whenever a comparison of activities that are in a constant ratio is to be made, the result becomes very much clearer if it is plotted with concentrations converted to their logarithms or alternatively the scale of doses is made logarithmic. This is because the logarithmic operator has the property of turning multiplication into addition. In FIGURE 1.2 it can be seen that the log dose–response curve of acetylcholine is now S-shaped and that the middle section of the curve is very nearly straight. The curve for propionylcholine is identical in shape but displaced to the right. It is now obvious that the response to propionylcholine is similar to that of acetylcholine but weaker. Log dose–response curves are almost universally used for plotting the results of pharmacological measurements for three main reasons:

1. Similar substances give parallel curves so that potency is easy to measure.
2. If only the middle response range is used, a straight line provides a reasonable fit for the data; this is very useful when only two or three points have been obtained.
3. A logarithmic scale gives equal weighting to all dose levels and allows a wide range

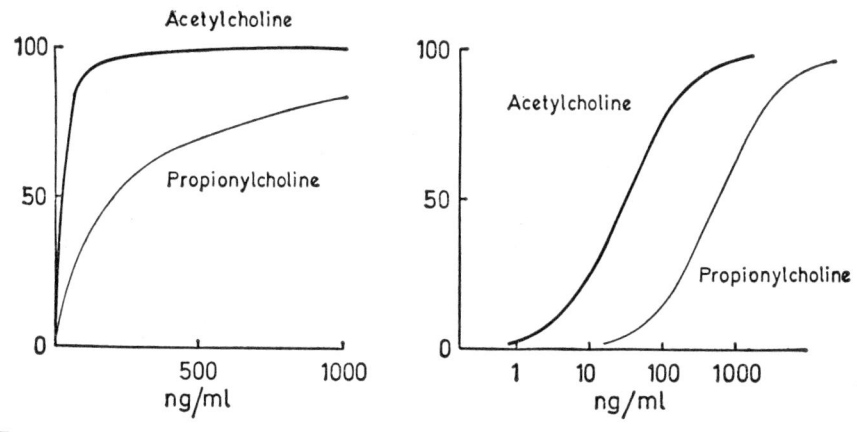

FIG. 1.2. Dose–response curves obtained on the guinea-pig ileum. The abscissa shows the contraction as a percentage of the maximum obtainable. In the left-hand graph the dose of drug is shown on a *linear* scale; in the right-hand graph on a *logarithmic* scale.

of doses to be plotted in a single graph without undue compression of any values.

$$CH_3-COO-CH_2-CH_2-\overset{+}{N}{\diagdown}_{CH_3}^{CH_3}{\diagup}^{CH_3}$$
Acetylcholine

$$H-COO-CH_2-CH_2-\overset{+}{N}{\diagdown}_{CH_3}^{CH_3}{\diagup}^{CH_3}$$
Formylcholine

$$CH_3-CH_2-COO-CH_2-CH_2-\overset{+}{N}{\diagdown}_{CH_3}^{CH_3}{\diagup}^{CH_3}$$
Propionylcholine

FIG. 1.3

Continuing with our homologous series we find that butyrylcholine is even less active and that the maximum response is less than with acetylcholine or propionylcholine. Valerylcholine, however, produces no contraction. Formylcholine is active and has about a quarter the potency of acetylcholine.

We have learned from this experiment that acetylcholine is not unique in the aliphatic esters of choline in being able to produce a contraction of the smooth muscle of the intestine, that a maximum response can be produced if there is one carbon less or more although the potency is reduced, i.e. acetylcholine is the optimal compound. However, lengthening of the chain by more than two carbons leads to a complete loss of ability to cause contraction. Related homologous series can be made by changing the length of the alcohol chain or by replacing the methyl groups on the nitrogen with similar results, i.e. acetylcholine is the optimum structure but small changes can be made with loss only of potency.

We can make a more far-reaching change in structure by replacing some of the atoms in acetylcholine by other groupings. For instance we can systematically replace the oxygen atoms by hydrogens or methylenes as appropriate [TABLE 1.1]. It can be seen that these modified molecules are still active and indeed weak activity is still retained in the very simple substance tetramethylammonium.

So far we have applied simple chemical reasoning to the study of some structure activity series, but drugs are more often found as a result of screening, i.e. testing new compounds to find what kind of activity they have, and by this means quite unexpected compounds may be found to be active. TABLE 1.2 shows five such compounds all with activity comparable to acetylcholine, indeed in three cases considerably more active than acetyl-

General Pharmacology

TABLE 1.1

	Relative activity
$CH_3-CO-O-CH_2CH_2N(CH_3)_3$ Acetylcholine	100
$CH_3-CH_2-O-CH_2CH_2N(CH_3)_3$ Choline ethylether	8
$CH_3-CO-CH_2-CH_2CH_2N(CH_3)_3$ 4-ketopentyl trimethylammonium	0·5
$CH_3-CH_2-CH_2-CH_2CH_2N(CH_3)_3$ Pentyl trimethylammonium	0·5
$CH_3N(CH_3)_3$ Tetramethylammonium	0·1

TABLE 1.2

	Relative activity
Acetylcholine	100
Methyl dilvasene	1000
Muscarine	300
Methyl furmethide	300
Arecoline	100
Oxotremorine	50

choline itself. In the first three compounds it is easy to see a chemical resemblance to acetylcholine and in any case the terminal $CH_2N(CH_3)_3$ group is retained. In arecoline (an alkaloid from the betel nut) the resemblance is more tenuous and in oxotremorine remote. When the resemblance is so slight we must bear in mind the possibility that the drug is acting by a different mechanism.

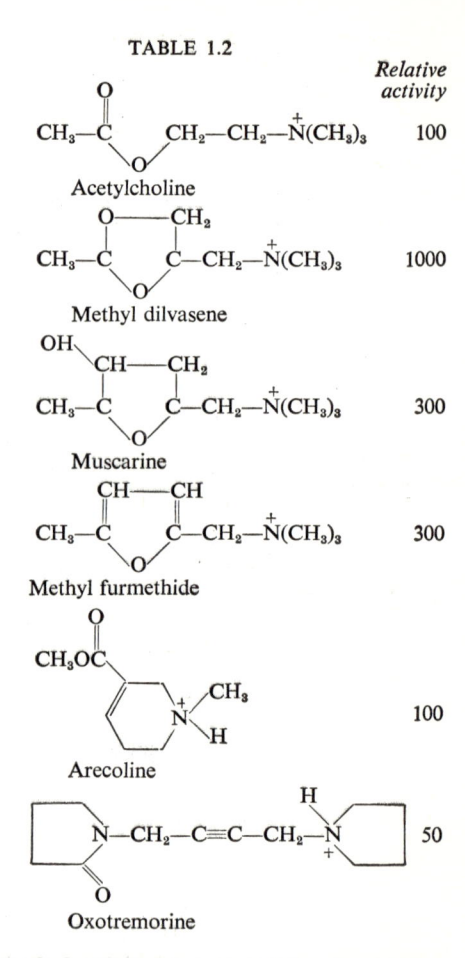

We mentioned at the outset that for drugs to produce an action they must react with some cellular constituent—this may be called a drug receptor—an idea first put forward by Ehrlich and by Langley. It will readily be appreciated that the strength of interaction of the drug with the receptor will be influenced by the chemical structure of the drug. What kind of chemical reaction occurs? The reactions familiar to us from organic chemistry are those in which covalent linkages are made or broken with the transfer of atoms from one reactant to the other. There are reasons for thinking that this kind of chemical reaction does not commonly occur when drugs react with their sites of action on the cell and the line of argument may be illustrated from the series of drugs just considered. Starting with acetylcholine we could consider the possibility that it acts by transference of its acetyl groups on to some reactive site in the cell, but we can see right away that this cannot be the case because we have found that a number of the substances having the same kind of pharmacological activity have no acetyl group or even no acyl group; further consideration of the chemical structures of these substances enables us to eliminate all the possible groups that might be transferred, or for that matter it is just as difficult to see how any group from the cell could be accepted by *all* in this group of drugs. We are therefore led to the conclusion that the reaction with the cell is not due to any covalent linkage but is due to the operation of other intermolecular forces (ionic, dispersion, dipolar, etc.) which do not lead to chemical change in the drug. These forces can lead to the formation of reversible complexes between a drug and other substances and we would expect that the stability of the complex would depend on how well the two components fit together, since this would determine how close the component atoms of the drug could fit with those on the combining site and hence the number and strength of the atomic interactions.

These ideas have led to the postulation of specific drug-combining sites in cells which are called drug receptors and to the idea that the potency of drug action is also dependent on how good the fit between the drug and the receptor is. We may imagine the receptor being complementary in shape and structure to that of the drug.

Similar ideas to this are current in biochemistry to explain the initial complex formed between enzymes and their substrates and in immunology to explain the complexes formed between antigens and antibodies. The drug receptor must have some additional property because when an agonist drug such as acetylcholine reacts with a smooth muscle cell the function of the cell is altered (for instance the permeability of the cell membrane to ions is altered, see Chapter 8). Recently several workers have succeeded in isolating from cell membranes a macromolecular structure probably a complex of protein and lipid of molecular weight about 40,000 which combines with acetylcholine and other agonists (and antagonists, see later) with affinities corresponding closely to the pharmacological activities deduced *in vivo*. Over the next few years we can expect that the study of such isolated receptors will lead to a better understanding of drug activity.

Up till this point we have taken as evidence of drug action only the agonist response seen as contraction of smooth muscle. However, some drugs, while not producing a direct response, will interfere with the response of an agonist. An example is seen in FIGURE 1.4.

In this experiment, after a preliminary dose–response, curve to acetylcholine had been obtained, the ileum was immersed in Ringer salt solution containing atropine sulphate. When acetylcholine in the doses used in the

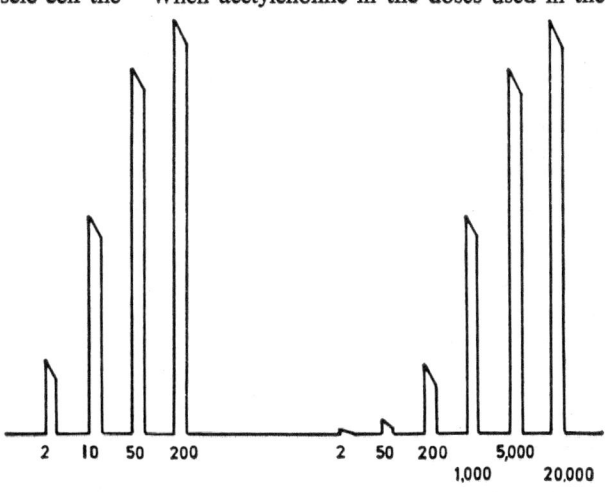

FIG. 1.4. The contractions of the ileum shown on the left part of the curve were produced by the concentrations of acetylcholine marked under each curve. After adding atropine, 0·2 ng./ml., to the fluid bathing the intestine larger doses of acetylcholine were required to produce effects equal to those produced before atropine was added.

preliminary run was tested again, no contraction was seen, but when the dose of acetylcholine was increased the muscle responded and with a large enough dose the maximum response was as large as before atropine was added. The new log dose–response curve for acetylcholine in the presence of atropine is parallel to the control curve but shifted to the right as though acetylcholine had become a weaker drug. If the concentration of atropine is increased the shift of the curve is correspondingly increased. If we test some others of the range of acetylcholine-like drugs mentioned previously in the presence of any particular concentration of atropine we find that their potencies are all reduced by exactly the same factor. The most likely explanation of these results is that while acetylcholine and the other agonist drugs of this series combine with the 'acetylcholine receptor' and lead to contraction, atropine combines with the same receptor without activating it. Thus, when atropine is present a proportion of the receptors are occupied by atropine molecules and are not available to react with acetylcholine, and hence the response to a particular dose of acetylcholine is reduced. No absolute proof of this hypothesis is available yet. However, if this were true, we might expect to see some resemblance chemically between atropine and acetylcholine, and the formula of atropine suggests there is some. It may be thought this is a little fanciful but the reader may be more convinced by the following facts. We saw earlier that valerylcholine did not produce contraction of the smooth muscle. However, if we add valerylcholine to the bath in a suitable concentration and then test the response to acetylcholine, we find it is reduced and indeed valerylcholine has similar antagonist properties to those displayed by atropine, although it is much less potent. In fact we find that when the group on the acyl part of acetylcholine is increased in size antagonists are regularly produced and with bulky aromatic acids such as benzilic acid very powerful antagonists may be produced. Since in these compounds the resemblance of the antagonist to acetylcholine is quite obvious, our original hypothesis about atropine seems less far-fetched. We will see in later parts of this book that many antagonists do bear a close resemblance to the chemical structure of the agonists which they antagonize. However, in other groups of antagonists the chemical resemblance may be much more remote, and it is likely in these cases that combination of the antagonist with the receptor depends mainly on association with portions of the receptor that are not involved in the association with the agonist.

One of the dilemmas of pharmacology is to explain just what it is that makes some members of a drug series agonists and some antagonists. There are two major theories current. The first theory assumes that both agonist and antagonist form complexes with the receptor and that the intensity of their actions is dependent on the amount of complex formed but that when an agonist reacts with a receptor it changes the spatial form (conformation) of the receptor, and this is responsible for the cellular changes that ensue, whereas the antagonist combines without such changes in conformation. This idea stems from studies on enzymes mainly in the protein synthesis paths in which Monod and his collaborators have interpreted substrate control in terms of conformational changes which they have called allostery. The best case in which direct evidence of whether conformation is altered when association occurs have been obtained, is in the reaction of the two anaesthetics xenon and cyclopropane with myoglobin and haemoglobin. Xenon forms a strong complex with myoglobin, and from X-ray crystallography of the complex it is known that no alteration in the structure of the myoglobin occurs. On the other hand, cyclopropane forms a complex with haemoglobin in which the structure of the protein is altered. In enzymology the best-documented example of a conformation change is in the proteolytic enzyme carboxypeptidase in which the tyrosine in position 248 moved by 14 Å, in atomic dimensions a very large distance, when the substrate was bound.

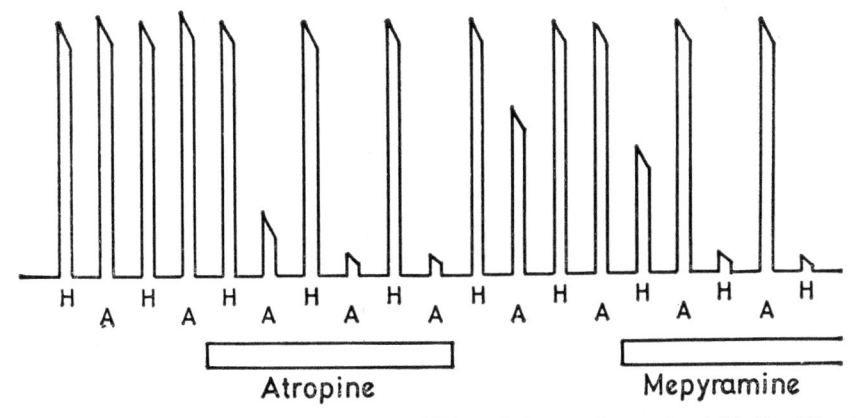

FIG. 1.5. The ileum was made to contract by addition of alternate doses of acetylcholine (A) and histamine (H). Atropine selectively antagonizes the acetylcholine effects and mepyramine the histamine effects.

The second explanation is based on the proposition that drug action results from the act of forming a complex with the receptor, so that the act of combination liberates a 'quantum' of action and the total activity produced by a drug depends on the rate at which drug-complexes are turned over. It was pointed out earlier that the agonist response appears rapidly, indeed at the neuromuscular junction where it is possible to apply agonists in a very localized fashion it is found that the latency of action is of the order of tens of microseconds. On the other hand antagonist actions are usually relatively slow, for instance after atropine action on the intestine has become steady, the half-time of recovery on replacing with fresh salt solution is of the order of 5–10 minutes. Antagonist–receptor complexes, therefore, turn over much more slowly than agonist–receptor complexes and this may explain their lack of agonist activity. Comparable situations exist with enzymes, for instance neostigmine is a very good inhibitor of acetylcholinesterase, but in fact is a very poor substrate with a low turnover rate.

These explanations may also be interpreted in terms of the formation of an intermediate state in the drug–receptor complex, which is the active state as far as agonist action is concerned; with agonists we would postulate that this forms readily, with antagonists it probably does not form at all.

The value of the receptor concept can be illustrated with some examples. Histamine can also cause contraction of the intestinal smooth muscle and produce a similar maximum response to that caused by acetylcholine and while its chemical structure bears little resemblance to acetylcholine, it is really no more dissimilar in structure than say oxotremorine. However, when we examine the response in the presence of suitable doses of atropine we find that histamine is not antagonized whereas acetylcholine and oxotremorine are. This suggests that histamine is combining with a different receptor; if this is so it ought to be possible to find an antagonist for histamine that does not affect the response to acetylcholine. Many such antihistamines are known of which mepyramine may be taken as an example. We have, in the use of selective antagonists, one of the most satisfactory and discriminating criteria for distinguishing between receptors and hence between groups of drugs [FIG. 1.5].

A further problem to be considered is whether receptors for a given drug are the same in all cells. Let us look at the action of the

TABLE 1.3

ACTIVITY RELATIVE TO ACETYLCHOLINE

THE RELATIVE POTENCIES OF A HOMOLOGOUS SERIES OF CHOLINE ESTERS IN CAUSING CONTRACTIONS OF THE GUINEA-PIG ILEUM AND THE FROG RECTUS ABDOMINIS MUSCLE.

	ILEUM	RECTUS ABDOMINIS
Formylcholine	25	10
Acetylcholine	*100*	*100*
Propionylcholine	5	400
Butyrylcholine	0·5	150
Valerylcholine	0	30

acylcholines on another tissue, the rectus abdominis muscle of the frog. Acetylcholine causes this striated muscle to go into contracture and so do some of the other acylcholines, whose activity is listed in TABLE 1.3 and compared with their activity on smooth muscle. In this series acetylcholine is not the most active member since both propionyl- and butyrylcholine are more active. Perhaps the most striking difference is with valerylcholine which is without agonist effect on the ileum but is a third as active as acetylcholine on the rectus. Similar differences apply to other compounds, for instance oxotremorine and muscarine are almost without activity on the rectus, whereas succinylcholine and nicotine, which are highly active on the rectus, are without effect on the ileum. These differences in structure–activity relationship suggest that the receptors for acetylcholine in the two tissues differ in structure and we readily find confirmation of this by using antagonists. Atropine is unable to block effects of acetylcholine on the rectus except in concentrations much higher than those that are effective on the ileum, but d-tubocurarine readily blocks the acetylcholine response on the rectus while being ineffective on the ileum.

There should be no difficulty in accepting the conclusion that there are two distinct types of receptor for acetylcholine corresponding to the muscarine-like and nicotine-like actions of acetylcholine first described by Dale. Further work has shown that while the main acetylcholine receptor on autonomic ganglion cells responds to agonists in the same general way as does that on striated muscle, they can be distinguished by antagonists so that there are in fact two closely related receptors in autonomic ganglia and skeletal muscle, both of which respond to nicotine-like drugs. The therapeutic value of selective antagonists will be readily appreciated; this permits the use of atropine to dry the mouth or speed up the heart without causing paralysis, or fall in blood pressure, and by contrast the use of gallamine to produce muscular paralysis in surgery without changes in cardiovascular function.

A further point of interest is seen in the action of acetylcholine on the heart auricles—acetylcholine slows the rate of beating and diminishes the force of contraction—an inhibitory action [see Chapter 6], and yet we find that the acetylcholine receptor on the heart appears identical to that on the ileum as judged by the structure-activity of agonists and the effect of antagonists. In these two tissues we have the same kind of receptor coupled to different effector systems—indicated by depolarization of the cell membrane of ileal smooth muscle cells, contrasted with hyperpolarization of cardiac muscle cells when exposed to acetylcholine.

The examples used in this discussion have been drawn from acetylcholine because the information available is extensive and the chemical problems relatively simple, but the principles enunciated apply equally well to other drugs.

The receptors may be like the acetylcholine receptor, bound to a cell membrane and mediating a change in cell permeability to ions that causes cell excitation. Other receptors may be specific enzymes. Good examples of this, which will be discussed in detail later, are cholinesterase, the enzyme concerned with the termination of action of acetylcholine after its release from nerve endings; carbonic anhydrase, the enzyme concerned with the provision of hydrogen ions in many secretory organs; and dihydrofolic reductase, an enzyme concerned in nucleic acid synthesis. Other receptors may be neither membrane bound nor enzymatic in nature; for instance, colchicine arrests cell mutations in metaphase and achieves this because the protein that composes the mitotic spindle has a receptor for colchicine and is unable to contract once colchicine has combined with it. It can be seen that the receptor concept is quite general and is indeed the central concept of pharmacology. The selectivity of drug action, i.e. the goal of producing drugs with a minimum number of side actions, depends on how selective it is possible to make the combination of drug with particular receptors. However, even if we came to have perfect selectivity the distribution of drug action could then depend on the way in which these receptors were distributed in the body. For instance, if the drug reacts with the muscarinic acetylcholine receptor it will affect those in the heart, the intestine, and the salivary glands and such differences as do occur will depend on the physiological responses produced. In general, if complete organ selectivity is required a different mode of action must be sought. An example of this is seen in drugs used to lower blood pressure; the first drugs used were ganglion blockers which block all autonomic ganglia, sympathetic and parasympathetic alike. Attempts to find drugs that would discriminate between these two sets of ganglia have been unsuccessful—the acetylcholine receptors in the two types of ganglia are identical. Improved pharmacological selectivity was achieved by changing the target to blockage of the postganglionic synapse where it is easy to find drugs that affect the sympathetic synapse whose transmitter is noradrenaline without affecting the parasympathetic synapse whose transmitter is acetylcholine.

There are a few instances where tissue selectivity can be produced by the distributional factors that will be discussed in detail in the next section. An example is as follows. Some synapses in the central nervous system are muscarinic in type. If we wish to block peripheral muscarinic receptors without affecting central muscarinic receptors we can use an atropine type drug with a quaternary ammonium group (atropine methonitrate or lachesine) since this cannot penetrate into the brain. On the other hand, if we use a highly lipid-soluble antagonist such as benzhexol we achieve a high concentration in the brain and are able to produce a selective action on the brain muscarinic receptor with a minimum of side-effects in the periphery; this action is useful in the treatment of Parkinsonism.

DISTRIBUTION OF DRUGS

We will start by considering the distribution after the intravenous injection of a drug which is in free solution in the plasma and which has an oil/water distribution coefficient of about one. Because of its high lipid solubility such a drug will be able to cross cell boundaries very rapidly and hence there will virtually be complete equilibration between the drug concentration in the plasma and in the tissue being perfused by the blood. Thus the rate at which the drug reaches the tissue will depend entirely on the tissue blood flow—this is called blood flow limited access. If all tissues were perfused at the same rate the concentration in the tissues would be the same, but some tissues, notably the brain, heart, kidneys, and liver, are perfused at high rates, whereas the subcutaneous fat and the bones are perfused at very low rates; skin and muscle are intermediate with rates depending on usage and ambient temperature. The rapidly perfused organs constitute only a small fraction of the body mass but rapidly acquire a drug concentration similar to that in the plasma. The concentration in the slowly perfused organs rises more slowly and as it does so, the concentration in the plasma and rapidly perfused organs falls, due to the redistribution of drug that occurs. This redistribution occurs with a half-time of 20–40 minutes so that it is effectively complete in 2 hours. This phenomenon has important consequences; for instance, if an intravenous anaesthetic is given quickly it will produce rapid effects on the central nervous system that will be waning in a few minutes, and have reached a steady level only after 2 hours (we are ignoring here any effects of

TABLE 1.4
BLOOD FLOW IN VARIOUS PARTS OF THE BODY

	MASS (KG.)	% BODY WEIGHT	BLOOD FLOW L/MIN.	% CARDIAC OUTPUT	TURNOVER TIME (MINUTES)
Well perfused					
Kidneys	0·3	0·5	1·25	23	0·25
Heart	0·3	0·5	0·25	5	1
Brain	1·4	2·2	0·75	14	2
Liver	2·6	4·1	1·50	28	2
			7·3	70	
Poorly perfused					
Skin	4	6·3	0·45	8	9
Muscle	30	48	0·83	16	35
Skeleton	13	21	0·2	4	65
Fat	11	17	0·15	3	70
Total		63	5·4		

metabolism or excretion on the blood level). Corresponding time curves will apply to the other rapidly perfused organs. If the drug has only a low solubility in lipids it will be able to cross the capillary walls with difficulty and will not readily cross the plasma membrane of tissue cells and will therefore be initially confined to the extracellular space. The consequence will be that the plasma level will be higher and will fall away more slowly. Even slower disappearance is seen when the drug is bound to plasma proteins. In this case only that fraction of the drug in the plasma which is unbound will be free to diffuse, so that in the case of drugs that are strongly bound to proteins the plasma level falls very slowly.

On the other hand, when drugs are much more soluble in lipids than in water, the subcutaneous fat acts as a very large reservoir into which the drug is slowly carried by the blood and from which it is only slowly released as drug removal occurs by other processes. The adipose tissue thus acts as a reservoir whose size is increased in proportion to the oil/water distribution coefficient and with which equilibration occurs with a half-time equivalent to the tissue mass × oil/water distribution coefficient/ blood flow. The plasma level may therefore be reduced to very low levels. Note that the fall in plasma concentration in the first 10–15 minutes after administration is not affected by high lipid solubility but it is in the later phases that the blood level continues to fall rapidly. This action is important in determining the relative brevity of the barbiturate thiopentone and the inhalational anaesthetic halothane. However, the concentration of the drug in the adipose tissue also takes a long while to be dissipated and with halothane the half-time of removal may be as much as a week. The highly lipid-soluble insecticide dicophane (DDT) may remain in the body fat for many months after administration.

ABSORPTION FROM THE TISSUES

When drugs are injected directly into the subcutaneous or muscular tissues the entry into the blood stream is determined in part by the volume injected; very small volumes permeate between the tissue cells and the drug is absorbed into the blood stream through the capillary walls. The rate of absorption is then governed by the same factors as in TABLE 1.4. However, most drugs are irritant and cause local hyperaemia which speeds their absorption. In general the half-times of absorption of drugs by these routes are of the order of 5–15 minutes. The absorption rate is modified by exercise in the case of intramuscular injection and by skin temperature in the case of

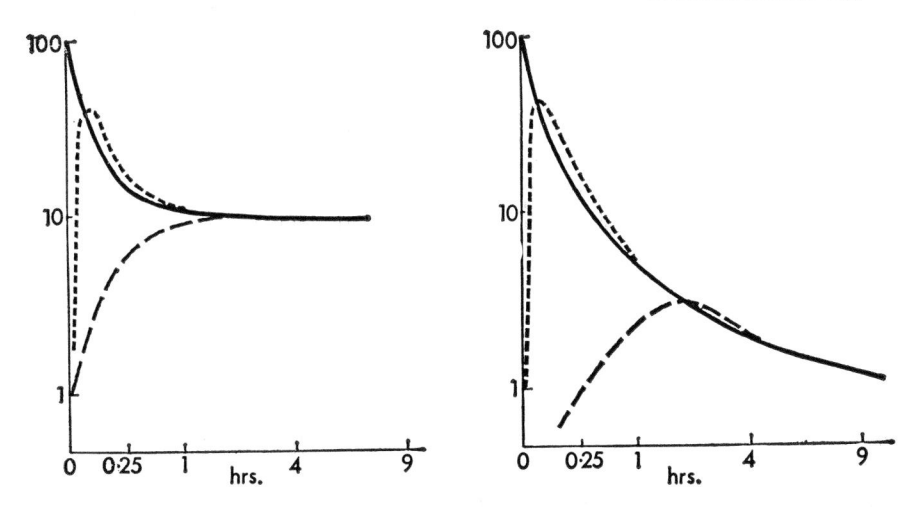

FIG. 1.6. Distribution of a drug after intravenous injection. The drug in the left-hand panel is equally soluble in oil and water and is not protein bound. That in the right-hand panel was about ten times as soluble in oil as in water.

——————— Concentration in the plasma.
- - - - - - - Concentration in rapidly perfused organs, i.e. brain, heart, liver, kidneys.
— — — — Concentration in slowly perfused organs, i.e. muscle, bone.

subcutaneous injection. Drugs which are vasoconstrictors slow their own absorption —this is true when adrenaline is injected subcutaneously, but since adrenaline dilates muscle vessels the absorption from intramuscular injection is fast. In traumatic shock when skin flow may be very small absorption from subcutaneous sites may be very slow, but may speed up when the patient is treated. When large volumes are injected part of the fluid injected is forced into lymph vessels and absorbed fast but the over-all absorption is generally slower than with small volumes. If the drug is injected as a suspension of a poorly soluble form, only the dissolved part is rapidly absorbed and the absorption of the remainder depends on its rate of dissolution. This may be quite slow, so that absorption of drug from suspensions is prolonged. The rate of dissolution depends both on the solubility of the drug in the tissue fluids and on the character of the insoluble particles. Small particles, because they have a large surface/mass ratio, dissolve more rapidly than large particles. These principles are used in preparation of 'delay' forms of drugs which are slowly absorbed and therefore give more prolonged blood levels. Good examples are the preparations of insulin [see Chapter 14]. Ordinary insulin is soluble and is rapidly absorbed so that the peak blood level is reached in about 10 minutes after subcutaneous injection. If, however, suspensions of the insoluble zinc salt of insulin are injected, the peak blood level is reached in about 2 hours when the particles are small (Semilente insulin) but may not be reached for 18–24 hours if the particles are large (Ultralente insulin). With penicillin, ordinary sodium benzylpenicillin, which is soluble in water, is very rapidly absorbed but the suspension of the procaine salt of benzylpenicillin is half absorbed in about 12 hours [see Chapter 16]. The very insoluble benzathine salt of benzylpenicillin takes several days to be absorbed. Oil solutions of lipid-soluble drugs are also relatively slowly absorbed—in this case the concentration in the tissue fluids determines the rate of absorption and this depends on the partitioning of the drug between the oil and the tissue fluid.

ADMINISTRATION BY MOUTH

Most drugs are absorbed when taken by mouth unless they are broken down in the alimentary canal (e.g. insulin). The rapidity of absorption and the site of absorption depend on chemical and physical properties of the drug.

The barrier to absorption is the cell wall of the epithelial cells lining the gastro-intestinal tract and the ease with which a substance can penetrate through these cells depends on its partition coefficient between the aqueous phase in the gut lumen and cell cytoplasm and the 'lipid' phase in the cell membrane. Substances that are highly hydrophilic, for instance quaternary ammonium ganglion blockers (e.g. hexamethonium), are very poorly absorbed, whereas the more lipophilic ethanol is absorbed very rapidly. A great many drugs are weak cations, i.e. in acid solution they are cations and in alkali they are uncharged. At the pH corresponding to the pK there are equal amounts of cation and uncharged form. The two forms differ in their partition co-efficients, the cation being hydrophilic and thus poorly absorbed whereas the uncharged form is more lipophilic and thus more readily absorbed. The over-all rate of absorption will thus depend on the proportion of un-charged form present and this will be determined by the pH. Such a drug will be almost wholly cationic in the stomach and hence not appreciably absorbed there, but in the more neutral pH of the intestinal contents enough uncharged form is present to ensure good absorption. Needless to say, as the uncharged form is absorbed it is replenished from the cationic form by re-equilibration.

In the case of anionic drugs (e.g. salicylates, barbiturates) the anion is poorly absorbed. Here the uncharged form predominates in the stomach so that absorption from the stomach may be quite significant although the major part of absorption is still in the small intestine.

As pointed out in connexion with absorption from the subcutaneous tissues, it is dissolved drug which is absorbed, so that insoluble drugs are slowly absorbed and the rate at which they are absorbed will be determined primarily by the rate of dissolution. It is therefore important that tablets of insoluble drugs should be composed of particles of the order of a few microns in diameter.

It is sometimes an advantage to coat tablets of drugs with protective coatings either to prevent dissolution in the stomach if they are liable to cause gastric irritation, or to prolong the period of absorption to give a longer effect. A typical 'enteric' coating is cellulose acetate phthalate which is insoluble in acid but dissolves quite rapidly in intestinal juice. In general, absorption of drugs taken by mouth begins in 15–60 minutes and reaches a peak in an hour or two so that oral administration produces less fluctuation in blood level than parenteral administration; a further difference is that since absorption from the intestine occurs into the portal venous system the drug must pass through the liver before reaching the general circulation. Since most of the drug metabolizing systems are concentrated in the liver, a higher proportion of the drug is metabolized when given by the oral route so that quite apart from the efficiency of absorption, less of the original drug reaches the general circulation and this means that doses must usually be higher to attain the same result when the drug is given by mouth.

A way round this is for the tablet of the drug to be sucked rather than swallowed. Dissolution occurs in the mouth and adsorption occurs through the buccal mucosa directly into the systemic circulation. This is a useful method of getting rapid absorption of readily meta-bolized drugs and is used in the case of glyceryl trinitrate in the treatment of angina and of isoprenaline in asthma. The main limitation to this method is the objectionable taste of most drugs and the high proportion of drugs that are surface anaesthetics.

ADMINISTRATION BY INHALATION

For volatile drugs administration by inhalation may have particular advantages, and notably the ease with which the concentration in the plasma and tissues may be controlled and this is exploited in inhalational anaesthetics [CHAPTER 2].

However, non-volatile drugs may also be administered by this route as fine mists or dusts; these are frequently used in the treatment of asthma (e.g. isoprenaline and cromoglycate). The purported objective here is to produce a local action and for this the particles must be fine enough to penetrate into the smaller bronchioles. There is considerable doubt whether the local action is the dominant one and the effectiveness of the drug given by this route rests more on rapid and efficient absorption from the large absorbing area made available.

DRUG EXCRETION

Most drugs are extensively metabolized so that excretion of the unchanged drug is not usually the rate-limiting step in the disappearance of the drug from the body. The main cases in which excretion is of paramount importance are the chemotherapeutics (sulphonamides, penicillin, streptomycin, tetracycline, etc.) and ganglion and neuromuscular blocking agents (hexamethonium, mecamylamine, tubocurarine, gallamine). Excretion by the kidneys depends first on glomerular filtration which applies only to free drug (i.e. not bound by plasma proteins). The subsequent handling in the tubules depends on whether the drug is uncharged or is a cation or anion. The permeability of the renal tubule to drugs is rather similar to that of the epithelium of the gut, i.e. uncharged drugs readily diffuse across the tubule whereas cations and anions do not. The clearance of a drug will depend therefore on its pK and the pH of the urine. For example, mecamylamine is a weak cation (pK_a 11·2). If the urine is alkaline a considerable fraction of the drug in the distal tubule is uncharged and diffuses back into the blood because its over-all concentration is higher in the tubule due to water reabsorption. The excretion of the drug will be small. If the urine is acid a much smaller fraction of the drug will be un-ionized and hence the reabsorption will be reduced and the rate of excretion increased. The duration of action of mecamylamine will therefore depend on the acid–base balance of the patient.

Penicillin and methonium compounds are especially rapidly excreted by the kidneys because of active secretion by the cells of the proximal tubule in addition to free filtration.

DRUG METABOLISM

Nearly all drugs are metabolized, and the metabolic products are usually less active pharmacologically and more soluble. While some metabolism occurs in the gut wall (e.g. tyramine) or in the blood (e.g. acetylcholine) the main site of drug metabolism is the liver. The processes are stereotyped and are largely confined to hydrolysis, demethylation, side chain or nuclear oxidation, and conjugation with glycuronic acid, sulphate, or glycine.

Oxidation and demethylation are carried out by microsomal enzymes that may show the property of induction, i.e. the production of the enzyme may be increased by drugs. A striking example of this is the metabolism of the barbiturate amylobarbitone in which oxidation of the isoamyl side chain is responsible for terminating its action. If amylobarbitone is injected intravenously into a rabbit in a dose large enough to cause loss of consciousness, the animal may take some 20 minutes before it attempts to regain its sitting posture. If the same dose is repeated daily the duration of the loss of righting is reduced on successive days until it reaches a minimum after about a week. At the same time it is found that the rate of disappearance of the drug from the blood stream is accelerated. If amylobarbitone is shaken with a homogenate of rabbit liver it slowly disappears due to metabolism. If the liver is obtained from rabbits that have received repeated conditioning doses of amylobarbitone the rate of metabolism is greatly increased. The amylobarbitone has induced the formation of an increased amount of the enzyme system causing side chain oxidation. In the case of slowly metabolized drugs this effect may be more dramatic, for instance a single dose of phenobarbitone induces a large increase in this enzyme system which only returns to the basal level over a period of about 2 weeks. Since the metabolic process is not specific to the drug inducing it this effect may affect other unrelated drugs too and this may be an unanticipated source of drug interaction in treatment. A well-known example is that metabolism of the anticoagulant dicoumarol is accelerated when the barbiturate oxidizing system is induced so that the extent of anticoagulation by this drug may be indirectly modified by the administration of phenobarbitone.

In a few instances metabolism of a drug may lead to the formation of a substance of greater pharmacological activity or toxicity. A simple example is methanol which is intrinsically of low toxicity but is metabolized to the very toxic substance formaldehyde. Another example is tremorine which has only weak pharmacological activity but is oxidized in the liver to oxotremorine which is a highly active parasympathomimetic substance causing cardiovascular effects and centrally induced tremor. Some drugs also produce their pharmacological effects by interfering with the metabolism of other drugs—for instance the antifolic, methotrexate, by inhibiting folic reductase prevents folic acid being reduced to tetrahydrofolic acid which is the active form for one carbon transfer, or the anticholinesterases by inhibiting cholinesterase prevent the normal removal of acetylcholine after its physiological release.

FURTHER READING

ARIËNS, E. J., and ROSSUM, J. M. VAN (1964) *Molecular Pharmacology*, London.

BARLOW, R. B. (1964) *Introduction to Chemical Pharmacology*, London.

BINNS, T. B. (1964) *Absorption and Distribution of Drugs*, Baltimore.

BLOOM, B. M., and LAUBACH, G. D. (1962) The relationship between chemical structure and pharmacological action, *Ann. Rev. Pharmacol.*, **2**, 67.

BURGER, A. (1970) *Medicinal Chemistry*, New York.

BURGER, A., and PARULKAR, A. P. (1966) Relationship between chemical structure and biological activity, *Ann. Rev. Pharmacol.*, **6**, 19.

HOLLAND, W. C., KLEIN, R. L., and BRIGGS, A. H. (1964) *Introduction to Molecular Pharmacology*, London.

KOROLKOVAS, A. (1970) *Essentials of Molecular Pharmacology*, New York.

KROMOR-BORISOV, N. V., and MICHELSON, M. J. (1966) Drug receptors, *Pharmacol. Rev.*, **18**, 1051.

PAPPER, E. M., and KITZ, R. J. (1963) *Uptake and Distribution of Anesthetic Agents*, New York.

PORTER, R., and O'CONNOR, K. (1970) *Molecular Properties of Drug Receptors*, London.

SHANKER, L. S. (1962) Passage of drugs across body membranes, *Pharmacol. Rev.*, **14**, 501.

SHANKER, L. S. (1964) Physiological transport of drugs, *Advanc. Drug Res.*, **1**, 72.

TRIGGLE, D. J. (1965) *Chemical Aspects of the Autonomic Nervous System*, London.

WILLIAMS, R. T. (1959) *Detoxication*, New York.

WILLIAMS, R. T. (1966) Symposium on receptors, *Advanc. Drug Res.*, **3**, 1–293.

2

CENTRAL NERVOUS SYSTEM DEPRESSANTS I

The drugs described in this chapter are probably the most important known to man. They include the general anaesthetics without which none but the most rudimentary surgery would be practicable. Although the mechanism and site of action of these compounds are still poorly understood, there have been notable advances in this field which now allow prolonged and complex surgery to be undertaken with excellent control of anaesthesia and its after effects.

EXPERIMENTAL METHODS FOR THE STUDY OF CENTRALLY ACTING DRUGS

An extremely wide range of techniques is now available for the study of centrally acting drugs. These techniques may be methods based simply on the observation of the whole organism or may involve sophisticated experiments which allow the effect of drugs on single nerve cells to be analysed.

The gross effects of drugs can be studied by direct observation of the movements of animals. No special skill or apparatus is needed to determine when an animal is anaesthetized or is convulsing but additional tests such as the recording of reflexes or the measurement of electrical activity in the brain usually provide valuable additional information.

Visual observation may be supplemented by automatic records of total activity by recording movements of a cage, or the floor of a cage, which is freely suspended and moves when the animal moves. A more satisfactory way of doing this is to arrange for movements of the animal to interrupt beams of light or infra-red rays and so signal movements. Drugs which alter behaviour, perhaps by reducing anxiety or stimulating exploratory activity, may be studied on animals placed in simple mazes.

The effects of drugs on reflexes can quickly be tested on frogs, by comparing reactions before and after the drug and by measuring the latent period and the duration of the effect. After strychnine, for instance, frogs give exaggerated responses to mild stimuli such as touching the skin.

More satisfactory ways for measuring the effect of drugs on reflex activity involve electrical and mechanical recording techniques. Early experiments made use of an automatic patellar tendon hammer and a myograph device for recording muscle shortening when the knee jerk reflex was evoked. Drugs were injected systemically and their effect on the characteristics of the reflex recorded. This type of experiment is rarely performed nowadays because the site of action of the drug cannot be properly localized. It is now much more convenient and informative to stimulate afferent nerves directly and to record the reflex responses evoked in nerves leaving the spinal cord. Drugs may be applied topically to the spinal cord or be given by close arterial injection and their effect on individual reflex pathways recorded. There are many variations of this basic type of experiment, the most recent being the introduction of methods for recording from single cells in the spinal cord and for applying drugs micro-electrophoretically to

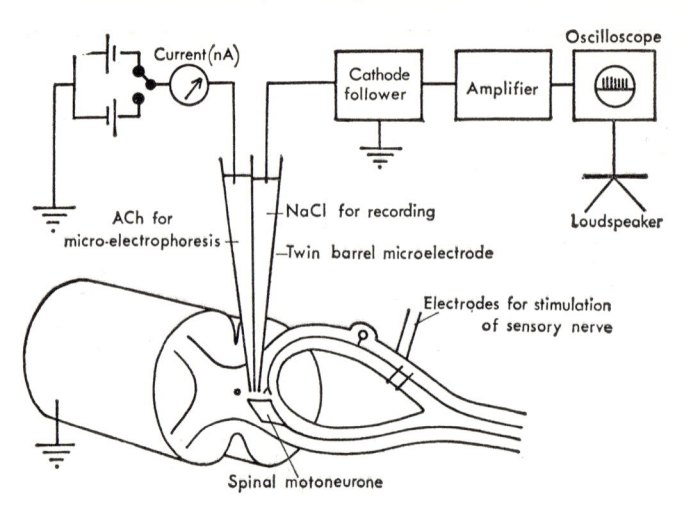

FIG. 2.1. Diagram of apparatus for recording from single nerve cells and for applying drugs by micro-electrophoresis.

these cells. Records are usually obtained from single cells by preparing glass micropipettes with tip diameters of a few microns. These pipettes are filled with a strong electrolyte solution, NaCl for extracellular recording, and are then coupled through a cathode follower to suitable amplifiers and display equipment. By moving the tip of the electrode through the tissue with a micromanipulator, the action potentials of individual cells are picked up, and displayed [FIG. 2.1].

To apply drugs to single cells, micropipettes are again used but they are filled with a strong solution of the drug to be tested. This drug must be at a pH which allows good ionization of the compound and the polarity of the charged ions must be known. If this pipette is now placed very near a nerve cell membrane and if a voltage, of the same polarity as the ionized drug, is applied to the drug solution, a current (measured in nA) will flow from the tip of the pipette and a small amount of the charged drug will be ejected. Numerous precautions have to be taken with this technique, a small 'braking' current must always be applied to the pipette to prevent the leakage of the drug by diffusion and controls must be performed to ensure that the electrophoretic current itself has no effect on the cells. It is usual for these micro-electrophoresis pipettes to be fused to at least one other micropipette so that electrical recordings may be made, and other drugs applied simultaneously, to the cell being studied. With this type of apparatus many detailed and valuable studies of the effect of drugs on reflex and nerve cell activity in the spinal cord and other parts of the CNS have been made.

Drug effects in the brain may also be studied by using electrodes which record the activity of whole populations of nerve cells. These electrodes, which need not be of very small dimensions, can be chronically implanted in the brain so that records are obtained from the conscious, free-moving animal.

The site of action of a drug may be determined by recording its effect before and after central lesions have been made. If the effect survives complete destruction of the nervous system it must, of course, be peripheral. If it does not survive then spinal, brain stem, and cerebral lesions can be produced in order to locate the approximate site of action. The central action of drugs can sometimes be determined, and their site of action located, by applying them locally. In this case the experiment is only convincing if very small doses are effective, since drugs which are given in this way may be absorbed by the blood stream and carried to a distant site of action. Drugs may be applied to the surface of the brain, to deep structures by micro-injection, or injected into cerebral blood vessels or the ventricles.

If a drug can be made radioactive it is sometimes possible to determine its distribution and predict its site of action, by making autoradiographs of brain sections after administration of the drug.

GENERAL ANAESTHESIA

Various drugs such as alcohol, opium, and hashish were amongst the first compounds used to reduce the pain of operations but effective general anaesthesia was only introduced in the nineteenth century. Although ether was known in the thirteenth century, it was only in the sixteenth century that its potential for relieving pain was suggested. This suggestion was forgotten and ignored until Sir Michael Faraday used ether for its anaesthetic power 200 years later. At about the same time, Sir Humphry Davy discovered the anaesthetic powers of nitrous oxide, but these discoveries were not immediately exploited. Only in 1846 when William Morton, an American dentist, used ether, first on dogs and then on man, for extracting teeth, did general anaesthesia begin to find wide acceptance. In 1847 Dr. James Simpson used chloroform to relieve labour pains and, despite opposition from many quarters, he persevered and then in 1853 the use of these agents gained a new respectability when Queen Victoria was given chloroform during the birth of her seventh child.

With early anaesthetics and anaesthetic techniques, the procedure of anaesthesia was both unpleasant and hazardous for the patient but advances in premedication and in the nature and purity of the anaesthetic compounds have now completely altered this picture. In addition, it is now possible to use much smaller doses of anaesthetic than before because separate drugs can now be used to secure the muscle relaxation required for surgery. Previously this was obtained by taking general anaesthesia to a very deep level. There is now a wide choice of anaesthetic compounds available and these include both volatile and non-volatile agents. Each type of agent tends to be particularly useful in a special situation and these are described under the appropriate headings for the individual anaesthetic agents.

THEORIES OF ANAESTHESIA

The mode of action of anaesthetics is still a matter for debate and, despite the advances made during the past decade in our knowledge of the functioning of nervous tissue, it is still impossible to decide the way in which anaesthetics act.

There is little doubt that anaesthesia is the result of a wide-spread depression of the CNS which is likely to arise from an action of the anaesthetic agent on either nerve axons, transmitter release from nerve terminals, or the excitability of postsynaptic membranes. It is difficult to obtain information about these possible sites of action by observing the action of anaesthetics on a complex structure like the brain, but experiments on peripheral tissues have shed some light on the problem.

Without doubt, all anaesthetics affect conduction in peripheral nerve axons but the concentrations of drug required to do this are much higher than those encountered in the brain during anaesthesia and, invariably, any associated synaptic junctions are much more vulnerable to the action of the anaesthetic. It has been convincingly demonstrated that anaesthetics block transmission through autonomic ganglia but the mechanism remains obscure although it is known that ether and chloroform, which block transmission, have no effect on the oxygen consumption of the tissue. Experiments on cells in the spinal cord have shown that ether diminishes reflex activity by reducing the evoked postsynaptic response to afferent nerve stimulation and by increasing the excitable threshold of the cell.

An effect of anaesthetics on transmitter release from nerve endings in the CNS is hard to measure directly but, on the guinea-pig intestine, volatile anaesthetics can block 80 per cent. of the transmitter output. If these experiments are considered in conjunction with experiments that show an increase in acetylcholine content in the brain during anaesthesia coupled with a fall in acetylcholine release from the cortex, it seems possible that anaesthetics may act by reducing transmitter release in the brain. Anaesthetics also reduce the sensitivity of the neuromuscular end-plate to applied acetylcholine and so anaesthetic action at peripheral synapses suggests two possible mechanisms for their action in the brain: (1) a reduction of transmitter release from nerve endings; and (2) a reduction in the sensitivity of postsynaptic membranes.

Various theories have been proposed which, if confirmed experimentally, might suggest how these changes at a synaptic level could be brought about by anaesthetic drugs.

The theories fall into two main groups, biochemical and physical. The first group suggests that volatile anaesthetics depress enzyme systems, and the second that they interact with cell membranes.

Anaesthetics do interfere with brain enzyme systems but high concentrations of drug are required and it is not possible to be sure that these effects actually cause anaesthesia. High concentrations of anaesthetics lower brain tissue oxygen consumption and it has been suggested that barbiturates, chloral hydrate, and urethane interfere with the citric acid cycle. However, this is not accompanied by the decrease in the production of energy-rich phosphate compounds that would be expected. It is also possible that these changes occur as a result of reduced neuronal activity, and are therefore not concerned with the initiation of anaesthesia.

A suggestion by McIlwain bridges biochemical and physical hypotheses. He suggests that depressant agents reduce ion movements across cells by an effect on the membrane and that this reduced activity allows a fall in tissue oxygen consumption and a rise, which can be observed, in phosphate energy stores. An action of some types of anaesthetics on the sodium carrier mechanism, which is activated during the generation of an action potential, has been observed and, provided that the ionic movements affected by anaesthetics are concerned in the regulation of transmitter release or postsynaptic excitability, the hypothesis seems quite reasonable.

The first important physical theory of anaesthetic action was suggested by the early work of Meyer and Overton who proposed that the depression of activity caused by an anaesthetic was directly related to its lipid solubility. Certainly the correlation of anaesthetic potency with lipid solubility is striking and it is now known that highly fat-soluble anaesthetics, such as chloroform and ether, do stabilize the cell membrane and so reduce its sensitivity to electrical and other types of stimulation.

Other theories go further than explaining a correlation, they attempt to describe a mechanism of action at the cell membrane. Mullins suggests that anaesthesia occurs when 'pores' in the cell membranes are blocked by anaesthetic molecules so preventing the movement of ions. The portion of the membrane containing the 'pores' is considered to be of a lipid nature and so the relationship between anaesthetic potency and lipid solubility might be explained.

An intriguing suggestion by Pauling is that anaesthetics are able to form microcrystals of ice (clathrates) within the central nervous system. The microcrystals might interfere with synaptic transmission or with the excitability of neuronal membranes. At body temperatures these microcrystals are not stable and Pauling suggests that they are stabilized by the charged side chains of proteins and solutes. There are modifications to this theory but all are proving difficult to test experimentally.

In 1939 Ferguson suggested that structurally non-specific drugs like general anaesthetics might have their potency determined by their thermodynamic activity. The thermodynamic activity is a measure of the number of molecules which are free to react with biologically important sites. The thermodynamic activity of a drug is not therefore necessarily determined by its concentration. A volatile anaesthetic given with oxygen has a thermodynamic activity proportional to the partial pressure of the drug divided by the saturated vapour pressure of the anaesthetic alone at the same temperature. The theory predicts that structurally non-specific drugs will have similar biological activity if their thermodynamic activities are arranged to be the same. This implies that the potency of a structurally non-specific drug is inversely proportional to its solubility in water. This hypothesis complements that of Overton-Meyer since high lipid solubility is not the only property which is associated with low solubility in water.

None of the theories of anaesthesia which have been described is completely satisfactory and they are now under close examination using the sophisticated physical techniques which are now available. These studies have been directed at the interaction of anaesthetic molecules with membranes, particularly the red blood cell membrane. At this site all anaesthetics produce qualitatively similar results—at low concentrations the cells become more resistant to haemolysis but at high concentrations they tend to lyse.

It seems likely that the anaesthetic molecules enter the membrane and the increased molecular packing produces membrane stabilization. If too many molecules enter then the structure becomes unstable and is labilized and it is found that anaesthetic potency of a compound correlates well with it, anaesthetic concentration causing half maximal stabilization. In order to determine just what alters in the membrane when an anaesthetic penetrates it, the membrane behaviour is being studied by spectroscopic techniques (nuclear magnetic resonance and electron spin resonance) which allow the behaviour of molecules within the membrane to be studied.

Although the cause of anaesthesia is likely to involve both the protein and lipid components of a membrane, advances in this subject are only likely to follow advances in our knowledge of membrane structure itself.

Neurophysiological approaches to the problem of the mechanism of action of anaesthetics have contributed evidence for the site of action of these compounds but little towards their mode of action, although they have resulted in the formation of many tentative theories of anaesthetic action. The most important piece of information to emerge has been that many anaesthetics exert their effect on the reticular formation, the brain stem network whose association with consciousness has been well demonstrated.

It is usually assumed that the reticular formation is particularly susceptible to the action of anaesthetics because of the abundance of synaptic connexions which are especially vulnerable to drug action, but evidence for this view is weak, the anaesthetics could also be acting directly on reticular cell bodies.

In whatever manner anaesthetics may act on the reticular formation, the final result seems to be a non-specific inhibition of ascending reticular influences to higher centres and it is this effect which is thought to produce unconsciousness and anaesthesia.

Studies of the effect of anaesthetics on cell membranes, the electrical activity and the metabolism of single cells in the CNS may soon begin to provide important evidence on the mode of action of anaesthetics, a subject upon which, at present, one can do little more than speculate.

THE SIGNS OF ANAESTHESIA

Four stages of anaesthesia can be observed when induction is slow. With rapidly acting intravenous anaesthetics the earlier stages are passed so quickly that they are not normally encountered.

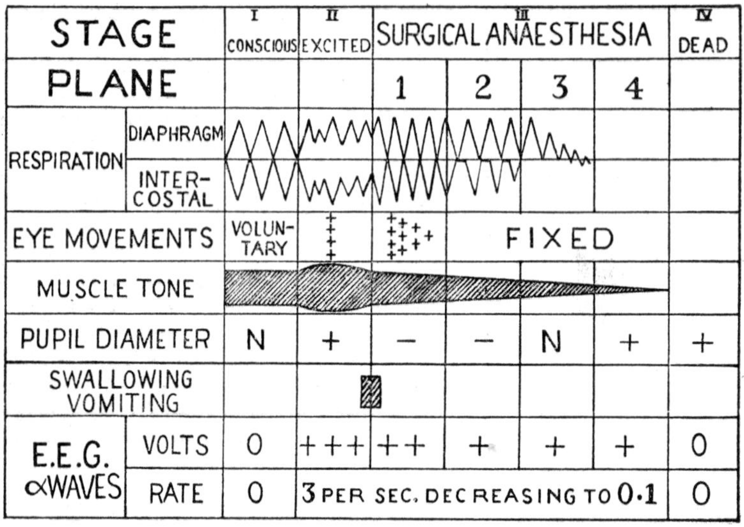

STAGE	I CONSCIOUS	II EXCITED	III SURGICAL ANAESTHESIA				IV DEAD
PLANE			1	2	3	4	
RESPIRATION DIAPHRAGM							
RESPIRATION INTERCOSTAL							
EYE MOVEMENTS	VOLUNTARY			FIXED			
MUSCLE TONE							
PUPIL DIAMETER	N	+	−	−	N	+	+
SWALLOWING VOMITING							
E.E.G. α WAVES VOLTS	0	+++	++	+	+	+	0
E.E.G. α WAVES RATE	0	3 PER SEC. DECREASING TO 0.1					0

FIG. 2.3. Effects of anaesthesia.

1. Stage of analgesia. The patient is conscious and can talk and obey commands. Awareness of pain is reduced towards the end of this stage.

2. Stage of excitement. This stage begins with loss of consciousness and extends to a level where surgery is possible. The patient can no longer exert control over himself, the pupils dilate and the pulse is rapid and strong. Muscular tone and movement may increase. This stage of anaesthesia is maintained for as short a period as possible.

3. Stage of surgical anaesthesia. Excitement disappears, respiration becomes regular, the pulse slows, and reflexes disappear. Reflexes are not all lost simultaneously, the reflexes controlling voluntary muscles go first. The conjunctival and eyelid reflexes are abolished and the cough and vomiting centres in the medulla become paralysed. The third stage of anaesthesia is sometimes subdivided in four planes.

4. Stage of respiratory paralysis. At this stage the medulla becomes severely depressed and the result is shallow, irregular respiration, a rapid pulse, a fall in blood pressure, and pupil dilatation. Death is due to a stoppage of respiration as the respiratory centres in the brain stem become paralysed.

THE ELECTROENCEPHALOGRAM AND ANAESTHESIA

Spontaneous electrical rhythms can be recorded from the brain of all living mammals. In a relaxed human subject, with eyes closed, the dominant frequency in the electrical waves is about 10 cycles per second but the administration of an anaesthetic causes marked, but reversible, changes in this rhythm and in the amplitude of the recorded waves.

During induction with most anaesthetics the pattern of the dominant rhythm (the high voltage α rhythm) becomes desynchronized and a high frequency, low voltage pattern emerges. This usually coincides with the stage of delirium in the subject.

As anaesthesia develops, the electroencephalogram again becomes synchronized and the voltage of the waves increases, with a well-defined rhythm which gradually becomes more complex as slow frequency waves are superimposed.

Further deepening of anaesthesia results in

diminution of the voltage and in the eventual disappearance of all electrical activity.

Although different anaesthetic agents may produce their own series of characteristic changes in the electroencephalogram it has been possible to correlate the concentration of a given anaesthetic in the arterial blood with the pattern of the electrical rhythm. The clinical signs of anaesthesia may lag behind the changes in the electroencephalogram, especially during induction and termination of anaesthesia, but nevertheless, the use of this technique has become a valuable aid in the control of anaesthetic depth especially when neuromuscular blocking drugs are employed which may mask some of the clinical manifestations of anaesthesia.

Several methods have been described whereby the electroencephalogram from the patient can be used to control, automatically, the amount of anaesthetic delivered so as to maintain a constant and predetermined depth.

PREMEDICATION

Before giving a general anaesthetic it is usually desirable to reduce anxiety and pain if these are present and also to produce sedation in the patient to allow a smooth induction of the anaesthetic. It is also an advantage to reduce bronchial and salivary secretion in order to prevent choking when the swallowing reflex becomes paralysed. The sedative drugs commonly used are morphine, papaveretum, and pethidine, the latter compound has no sedative action but relieves anxiety and produces a feeling of well-being.

Barbiturates are also used, but less frequently now than in the past, because their effect is somewhat unpredictable when given orally. Phenothiazine derivatives may also be employed and their anti-emetic properties may be of especial value in some patients.

Excessive salivary and bronchial secretions may be stopped by the use of an anticholinergic drug such as atropine, which blocks muscarinic receptors. The use of atropine-like drugs has the additional advantage of reducing reflex bradycardia mediated by the vagus. Vagal bradycardia is especially liable to occur with halothane and cyclopropane anaesthesia and this may lead to cardiac arrest. This effect may be abolished by the use of atropine-like compounds, although the release of catecholamines which occurs during cyclopropane anaesthesia may produce cardiac arrhythmias more readily when vagal tone to the heart is reduced. Hyoscine is often preferred to atropine because it is more effective in reducing secretions and has marked sedative properties of its own, although it is less effective in preventing vagal slowing of the heart.

Atropine-like compounds are usually given intravenously shortly before induction of anaesthesia, this has the advantage of ensuring that the patient is adequately atropinized during surgery and removes the discomfort to the patient of long periods of waiting with a dry mouth before the operation.

VOLATILE AND GASEOUS ANAESTHETICS

Volatile anaesthetics are absorbed from the lungs and largely excreted again unchanged. The passage of an anaesthetic like chloroform from the lungs to the blood is very rapid but many hours of absorption may be required before the body becomes saturated. This delay occurs because the gas passes slowly from the blood into other tissues and particularly into tissues rich in fat. In the early stages of administration the concentration of the anaesthetic in the venous blood is much less than in the arterial blood but both these concentrations increase and the difference between them becomes less. As the concentration in the blood rises the rate of absorption by the tissues gradually decreases until the blood is in equilibrium with the concentration of the anaesthetic which is used. Excretion is rapid at first, so that when administration ceases the blood concentration falls to about half its original value in 5 minutes.

The solubility of an inhalation anaesthetic in blood is important because it largely determines the rate of induction and recovery from anaesthesia. With gases of low solubility the tension rises quickly in the blood and therefore acts rapidly on the brain.

TABLE 2.1. PARTITION COEFFICIENTS OF SOME GASES AT BODY TEMPERATURE

	BLOOD/GAS	TISSUE/BLOOD BRAIN	FAT
Nitrogen	0·01	1·1	5·2
Cyclopropane	0·46	..	20·0
Nitrous oxide	0·47	1·0	3·0
Halothane	2·3	2·6	60·0
Chloroform	7·3	1·0	68·5
Trichlorethylene	9·0	..	107
Diethyl ether	15	1·14	3·3

THE VOLATILE AND GASEOUS ANAESTHETIC AGENTS

Halothane (CHBrCl.CF$_3$)

Halothane is a colourless liquid with a sweet, non-irritant odour. It is non-flammable and not explosive alone or in mixture with air or oxygen. It is now used in about 70 per cent. of all operations requiring general anaesthesia.

The stage of excitement during induction is brief and recovery from full anaesthesia is rapid and not unpleasant.

Halothane tends to lower blood pressure, probably by a combination of effects including the block of sympathetic ganglia, increase in vagal tone, direct myocardial depression, central vasomotor depression, and an increase in afferent discharge from the baroreceptors.

The most common arrhythmias associated with halothane anaesthesia are nodal rhythm and ventricular extrasystoles. Catecholamines should not be injected during anaesthesia because halothane is known to sensitize the myocardium to these compounds.

Halothane potentiates the action of curare-like drugs but antagonizes the effect of suxamethonium. There have been some reports of liver damage following the use of halothane but the incidence of the complication is ex-

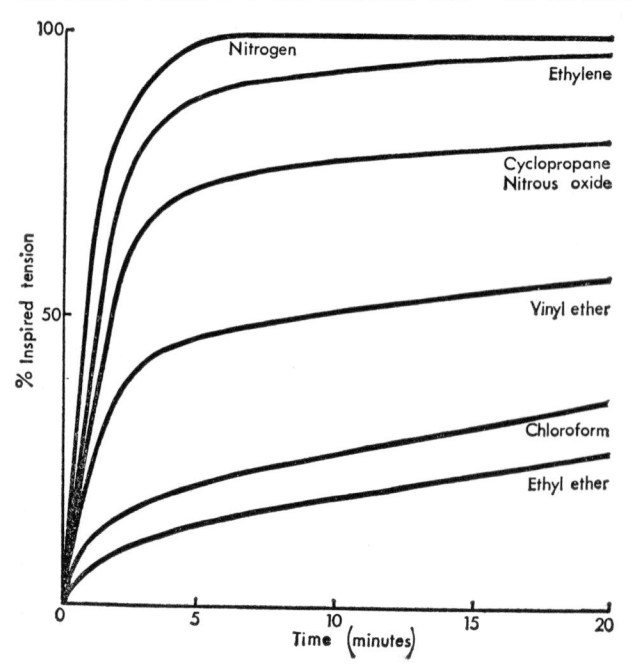

FIG. 2.2. The effect of the blood solubility of anaesthetic gases on their alveolar or arterial uptake curves. The rate of induction and recovery with these anaesthetics is largely a function of their solubility in blood.

tremely low and is often referable to a previous history of liver disease.

Methoxyflurane

Methoxyflurane is a non-flammable gas which is not explosive when mixed with oxygen and is stable in contact with soda lime. Because it has a low vapour pressure, induction is slow but when used with thiopentone this disadvantage is overcome. Methoxyflurane produces good muscular relaxation. Although the use of this anaesthetic is contra-indicated in the presence of liver disease and, like halothane, it may occasionally produce a fall in blood pressure and respiratory depression, it is regarded as a safe anaesthetic and is in wide use.

Fluoroxene

Fluoroxene is a new volatile anaesthetic which is flammable and explosive. It must be used in a closed-circuit system and is suitable for the induction of light anaesthesia.

Diethyl Ether (Anaesthetic Ether ($CH_3CH_2)_2O$)

Apart from nitrous oxide, ether is the oldest volatile anaesthetic still in use. Ether is a volatile (boiling point 35° C.), colourless liquid, with a pungent smell. It decomposes in air and in the presence of light and heat. Mixtures of ether with air, oxygen, or nitrous oxide are dangerously flammable and explosive.

An unexpected property of ether is that it has a neuromuscular blocking action and reduces the contraction of skeletal muscle evoked by nerve stimulation or by the close-arterial injection of acetylcholine. This effect is similar to that obtained by curare-like compounds whose action it potentiates. Before the introduction of neuromuscular blocking drugs, this effect of ether in producing a reduction of muscle tone made it a popular anaesthetic but its use has diminished in recent years.

Ether is a safe and versatile anaesthetic and, although it is not now used alone in major surgery, it is still used for short operations after anaesthesia has been induced by some other agent.

Ethyl Chloride (C_2H_5Cl)

The boiling point of ethyl chloride is 12·5° C. so that this substance is a gas at ordinary temperatures and pressures but a liquid if kept under slight pressure. It is slightly soluble in water and is flammable and forms explosive mixtures with air and with oxygen.

Ethyl chloride has been used as a general anaesthetic since the beginning of the century and for local analgesia by virtue of its cooling effect when applied locally.

It is still used as the sole anaesthetic for short operations on children and for the induction of anaesthesia prior to the use of another anaesthetic but it is being increasingly replaced by safer compounds.

Nitrous Oxide (N_2O)

Nitrous oxide was the first general anaesthetic to be used. It is a colourless gas, heavier than air, with a faint sweet smell. It is not flammable but, like oxygen, it supports combustion.

Nitrous oxide is a weak anaesthetic and is therefore commonly used in conjunction with analgesics or for the maintenance of anaesthesia after the administration of a rapidly acting barbiturate.

The gas can only be given in concentrations up to 80 per cent. with oxygen; higher concentrations than this produce hypoxia which may result in damage to the CNS.

When used without other drugs, an 80 per cent. mixture of nitrous oxide with oxygen does not usually produce more than second stage anaesthesia.

The gas may be used alone for very brief operations and it is used, in a 35–50 per cent. mixture with oxygen, as an analgesic in obstetrics.

There is little difference in the analgesic action of nitrous oxide when mixed with air instead of oxygen and this suggests that hypoxia is not responsible for the analgesic effect of nitrous oxide inhalation.

Cyclopropane

Cyclopropane is a colourless gas which is heavier than air, explosive, and flammable.

It is a potent but expensive anaesthetic gas and was extensively used until the advent of balanced anaesthetic techniques.

Cyclopropane is usually given from a closed-circuit anaesthetic machine and it acts rapidly after a not unpleasant induction.

The gas is safe but, because it is potent and rapidly absorbed, it is easy to give an overdose. Recovery from the anaesthetic is rapid but may be followed by restlessness due to a lack of analgesic activity during the recovery phase.

Apart from the risk of explosion it is a useful anaesthetic especially as it allows good oxygenation and has no serious toxic actions.

ANAESTHETIC SOLUTIONS

Various attempts have been made to produce anaesthetics that could be given in solution either intravenously or rectally. It is not usually considered safe to produce full and prolonged anaesthesia by a single dose in this way because the appropriate dose varies in an unpredictable way for different individuals. A dose which is large enough to produce surgical anaesthesia in a reasonable proportion of people would be fatal for some, and once the anaesthetic has been administered, it is impossible to recall it. On the other hand, some barbiturates are quickly taken up by body fat or are very rapidly destroyed in the body, so that it is possible to inject them more or less continuously throughout the operation and to control the depth of anaesthesia by controlling the rate of infusion.

Thiopentone Sodium (Sodium Thiopental)

This is the most widely used intravenous anaesthetic. It acts rapidly and is used to induce anaesthesia. Because thiopentone acts so rapidly the classical stages of anaesthesia are rarely seen and the first signs of an overdose may be apnoea.

Thiopentone is not an analgesic and it cannot therefore be used by itself for painful operations. The drug is highly fat soluble and this means that it will have a rapid onset of action. It also means that, despite the fact that it is only metabolized slowly in the liver and other body tissues, there will be a rapid recovery from its effects because it will be taken up in body fat. This explains why rapid recovery from the anaesthetic may follow several repeated injections of the drug up to a point when no more can be stored in the fat. A further dose then gives prolonged anaesthesia and recovery only occurs as the drug is destroyed.

FURTHER READING

BRAZIER, M. A. B. (1961) Some effects of anaesthesia on the brain, *Brit. J. Anaesth.*, 33, 194.

EGER, E. I. (1962) Atropine, scopolamine and related compounds, *Anesthesiology*, 23, 365.

FAULCONER, A., and BICKFORD, R. G. (1960) *Electroencephalography in Anesthesiology*, Springfield, Ill.

GILLESPIE, N. A. (1943) The signs of anaesthesia, *Curr. Res. Anesth.*, 22, 275.

MULLINS, L. J. (1954) Some physical mechanisms in narcosis, *Chem. Rev.*, 54, 289.

PAPPER, E. M., and KITZ, R. J. (1963) *Uptake and Distribution of Anesthetic Agents*, New York.

PATON, W. D. M., and SPEDEN, R. N. (1965) Uptake of anaesthetics and their effect on the central nervous system, *Brit. med. Bull.*, 21, 44.

SHEARER, W. M. (1961) The evolution of premedication, *Brit. J. Anaesth.*, 33, 219.

3

CENTRAL NERVOUS SYSTEM DEPRESSANTS II

THE drugs described in this chapter all have important and often strong depressant actions on the CNS. In sufficiently large doses, most of them will produce anaesthesia by a non-specific depression of the nervous system, but their main usefulness is found in a specific depression of certain central functions obtained with lower, and sometimes very small, doses.

Like other compounds which act directly on the nervous system, our knowledge of their mode of action is meagre.

HYPNOTICS AND SEDATIVES

Sleep is as necessary as food, and lack of it is a serious complication of disease. A hypnotic is a drug which produces sleep, and a very large number of hypnotics are available, but none of them should be used if the patient can be got to sleep by more simple means because dependence upon a hypnotic may become a habit which is difficult to break.

The difference between a hypnotic effect and general anaesthesia is largely a matter of degree. Any hypnotic given in a large dose causes general anaesthesia, but few drugs are used for both purposes because few drugs have the necessary combination of properties.

Many drugs have some degree of hypnotic activity but their predominant effect may be another type of CNS inhibition and this determines their classification. One can then talk of the hypnotic effects of such a drug but not of the drugs themselves as hypnotics.

Sedatives are agents used to relieve tension and anxiety and make sleep more possible, and they should not, as hypnotics do, actually make the patient sleepy. They act by causing a mild degree of cortical depression. Sedative drugs are usually the common hypnotic agents given in small doses throughout the day.

BARBITURATES

The formulae of a number of barbiturates are shown in TABLE 3.1. They are derivatives of barbituric acid in which all the substituted groups are H. Barbituric acid may be regarded as a derivative of malonic acid (COOH . CH$_2$. COOH) and urea and it is therefore sometimes called malonylurea. Barbituric acid is not itself a hypnotic but substitution of various organic radicals for the hydrogen atoms on C$_5$ gives compounds with hypnotic actions, the barbiturates.

Replacement of the oxygen atom on C$_2$ by a sulphur atom gives thiobarbituric acid, the basis of the thiobarbiturates.

Barbiturates are almost insoluble in water but possess weak acidic properties because they exist as an equilibrium mixture of keto (–CO–NH–) and enol (–C(OH):N) forms. The hydrogen of the enol form can be substituted by sodium or other metals to form soluble salts.

Certain features of the structure of the barbiturates allow some generalization of their actions to be made. If the alkyl groups on C$_5$ are increased in length the potency increases

TABLE 3.1. DERIVATIVES OF BARBITURIC ACID

$$\begin{array}{c} R_1 \\ R_2 \end{array} \!\!\!\! \diagdown\!\!\!\! \begin{array}{c} (6) \\ C \\ (5) \end{array} \!\!\!\! \diagup\!\!\!\! \begin{array}{c} CO-NH \\ CO-N \\ (4) \end{array} \!\!\!\! \diagdown\!\!\!\! \begin{array}{c} CO \\ (2) \\ | \\ R_3 \end{array}$$

DURATION OF ACTION	TRADE NAME	R_1	R_2	R_3	MAIN USE
'Long' Acting (longer than 8 hours)					
Barbitone	Veronal	Ethyl	Ethyl	H	Hypnotic
Phenobarbitone (Phenobarbital)	Luminal	Ethyl	Phenyl	H	Hypnotic, sedative, anticonvulsive
'Short' Acting (up to 8 hours)					
Amylobarbitone (Amobarbital)	Amytal	Ethyl	Isoamyl	H	Sedative, hypnotic, premedicant
Allobarbitone	Dial	Ethyl	Allyl	H	Sedative, hypnotic
Butobarbitone	Soneryl	Ethyl	n-butyl	H	Sedative, hypnotic
Cyclobarbitone	Phanodorm	Ethyl	Cyclohexenyl	H	Sedative, hypnotic
Pentobarbitone (Pentobarbital)	Nembutal	Ethyl	1-methylbutyl	H	Sedative, hypnotic, premedicant
Quinalbarbitone (Secobarbital)	Seconal	Allyl	1-methylbutyl	H	Hypnotic, premedicant
'Very Short' Acting (I.V. Injection)					
Hexobarbitone	Evipan	Methyl	Cyclohexenyl	1-methyl	Anaesthetic
Methohexitone	Brevital	Allyl	1-methyl-pentynyl	H, S replaces O on C_2	Anaesthetic, hypnotic
Thiopentone Sodium (Thiopental)	Pentothal	Ethyl	1-methylbutyl	H, S replaces O on C_2	Anaesthetic
Thialbarbitone	Kemithal	Allyl	Cyclohexenyl	H, S replaces O on C_2	Anaesthetic

but the duration of action is reduced. A similar change in effect occurs if the alkyl groups on C_5 are substituted by alicyclic, branched or unsaturated side chains and by the attachment of an alkyl group to one of the nitrogen atoms of the ureide. Anticonvulsant properties appear in the barbiturates when a phenyl group is present on C_5 and are more marked in straight-chained alkyl derivatives than in those with branched chains.

Most barbiturates, except hexobarbitone and thiopentone, are absorbed when given orally and most of them may also be given intravenously. They are excreted in the urine partly unchanged, although most of them are also metabolized in the liver.

It has been usual to classify barbiturates according to their duration of action but this arbitrary division is not based on measurement in man and cannot be regarded as satisfactory. It is now known that hypnotic barbiturates fall only into the longer and shorter acting groups and even this classification may not be valid because there is evidence that the incidence of hangover with phenobarbitone is no greater than with quinalbarbitone.

Except for barbitone and phenobarbitone, equilibrium between the brain and the plasma is quickly attained. The fat depots of the body are important repositories for some barbiturates, particularly short acting ones like thiopentone.

The classical barbiturates are broken down by oxidation of their alkyl side chains and produce hypnotically inactive compounds. N-methyl derivatives, such as hexobarbitones, are demethylated to give hypnotically active barbiturates and these quickly appear in the urine.

Thiobarbiturates undergo desulphuration to give barbiturates with activity similar to that of the parent compound and these can be found in plasma and must therefore play a part in the anaesthetic and post-anaesthetic action of thiobarbiturates.

Barbiturates are used as sedatives, hypnotics, basal narcotics, anaesthetics, and anticonvulsants, the appropriate compound being chosen on the basis of its duration of action [see TABLE 3.1]. With the exception of the very short acting compounds, most of the derivatives can be used as hypnotics but those in most common use are phenobarbitone, amylobarbitone, pentobarbitone, and quinalbarbitone.

Those who take barbiturates regularly are liable to become physically dependent on them and withdrawal symptoms may be observed following prolonged use of the drugs. The first dose may weaken the memory so that the patient forgets he has taken a dose and takes more. Overdosage may cause incoordination and prolonged sleep or profound anaesthesia with paralysis of the respiration. Barbiturate poisoning produces cyanosis and markedly depressed respiration which may result in respiratory failure followed by cardiovascular collapse and death. The most important way to treat barbiturate poisoning is by instituting artificial respiration and clearing the stomach contents if the drug has only recently been taken. If the drug has been absorbed, it may be advisable to produce forced diuresis.

When the barbiturate overdosage is not too great the depression of respiration may be treated with a compound such as bemegride which appears to antagonize the action of barbiturates on the medullary respiratory centres. The slow-acting barbiturates like barbitone and phenobarbitone have a cumulative action when taken every day. Barbiturates should be used with caution in severe liver and kidney disease as metabolism and excretion will be delayed.

Tolerance to barbiturates develops when they are taken repeatedly due to the activation of liver enzyme systems which metabolize the drug so reducing the effect of a given dose.

NON-BARBITURATE HYPNOTICS AND SEDATIVES

Various halogen derivatives are used as anaesthetics, basal narcotics, and hypnotics. They are all liable to cause toxic effects and should be avoided in patients who are liable to ketosis or who have damaged livers.

Chloral Hydrate ($CCl_3CH(OH)_2$)

This was the first hypnotic, having been introduced in 1868 by Liebreich, who knew that alkaline solutions liberated chloroform, and hoped that the same change would occur in the body. It is now known that chloral hydrate is reduced in the body to trichlorethylalcohol ($CCl_3.CH_2OH$), and that it is this substance which is active in the body. It combines in the liver with glycuronic acid to form urochloralic (chloraluric) acid ($CCl_3.CH_2O(CHOH)_5.COOH$). Urine containing urochloralic acid acquires the power of reducing Fehling's solution. Chloral hydrate is widely used, especially in the elderly and in children, as a hypnotic which is taken by mouth and causes sleep in about half an hour, and lasts 6–8 hours. It is especially valuable in manic states and to treat delirium tremens. Chloral hydrate should be well diluted before administration because it irritates the gastric mucosa and may cause nausea and vomiting.

Dichloralphenazone is a combination of chloral with phenazone that is also used as a hypnotic.

Glutethimide

Glutethimide is a piperidinedione derivative with actions rather similar to the barbiturates. It is a CNS depressant with strong hypnotic

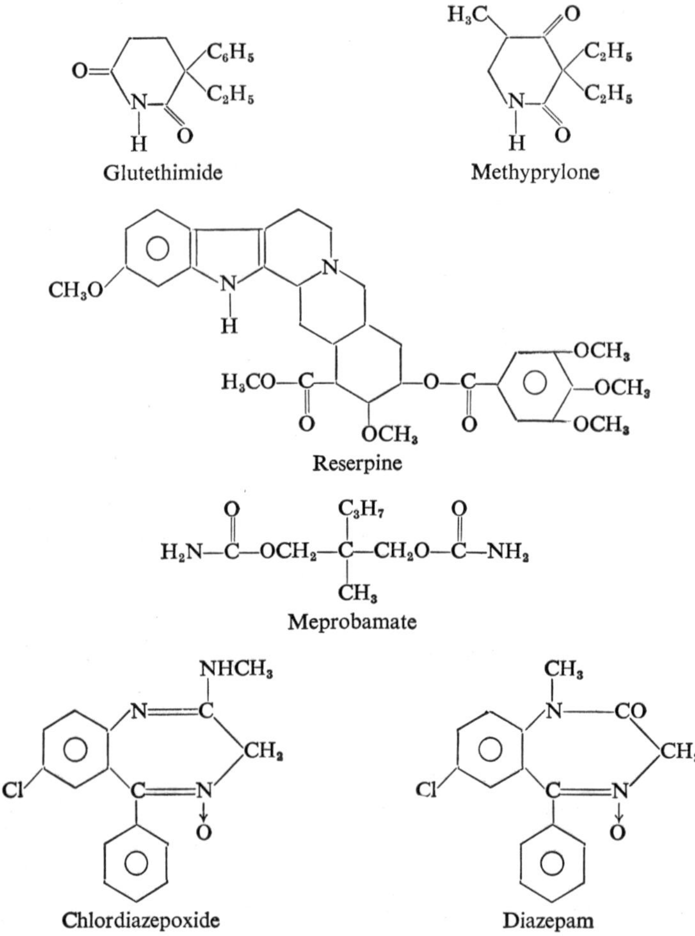

FIG. 3.1. The structures of some hypnotic and tranquillizing drugs.

Glutethimide

Methyprylone

Reserpine

Meprobamate

Chlordiazepoxide

Diazepam

activity and was introduced in the hope that it would prove less addictive than the barbiturates, but several cases of withdrawal symptoms, following discontinuance of the drug, have been reported and it must be considered a drug of addiction. It resembles phenobarbitone structurally and quinalbarbitone in its onset and duration of action. It is well tolerated and relatively non-toxic. It forms a useful alternative to barbiturates as a hypnotic.

Methyprylone

Methyprylone is used as a sedative and mild hypnotic, it acts within an hour and its effects last about 6 hours. Little is known about its side-effects but in normal dosage they appear to be absent.

Bromides

The bromides have a general depressant effect on the central nervous system with specific anticonvulsant activity. Their hypnotic and analgesic effects are weak in normal doses.

They are readily absorbed from the small intestine and are only excreted slowly in the urine. Complete elimination of the drug may not take place for 6 weeks or more and therefore their action is cumulative.

Bromides are not normally preferred to barbiturates and are no longer used except in some proprietary preparations.

ANTICONVULSANTS

The term 'epilepsy' describes a variety of disorders which may involve loss of consciousness, convulsions, and changes in the electroencephalogram.

The three major types of epilepsy are: (1) grand mal, in which major convulsions occur; (2) petit mal, in which there may be loss of consciousness with only mild convulsion and autonomic disturbance; and (3) psychomotor epilepsy in which there may be various types of confused behaviour.

The initiation of epileptic seizures appears to be due to a suppression of central inhibition and the development of abnormal nerve impulse activity in small feed-back loops, possibly as a result of enhanced post-tetanic potentiation (P.T.P.) effects in these circuits.

It seems that the most important action of anticonvulsants is to lower the excitability of certain central neurones and so diminish the excessive firing which would otherwise result in a seizure.

Most anticonvulsants are related to phenobarbitone, which is itself the oldest and best-tried anticonvulsant. Considerable efforts have been made to produce more potent anticonvulsants, without the disadvantages of barbiturates, by making small changes in the basic barbiturate molecule.

Most of the anticonvulsants contain a common basic ring structure and in all drugs except a few which are used for petit mal epilepsy only, the addition of a phenyl ring to the nucleus is essential for activity. The effect of structural changes on the central actions of these compounds can be followed in TABLE 3.2.

None of the anticonvulsant drugs at present in use are ideal because of their side-effects and because their action is not always predictable. These difficulties would be largely overcome if a drug were developed which could specifically potentiate central inhibitory processes. It is now known that γ-amino butyric acid is an inhibitory transmitter in parts of the brain including the cerebral cortex [see CHAPTER 4] and drugs which pass the blood–brain barrier and then mimic or potentiate its action may be highly effective anticonvulsants. It is already known that if γ-amino butyric acid itself, which does not pass the blood–brain barrier, is injected in very small amounts directly into the cerebral ventricle in man, it has a dramatic effect in alleviating the symptoms of epilepsy and produces no side-effects.

Phenobarbitone (Phenobarbital)

This was the first effective anticonvulsant known and is still in wide use. The upper dose limit is set by the appearance of sedation but this can be offset by combining the drug with a central stimulant like amphetamine.

Phenytoin (Diphenylhydantoin)

Phenytoin was developed in 1938 as a result of a planned search for a drug to diminish convulsions during electro-shock therapy. The drug is important because it is not a sedative and is particularly effective in suppressing electrically evoked convulsions in sub-hypnotic doses.

The mode of action of phenytoin appears to be to limit the spread of an epileptic focus rather than to increase the seizure threshold.

TABLE 3.2. THE STRUCTURES OF SOME ANTICONVULSANTS

Phenobarbitone. General anticonvulsant—sedative.

n-Methylphenobarbitone. General anticonvulsant—less sedative.

Phenytoin. Anticonvulsant, grand mal and psychomotor epilepsy—not sedative.

Troxidone. Anticonvulsant, petit mal—not sedative.

Phenacemide. Anticonvulsant, psychomotor epilepsy.

It is known that the drug is able to reduce P.T.P. in the spinal cord and a similar stabilizing action in higher centres could prevent the spread of epileptiform seizures. In petit mal attacks, where P.T.P. is thought not to be involved, this drug is ineffective. Phenytoin is well absorbed from the intestine and mostly destroyed in the body. Toxic effects are common and some may be serious. The less serious effects include dizziness, nausea, and skin rashes. The more serious complications are megaloblastic anaemia, morbilliform rash with fever, exfoliative dermatitis, and gingival hypertrophy.

Troxidone (Trimethadione)

The alkyl substituents in this compound confer a selective action on petit mal epilepsy and, unlike phenytoin, it has a marked effect on the electroencephalogram. Troxidone is a toxic drug and may cause rashes, photophobia, and, occasionally, agranulocytosis and aplastic anaemias.

Phenacemide

Phenacemide is used in the treatment of psychomotor epilepsy but only if other treatment fails because it is potentially toxic to the liver and bone marrow.

TRANQUILLIZING DRUGS

Tranquillizing drugs have been called the drugs of civilization and as modern society proceeds so the demand for these compounds rises.

Although their increasing and often indiscriminate use may be deplored, there is no doubt that they have revolutionized the treatment of the mentally ill and transformed the lives of many people who would otherwise have been condemned to institutions.

These drugs are used to treat conditions of fear, anxiety, and violence and have a particular use in the alleviation of the symptoms of schizophrenia and allied disorders. They do not have significant hypnotic or anaesthetic actions.

The tranquillizing compounds may be classified into two main groups, the major and the minor tranquillizers.

Major tranquillizers.
  Rauwolfia derivatives, i.e. reserpine.
  Phenothiazine derivatives, i.e. chlorpromazine, promazine, triflupromazine.
Minor tranquillizers.
  Propanediol derivatives, i.e. meprobamate.
  Benzodiazepine derivatives, i.e. chlordiazepoxide, diazepam.

MAJOR TRANQUILLIZERS

Rauwolfia Derivatives

Reserpine is the most important of the many alkaloids found in extracts of the climbing shrub known as *Rauwolfia serpentina* which has long been used in India for treating snake bites, hypertension, insomnia, insanity, and noisy children.

In recent times reserpine was used to relieve hypertension but the calming effect of this drug led to it being used as an effective tranquillizer. It is absorbed from the intestine and is commonly given by the mouth. Its action develops slowly during 2–4 hours and may last several days, even when the drug is injected intravenously, but the highest concentration in the brain is found comparatively soon, before any obvious effects on the whole animal are seen. It is hydrolysed in the body to methyl reserpate which appears in the urine.

It is generally agreed that the tranquillizing action of reserpine is quite different from the sedative action of barbiturates. Its mode of action is not known but what is known is that it depletes the brain of 5-hydroxytryptamine and noradrenaline, the latter to about 10 per cent. of its original level within 4 hours and for about 8 hours, but it is unlikely that these effects alone are responsible for the tranquillizing action of reserpine.

Reserpine has a prolonged sedative action without narcosis and is not an anticonvulsant. It inhibits the activity of sympathetic but not parasympathetic centres and as a result there is a fall of body temperature, constriction of the pupil, a fall in blood pressure, loss of pressor reflexes, and diarrhoea. The central side-effects of reserpine include fatigue, nervousness, insomnia, nightmares; tolerance and addiction do not occur. There is now little doubt that reserpine may also produce suicidal tendencies in some patients and for this reason it is not now in wide use.

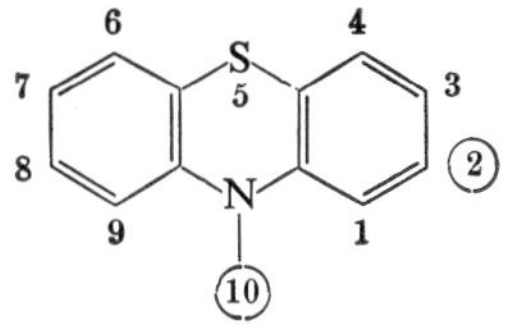

FIG. 3.2. The phenothiazine nucleus.

Phenothiazine Derivatives

This group forms the largest and most important group of major tranquillizers. They are all based on the phenothiazine nucleus, differing only in their substituents at positions 2 and 10. These compounds share the same general properties but differ quantitatively in their tranquillizing potency and side-effects.

There are many phenothiazine derivatives in addition to those shown in TABLE 3.3 but the

TABLE 3.3. PHENOTHIAZINE DERIVATIVES

	10	2	TRANQUILLIZING POTENCY
Chlorpromazine	$(CH_2)_3$—$N(CH_3)_2$	Cl	1·0
Promazine	$(CH_2)_3$—$N(CH_3)_2$	H	0·5
Triflupromazine	$(CH_2)_3$—$N(CH_3)_2$	CF_3	4
Trifluoperazine	$(CH_2)_3$—N⟨ ⟩NCH_3	CF_3	10

most important changes that may be made to the phenothiazine nucleus are illustrated by these examples. The most potent tranquillizers have a three-carbon chain attached at position 10 and the addition of a fluorine radical or a piperazine ring as in trifluoperazine raises their potency still further.

Chlorpromazine. This substance was first used in Paris in 1951 by Laborit and Huguenard to lower the body temperature and so cause 'artificial hibernation' during operations.

The most important effect of chlorpromazine is to cause tranquillization and in normal dosage it does not affect higher mental function.

It is widely used in mental hospitals to treat seriously disturbed patients and is often so effective they can return home. Like reserpine it increases the action of hypnotics, but unlike reserpine it does not reduce the amounts of 5-hydroxytryptamine and noradrenaline in the brain. It has an anti-emetic action on the vomiting centre in the medulla and it antagonizes the actions of various drugs on this centre. It has little or no action on motion sickness.

Its main peripheral action is to antagonize the α-receptor actions of catecholamines [CHAPTER 7]. It has local anaesthetic action and has an effect like that of quinidine on the heart. It does not block autonomic ganglia and in spite of its chemical similarity to promethazine, it has practically no atropine-like or antihistamine-like action.

Its effect on the circulation may be largely due to depression of the central and peripheral sympathetic nervous system. Under its action the blood pressure is low, the skin warm and dry, and the pulse rapid. It causes a marked reduction in temperature, partly due to cutaneous vasodilatation and partly due to the inhibition of shivering. The fall in temperature causes a fall in the metabolism of the tissues and this may protect them from harm when their circulation is depressed during operations, and in some other conditions where shock may occur. Some of the sedative effects may be secondary to the fall of temperature.

A single large dose may cause postural hypertension. Repeated doses may cause excessive sedation, Parkinson-like tremor, various allergic effects, leucopenia, and obstructive jaundice, the latter effect being the result of hypersensitivity in a few people to the drug.

Minor side-effects include a dry mouth, constipation, and urinary frequency.

Promazine and trifluoperazine have similar actions to chlorpromazine.

MINOR TRANQUILLIZERS

Propanediol Derivatives

These compounds are used for the treatment of anxiety states; they are not effective in the treatment of psychoses.

Meprobamate. Meprobamate blocks neuronal conduction in the hypothalamus and spinal cord and it produces mild tranquillization without drowsiness. It is used in the treatment of neuroses, alcoholism, and anxiety states but it does carry a serious addiction risk. It also reduces tolerance to ingested alcohol.

Mephenesin is a muscle relaxant and an interneuronal blocker. It is not a very effective tranquilliser but it has few side-effects. Mephenesin carbamate is more widely used than mephenesin because it is more slowly absorbed from the gastro-intestinal tract and has a longer duration of action.

Benzodiazepines

Chlordiazepoxide and Diazepam. These compounds form a new chemical class of tranquillizer. Chlordiazepoxide was the first to be used and diazepam, a more potent compound, was then introduced. These drugs are widely used for a variety of conditions, particularly anxiety states, to secure muscle relaxation, and in the rehabilitation of alcoholics. The tranquillizing effect of these chemicals was first used to tame tigers but they are now more extensively used on man.

They block electroencephalogram arousal patterns following stimulation of the reticular formation and reduce after-discharges in higher centres but, like all tranquillizers, their precise mode of action is unknown.

A great advantage of these drugs is that, although they are rapidly absorbed from the gut, their action is prolonged, the plasma half-peak concentration occurring after about 24 hours.

Unpleasant side-effects are only seen in very high doses when drowsiness and ataxia may be apparent. There is little, if any, development of tolerance or addiction and the drugs are safe, 2·25 G. having been taken over 24 hours without death.

ALCOHOL (C_2H_5OH)

Alcohol is an anaesthetic, a disinfectant, a protein precipitant, a local irritant and, in discreet doses, it may also be regarded as a valuable minor tranquillizer.

Alcohol is rapidly absorbed from the stomach and if any reaches the intestines it is rapidly absorbed from there. It can also be absorbed as a vapour through the lungs. Once absorbed, alcohol is quickly distributed throughout the body water.

Up to 98 per cent. of the alcohol that enters the body is completely oxidized, the rate at which this oxidation takes place is related more to body weight than to the concentration of alcohol present. About 10 ml. of alcohol can be oxidized by a normal adult per hour.

Primary oxidation of alcohol by alcohol dehydrogenase occurs in the liver where acetaldehyde is formed which is then converted to acetyl CoA. This is then further oxidized through the citric acid cycle or utilized in the synthesis of tissue constituents.

Alcohol which is not oxidized in the body is excreted almost entirely through the kidney and lungs. As the amount of alcohol removed from the body in this way comprises only a small part of that ingested the use of diuretics does little to remove the signs of intoxication.

Action of Alcohol

The effect of alcohol on the CNS tends to overshadow the numerous actions of this drug on other tissues.

Contrary to popular opinion, the action of alcohol on the CNS is mainly inhibitory and the apparent excitatory action of this drug results from the depression of inhibitory systems in the higher centres of the brain. These higher centres normally exert an inhibitory influence enabling the organism to behave sensibly. When these centres are suppressed the cruder instincts appear to be released and behaviour becomes more spontaneous, more childlike, and less critical.

Human alcohol intoxication is commonly divided into four stages:

1. In the first stage there is a slight loss of efficiency, a dulled critical ability, and spinal reflexes are slower and weaker but the subject feels pleased with himself.

2. In the second stage, the novice drinker loses all self-control, the hardened drinker speaks and moves with exaggerated care.

3. In the third stage the subject is unconscious with a flushed face, active sweat glands, red eyes, and dilated pupils.

4. In the fourth stage there is danger of death from paralysis of the respiratory and vasomotor centres in the medulla.

Alcohol affects the electroencephalogram, causing a slowing of the dominant rhythm and this has been used as a guide to the state of intoxication.

The mechanism of action of alcohol on cells in the CNS is obscure. It does seem to have a non-specific depressant action on the excitability of all neurones and this may be through a local anaesthetic action.

Serious additive effects are known to occur when alcohol is taken in addition to various psychotropic drugs. Chlorpromazine, for instance, greatly increases the expected impairment of judgement and co-ordination following alcohol ingestion.

Alcohol causes an increase in blood flow through the skin, probably by direct inhibition of the vasomotor centre. This leads to a feeling of warmth and a fall in body temperature. In reasonable doses, alcohol does not appear to have any direct effect on cardiac output, coronary or cerebral blood flow.

The increase in peripheral blood flow following alcohol ingestion causes a fall in body temperature and this may be aggravated by the occurrence of sweating. As with general anaesthetics, large doses of alcohol may inhibit the central temperature regulating mechanisms and so cause a pronounced fall in body temperature.

Alcohol produces diuresis partly because of the extra fluid that is ingested and also by a direct action inhibiting the release of antidiuretic hormone from the posterior pituitary. The diuretic effect is proportional to the level of circulating alcohol in the blood and is usually only seen as the alcohol level rises.

Chronic Alcohol Poisoning

The constant drinking of alcohol injures the CNS so that the drinker becomes careless, untidy, forgetful, and irritable. At the same time he acquires a certain amount of tolerance so that large quantities of alcohol have no apparent effect on him. This is mainly due to a real insensitivity of the nervous system, and to the fact that the persistent drinker has much practice in concealing the effects of drink. As time goes on the drinker becomes more irritable and more anxious and may eventually develop delirium tremens. In this condition he is very restless and may suffer a variety of hallucinations. This condition may eventually lead to permanent mental disturbance or to death.

Chronic alcoholism has many ill effects, some of which are due to associated factors such as vitamin deficiency. The stomach shows chronic gastritis; the kidneys show fatty changes and hypertrophy of connective tissue, and cirrhosis of the liver may occur. One of the most important effects is neuritis involving both sensory and motor nerves and causing loss of sensation in the skin and loss of power in the muscles. This neuritis is due to a deficiency of aneurine and can be cured by the injection of this substance. The diet of chronic alcoholics is usually deficient in this vitamin and absorption is poor.

Tetraethylthiuram disulphide (disulfiram, *Antabuse*) is a drug now used to treat cases of chronic alcoholism. This substance was originally tested as an anthelminthic but when first tested on man it was noticed that it produced disturbing and unpleasant symptoms when alcohol was ingested. Given by itself disulfiram is relatively non-toxic but it greatly alters the intermediate metabolism of alcohol by inhibiting the oxidation of acetaldehyde in the liver thus allowing the concentration of this substance in the body to rise. The symptoms of acetaldehyde poisoning include excessive flushing, headaches, palpitations, giddiness, and nausea and are so unpleasant that alcohol will be avoided as long as disulfiram is present.

ANALGESICS

Pain saves many lives, since it compels those who can, to avoid harm and to seek treatment when harm has been done. The relief of pain is always desirable, but the use of drugs for this purpose is dangerous if it makes diagnosis more difficult, or if it is allowed to take the place of more fundamental treatment.

Pain can be relieved by general anaesthetics,

local anaesthetics, counter-irritants, or by various drugs which act centrally without producing general anaesthesia. The best known of these are morphine and its derivatives, but various synthetic drugs are equally effective, and the antipyretics [CHAPTER 10] have a weak action of the same kind.

Painful stimuli cause a number of reactions, such as a sudden intake of breath, withdrawal from the source of pain, vocalization, a fall of blood pressure, and the psycho-galvanic reflex, which consists of changes in the electrical resistance of the skin. It is difficult to compare the relative potency and effectiveness of different analgesics because it is not easy to assess pain quantitatively. Weakly painful stimuli can be applied by a measured prick with a needle, heat, cold, or electric shocks which produce some unconditioned responses, such as the sudden intake of breath, without enough pain to disturb the animal. Analgesics such as morphine diminish these effects and their action can be measured in this way.

Another method of studying analgesics involves experiments on man. The pain may be due to disease or produced artificially. Painful agents used include ischaemia, pressure, and electrical currents and the effect may be judged by the man's response or description of his sensations. Such experiments are said to be subjective and are notoriously difficult, since the result may be affected by a multitude of factors.

OPIUM

Opium consists of dark resinous lumps, made by drying the milky juice that exudes when an incision is made in unripe seed capsules of the Oriental poppy (*Papaver somniferum*). It contains about twenty-five different alkaloids, the most important of which are morphine (3–20 per cent.), codeine (methylmorphine) (0·3–0·4 per cent.), narcotine (2–8 per cent.), and thebane (0·2–0·5 per cent.). The other alkaloids, including narceine and papaverine, constitute just over 1 per cent. of the drug.

MORPHINE

Morphine [TABLE 3.4] is the most important alkaloid in opium; it is readily absorbed when eaten, smoked, or injected. Its effects are seen in about half an hour and begin to pass away after 3–5 hours but may last for at least 12 hours. It is mostly oxidized, mainly in the liver, and a certain amount is excreted into the stomach and probably into other parts of the alimentary canal.

TABLE 3.4. THE STRUCTURE OF SOME MORPHINE-LIKE COMPOUNDS AND THEIR ANTAGONISTS

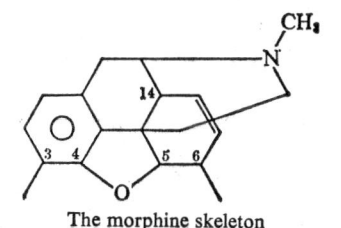

The morphine skeleton

	Substituents on morphine skeleton			
	3	4–5	6	N–
Morphine	HO	O	HO	CH_3
Codeine	CH_3O	O	HO	CH_3
Diamorphine	CH_3COO	O	CH_3COO	CH_3
Dihydromorphinone	HO	O	=O	CH_3
Levorphanol	HO	—	H	C_3H_5
Metopon	CH_3O	O	=O	CH_3
Nalorphine	HO	O	HO	C_3H_5
Levallorphan	HO	—	H	C_3H_5

Morphine exerts its most important effects on the CNS where it causes depression and excitation of certain centres. It depresses the cerebral cortex and reduces the powers of concentration, fear, and anxiety. Pain, particularly prolonged, as opposed to acute pain, is reduced and this produces a great feeling of contentment.

The effect on the cerebellum is mainly depressant and there may be motor incoordination. Various centres in the medulla are affected. The vomiting centre and the associated centres for salivation, sweat, and bronchial secretion are stimulated at first, though become depressed by large and subsequent doses. The sweating is associated with vasodilatation of the skin vessels, so that morphine increases heat loss and is a mild antipyretic.

The respiratory centre and the cough centre are depressed. The respiration is slow and deep and may be periodic. Large doses kill by stopping the respiration altogether. The parasympathetic portion of the oculomotor nucleus is stimulated and the pupils become constricted and, in morphine poisoning, may be of pinpoint size. Other effects mediated via the CNS include a feeling of heaviness in the limbs, a dry mouth, itching, and the reduction of hunger sensations.

Little is known about how morphine exerts these effects on the CNS. It does inhibit the hydrolysis of acetylcholine and in low concentrations it reduces the release of acetylcholine from nerve endings in the guinea-pig intestine. If acetylcholine is a neurotransmitter in the brain this may have some bearing on the action of morphine. Morphine also blocks the action of 5-hydroxytryptamine at peripheral sites and although there are indications that this chemical may be concerned in central transmission, it is again not possible to say if morphine works by this kind of action.

Morphine does not affect the excitability of sensory nerve endings nor does it affect axonal conduction but polysynaptic reflexes are affected more readily than monosynaptic, suggesting it may be the multineurone networks in the brain that are particularly vulnerable to its presence. It has also been suggested that the effect of morphine on the sensation of pain resembles the result of prefrontal lobotomy and there is electrophysiological evidence to suggest that morphine does alter the association between the frontal lobes and the rest of the brain.

Of the more peripheral actions of morphine, constipation is one of the most important. The constipation produced is unaffected by denervation of the intestine or by atropine, and is largely due to an increase in the tone of the gut and sphincters and an inhibitory action on Auerbach's plexus. Other factors which probably increase this action of morphine are inhibition of the secretion of the intestinal glands and depression of the reflexes responsible for defaecation.

Morphine also causes retention of both urine and bile by closing the sphincters. It raises the pressure in the common bile-duct and may cause biliary colic. It should therefore not be used in the treatment of pain due to biliary colic.

Tolerance and Dependence

Tolerance to morphine occurs and, over a period of time, the dose taken has to be increased to produce the same degree of effect. Tolerance in man usually takes 2–3 weeks to acquire on normal therapeutic doses and it applies only to the depressant action of the drug, the respiratory depression shows tolerance but the effect on the pupil and on the intestine continues unabated. People receiving morphine regularly are liable to become physically dependent on the drug. When this has occurred, withdrawal of the drug produces symptoms within 15–20 hours. In addicts, the morphine antagonist nalorphine [p. 38] can produce withdrawal symptoms within 30 minutes. The withdrawal symptoms commence with yawning, sweating, and running of the eyes and nose. There will then be restlessness for 18–24 hours. After this period there is mydriasis, 'goose flesh', cramp, nausea, insomnia, vomiting, and diarrhoea. Tolerance to morphine is rapidly lost during this period and the withdrawal symptoms may be terminated by a suitable dose of morphine.

MORPHINE-LIKE COMPOUNDS

Pethidine (Meperidine)

Pethidine is a piperidine compound and has many properties in common with both morphine and atropine. This drug has a slightly higher analgesic potency than codeine. It causes euphoria and may lead to physical dependence. Its actions differ in many ways from those of drugs in the morphine group. It is not an effective sedative or hypnotic and its direct effect on smooth muscle is inhibitory; it does not constrict the pupil or cause constipation. On the other hand, like morphine, it closes the sphincter of Oddi and thus increases the pressure in the gall-bladder, so that it should not be used in the treatment of biliary colic. Tolerance is not as complete as with morphine and with the doses that some addicts take, convulsions may occur.

Pethidine is used for acute pain in pre- and post-operative stages and for chronic pain associated with cancer. It may be used as a premedicant, in the early stages of labour, for incomplete anaesthesia during minor surgical procedures, and to produce basal narcosis in conjunction with drugs like chlorpromazine and promethazine. It is particularly useful in pulmonary and cardiac surgery because it depresses cardiac and bronchial reflexes.

Codeine

The actions of codeine are much weaker than those of morphine and it is less likely to cause unpleasant side-effects and, even in large doses, it does not depress respiration. It is not as addictive as morphine and unlike morphine, is not destroyed in the body, but is mostly excreted in the urine. It is used to treat minor pain and as an antitussive agent.

Pholcodine

Pholcodine resembles codeine in suppressing cough and is particularly useful in the treatment of unproductive cough. It is less toxic than codeine, does not cause constipation, and is well tolerated by children.

Diamorphine (Heroin)

Diamorphine is a slightly more powerful analgesic than morphine with fewer side-effects. Diamorphine is used nowadays only to relieve very severe pain, usually in a terminal illness.

Dihydromorphinone

Dihydromorphinone is a synthetic derivative of morphine with a similar but weaker analgesic activity. It may be used as a substitute for morphine and unpleasant side-effects are said to be less severe.

Levorphanol

Levorphanol acts like morphine but its effect is more prolonged. It has little hypnotic activity and anxiety is not relieved. Levorphanol is used for the relief of severe pain. Its lack of sedative action is an advantage in some patients.

Methadone

Methadone is a strong analgesic of similar potency to morphine but it has less sedative and euphoric action. Tolerance to the analgesic, sedative, and respiratory depressant effects has been observed. It is a drug of addiction. It is used to treat severe pain and in premedication. It is also used to treat morphine dependence because it may be withdrawn with few unpleasant consequences.

Phenazocine

Phenazocine is a synthetic analgesic with similar actions and uses to morphine but it is effective in smaller doses and has a more prolonged action. It was developed in the hope that it would be less addictive than morphine but this hope has not been fulfilled.

Etorphine

Etorphine is a new synthetic agent which is from one thousand to eight thousand times more potent than morphine. It has a powerful central depressant action which can be antagonized with nalorphine.

ANTAGONISTS OF MORPHINE ACTION

Nalorphine

This is a competitive antagonist of morphine and is used as an antidote not only for morphine but also for synthetic substitutes such as pethidine and methadone. Structurally it only differs from morphine in the replacement of the methyl radical attached to the nitrogen atom with an allyl group.

The actions of nalorphine alone are similar to those of morphine. Respiration and blood pressure are depressed and it has a slight sedative, but little analgesic, action.

When respiratory depression is established with morphine the administration of nalorphine will stimulate breathing. This probably occurs because nalorphine competes successfully with morphine for receptor sites in the respiratory centre, and while alone it would depress respiration, it would do so less than morphine so the net result is a reduction in the morphine depression.

Nalorphine can be used to establish whether addiction to morphine-like drugs is present because withdrawal symptoms will quickly follow the injection of nalorphine to the addict.

Levallorphan

Levallorphan is a morphine-like compound having the same relationship to levorphanol as nalorphine has to morphine.

Like nalorphine this compound antagonizes respiratory depression due to morphine-like drugs and will prevent respiratory depression if given with them. It also reduces the analgesic action of these drugs so the agonist and antagonist are not normally given together.

ANTIPYRETIC–ANALGESICS

These are considered, with their role in lowering body temperature, in CHAPTER 10.

FURTHER READING

BOVET, D., LONGO, V. G., and SILVESTRINI, B. (1957) Electrophysiological methods of research in the study of tranquillizers. Contribution to the study of the reticular formation, in *Psychotropic Drugs*, Amsterdam.

DOMINO, E. F. (1962) Sites of action of some central nervous depressants, *Ann. Rev. Pharmacol.*, **6**, 217.

FIELDS, W. S. (1957) *Brain Mechanisms and Drug Action*, Springfield, Ill.

LASAGNA, L. (1954) A comparison of hypnotic agents, *J. Pharmacol. exp. Ther.*, **111**, 9.

MILLICHAP, J. P. (1965) Anticonvulsant drugs, in *Physiological Pharmacology*, ed. ROOT, W. S., and HOFMANN, F. G., Vol. 2, New York.

SPINKS, A. (1963) Anticonvulsant drugs, *Progr. Med. Chem.*, **3**, 261.

STEINBERG, H. (1964) *Animal Behaviour and Drug Action*, London.

4

CENTRAL NERVOUS SYSTEM STIMULANTS

THE drugs described in this chapter excite both mental and motor activity but they often act in very different ways to achieve these ends.

Many of these compounds have more than one type of action on the nervous system but they are classified, and will be discussed here, under the heading of their most important action.

These compounds may act directly on the CNS by increasing the effectiveness of excitatory synaptic signalling or they may work by reducing central inhibition. There are numerous ways in which these changes may be effected by stimulant drugs and it is only in recent years that details of some of these actions are beginning to be understood. There are now plausible explanations for the actions of some convulsants and it is likely that this understanding will aid studies on the actions of other stimulant compounds.

ANTIDEPRESSANTS

Drugs in this class are used widely for patients who are socially maladjusted, apathetic, and depressed. They may be divided into four major classes: (1) the direct stimulants; (2) monoamine oxidase inhibitors; (3) dibenzazepine derivatives; and (4) xanthine derivatives.

DIRECT STIMULANTS

Amphetamine

Amphetamine increases the speed of mental arithmetic, delays fatigue, and produces a general feeling of well-being. It stimulates respiration and is used to treat poisoning by depressant drugs and as an adjuvant in the treatment of mild depressive neuroses. It helps to reduce obesity by reducing the appetite. Amphetamine has, like adrenaline, α and β peripheral actions and a powerful direct stimulant action on the CNS, particularly in the region of the reticular formation. This stimulant action occurs even when brain catecholamines have been depleted by reserpine and in the presence of monoamine oxidase inhibitors.

Amphetamine and amphetamine derivatives are now in wide use with and without medical supervision. This has led to considerable problems because of the addictive nature of these compounds. These drugs should only be taken for short periods and always under medical supervision. There is now good evidence that this class of compound may precipitate dangerous psychoses in some types of patient.

Dexamphetamine (Dextro Amphetamine)

This is the dextro-isomer of amphetamine and it is three to four times as potent as the L-isomer. It has similar pharmacological actions to amphetamine but its central effects, in relation to its peripheral actions, are stronger than those of amphetamine. The side-effects of this drug are as dangerous as those of amphetamine.

Dexamphetamine is often mixed with a CNS depressant, usually a barbiturate, and is officially used in this form to treat obesity. It is in this form that the drug is taken unofficially for its CNS stimulant activity. A common mixture is that of dexamphetamine with amylobarbitone (*Drinamyl*, *Dexytal*, 'Purple Hearts').

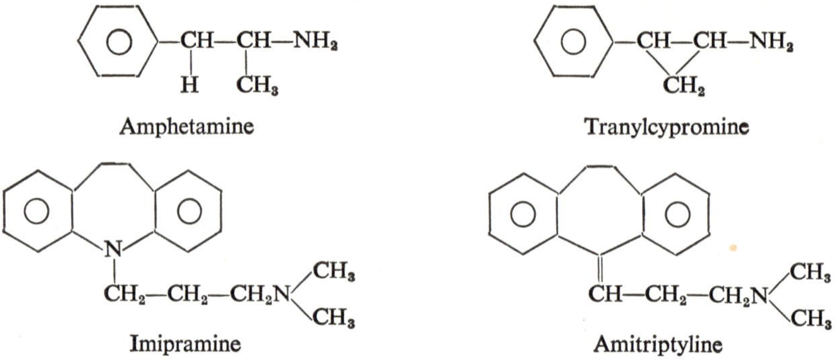

Amphetamine

Tranylcypromine

Imipramine

Amitriptyline

Fig. 4.1. The structures of some antidepressant compounds.

MONOAMINE OXIDASE INHIBITORS [Fig. 4.2]

The drugs in this section are all antidepressants and inhibit monoamine oxidase but there is little evidence to suggest any link between these two actions. It is possible that these compounds have a central action quite distinct from their ability to block monoamine oxidase systems.

The early monoamine oxidase inhibitors were hydrazine derivatives and were highly toxic and are therefore no longer in use (iproniazid, pheniprazine) but modifications to the structure of iproniazid have yielded less toxic hydrazines which are only slightly less effective as antidepressants (isocarboxazid, nialamide, phenelzine). Tranylcypromine, a monoamine oxidase inhibitor which is not a hydrazine derivative, has also been developed.

Iproniazid, Pheniprazine, Isocarboxazid, Nialamide, Phenelzine

These compounds are all derivatives of hydrazine and inhibit monoamine oxidase. Iproniazid was originally introduced as an antitubercular drug but its stimulating action on the CNS led it to be used for this action. This resulted in the development of related compounds with similar central actions but fewer toxic side-effects. The most serious side-effects encountered with iproniazid result from over-stimulation of the nervous system and include manic symptoms

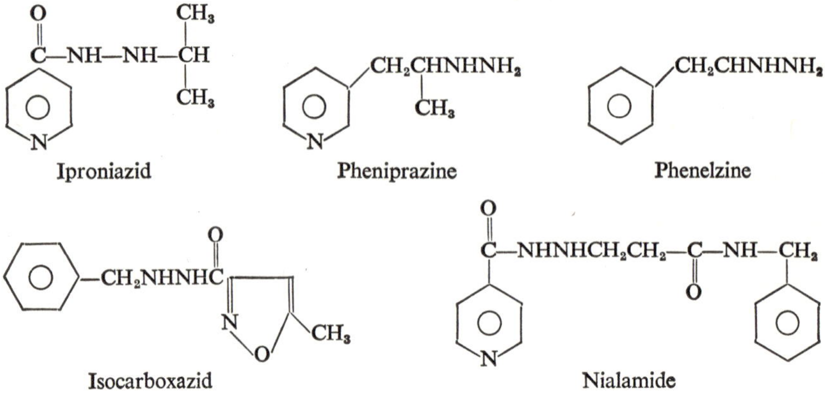

Iproniazid

Pheniprazine

Phenelzine

Isocarboxazid

Nialamide

Fig. 4.2. Hydrazine derivatives which are antidepressants.

and insomnia. Liver damage and hypertension may also occur. Isocarboxazid has a more delayed onset of action but its side-effects are less serious than those of iproniazid. Phenelzine may cause hypertension as may pheniprazine but this latter drug is a more effective monoamine oxidase inhibitor than iproniazid and is quicker acting and less toxic.

Tranylcypromine

This compound is not a hydrazine derivative but inhibits monoamine oxidase. Caution has to be exercised in the use of all the compounds which inhibit monoamine oxidase because serious complication can ensue when patients under their influence eat certain foods containing large amounts of tyramine [see CHAPTER 7].

DIBENZAZEPINE DERIVATIVES

These drugs are now the most widely used ones for the treatment of mental depression. They were discovered in 1958 during clinical trials of phenothiazine tranquillizers. It was found that one compound, imipramine, had a low tranquillizing potency but that it helped certain types of depressed patients.

This is remarkable since imipramine only differs from promazine, a useful tranquillizer, by the replacement of the sulphur atom which links the benzene rings, by a CH_2—CH_2 chain.

Imipramine, Desmethylimipramine

These compounds have only very weak monoamine oxidase inhibitory activity and, not surprisingly, they share many common properties with the phenothiazines, having some local anaesthetic action and mild atropine-like and antihistamine effects. The way in which they stimulate the nervous system is unknown but, unlike amphetamine, they are ineffective if brain catecholamines have been depleted by reserpine.

It has been demonstrated that imipramine has a cocaine-like effect on sympathetic nerve terminals and prevents the re-uptake of noradrenaline. This greatly reduces the inactivation of noradrenaline and therefore potentiates its action and this may account for the stimulant action of the drug on the CNS.

Amitriptyline

Amitriptyline is chemically and pharmacologically related to imipramine. It has atropine-like properties and the side-effects of its use include a dry mouth, tachycardia, blurred vision, and constipation.

Although imipramine, desmethylimipramine, and amitriptyline are all mild tranquillizers their clinical usefulness is found as antidepressants. It may be that the removal of anxiety from patients with some kinds of depression is sufficient to relieve the illness.

XANTHINE DERIVATIVES

Caffeine, Theobromine, Theophylline

The xanthine derivatives [FIG. 4.3] have many pharmacological properties in common. They stimulate the CNS, act on the kidney to produce diuresis, stimulate cardiac muscle, and relax smooth muscle [CHAPTER 8]. Although they share these properties it is usual to find

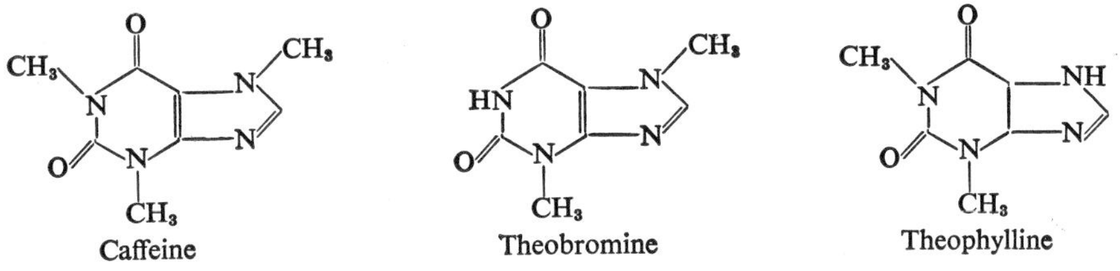

FIG. 4.3. The structures of some xanthine derivatives.

TABLE 4.1

	CNS AND RESPIRATORY STIMULATION	SMOOTH MUSCLE RELAXANT	DIURESIS	CARDIAC STIMULATION	SKELETAL MUSCLE STIMULATION
Caffeine	+++	+	+	+	+++
Theobromine	+	++	++	++	+
Theophylline	++	+++	+++	+++	++

that they are not all equally effective for each type of action.

The effectiveness of the pharmacological actions of each compound are shown in TABLE 4.1.

Caffeine is completely absorbed from the small intestine and most of it is oxidized to urea and carbon dioxide. Some is excreted as methyl-uric acids and some as methyl-xanthines and a very small amount is excreted in the urine unchanged. None of the xanthines are completely demethylated so there is no increase in the excretion of uric acid.

Caffeine is a strong CNS stimulant, theophylline is less powerful, and theobromine has only a weak action. Caffeine excites the CNS at all levels but the cortex appears most vulnerable and the spinal cord least vulnerable. Its main effect is to produce clear thought and to reduce drowsiness and fatigue. It increases the motor effects of conditioned reflexes and improves the higher functions of the brain such as those involved in mental arithmetic. These effects may be obtained with about 100–250 mg. of caffeine, the amount contained in one or two cups of coffee.

The xanthines also stimulate the respiratory, vagal, and vasomotor centres in the medulla. Caffeine is a particularly effective respiratory stimulant and it is used for this purpose. If very large doses are injected they cause strychnine-like convulsions by stimulating the spinal cord.

It has been known for some time that the methylxanthines have marked effects on cellular metabolism. Caffeine increases the oxygen consumption and lactic acid output of skeletal muscle and the twitch strength is increased. This may occur because methylxanthines, especially theophylline, are competitive inhibitors of phosphodiesterase, an enzyme that inactivates cyclic 3′, 5′ AMP. The concentration of cyclic AMP rises and tissue glycolysis therefore increases. In this way metabolic activity may be increased and may account, at least in part, for the stimulant action of these drugs on the nervous system.

These compounds are used therapeutically for their actions on the myocardium, smooth muscle, and CNS. Caffeine is mostly used only as a CNS stimulant while theobromine and theophylline are used most frequently for their effects on the myocardium.

CONVULSANTS AND ANALEPTICS [FIG. 4.4]

These drugs may produce stimulation of many regions of the CNS but their most important actions are often on the medulla.

Drugs which are used specifically to produce convulsions are called convulsants. Therapeutically they have limited applications although leptazol has been used in place of electro-convulsive therapy.

Drugs which overcome depression of the CNS due to overdoses of barbiturates, morphine, and similar compounds are known as analeptics. Their most important action is to stimulate centres in the medulla, but a sufficiently high dose of any of these drugs will produce generalized convulsions.

The mechanism of action of a few convulsants is now beginning to be understood. It appears that they have no important direct

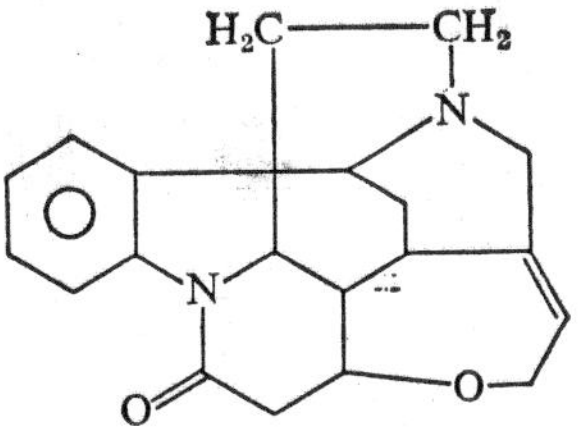

Strychnine

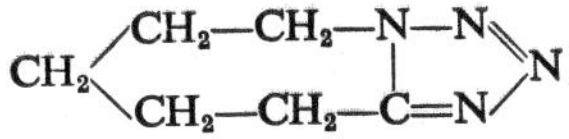

Leptazol

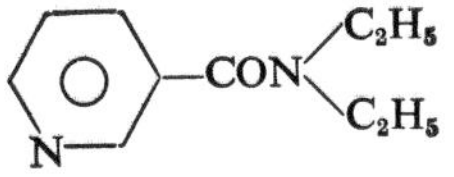

Nikethamide

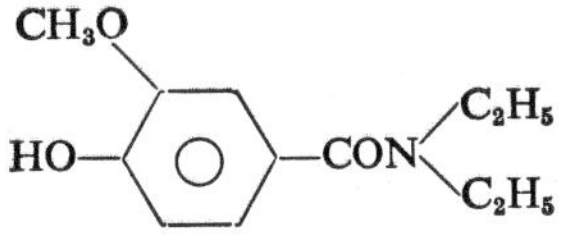

Ethamivan

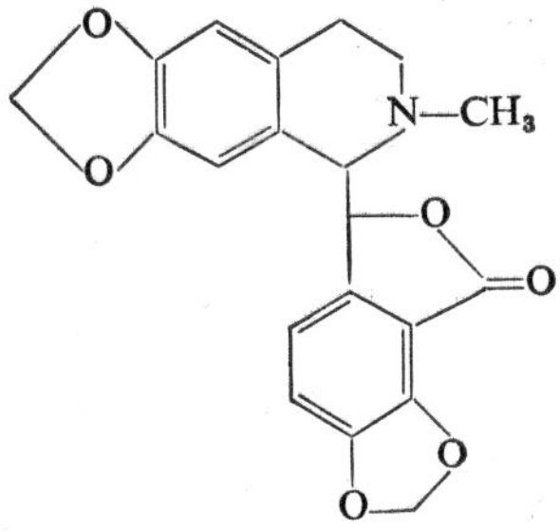

Bicuculline

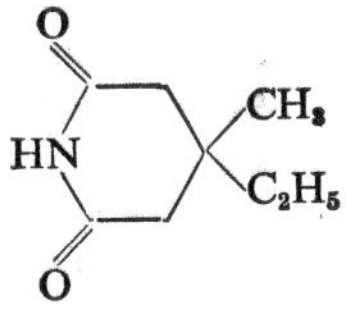

Bemegride

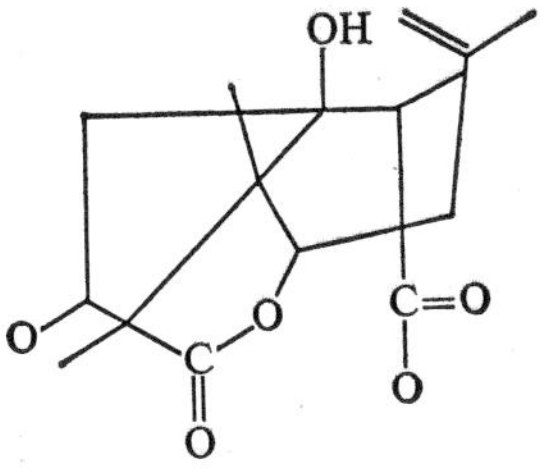

Picrotoxin

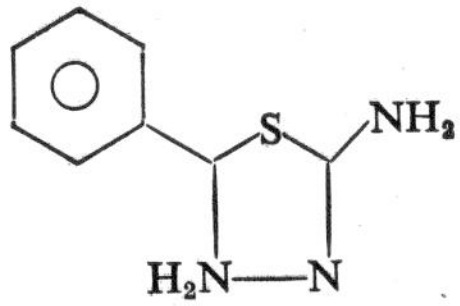

Amiphenazole

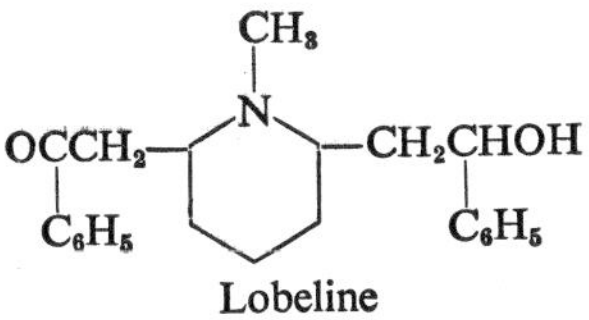

Lobeline

FIG. 4.4. The structures of some convulsants and analeptics.

stimulant action but that they work by antagonizing the action of natural inhibitory transmitters at central synapses. These effects are so clear for certain convulsants, e.g. strychnine, bicuculline, and picrotoxin, that central inhibition at various sites is now often described in terms of the convulsants that do or do not antagonize them.

Strychnine

Strychnine has no important therapeutic value but has proved useful in the investigation of the mode of action of convulsant drugs. Its mechanism of action on the CNS is better understood than that of any other stimulant compound.

Action. Strychnine's most striking effects are on the CNS and consist of the stimulation, followed by the depression of reflexes. After strychnine the motor effects of spinal reflexes are increased and the latent period is diminished. Reflexes become more generalized and, after large doses, small sensory disturbances will send all the voluntary muscles in the body into violent and painful convulsions.

The main site of action of strychnine is on the spinal cord and convulsions occur after removal of the rest of the nervous system. This action of strychnine has been analysed in considerable detail by Sir John Eccles and his co-workers, and it is known that strychnine does not excite directly but acts by inhibiting inhibition. This has been discovered by recording intra- and extracellularly from spinal motoneurones and stimulating inhibitory afferent nerves to these cells. Strychnine was given intravenously or by micro-electrophoretic application directly on to the motoneurones. It was found that strychnine did not alter membrane potentials, or the excitability of motoneurones, but that it did reduce the membrane hyperpolarization (inhibitory postsynaptic potential) generated by stimulation of the appropriate inhibitory afferent nerve.

This inhibitory postsynaptic potential can be exactly mimicked by glycine and by γ-amino butyric acid (GABA) when these compounds are applied to the motoneurones by micro-electrophoresis. From this information it could be argued that either or both these compounds are natural postsynaptic inhibitory transmitters but strychnine, which blocks natural postsynaptic inhibitory potential, only antagonizes the action of glycine and not that of GABA. This evidence, together with recent information concerning the regional distribution of glycine, its uptake with nerve tissue, and its release, makes it very likely that it is an important postsynaptic inhibitory transmitter.

In addition to having no effect on GABA inhibition, strychnine does not affect presynaptic inhibition in the spinal cord and so it

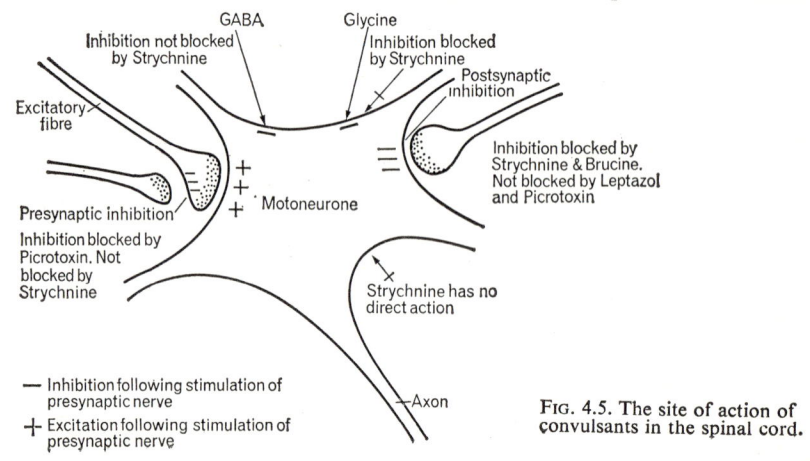

FIG. 4.5. The site of action of convulsants in the spinal cord.

is unlikely that either GABA or glycine mediates this effect.

In the brain strychnine does not antagonize postsynaptic inhibition and this suggests that the inhibitory transmitter is different to that in the spinal cord.

Strychnine has an excitatory action on the medulla, where it will stimulate the vasomotor and vagal centres. It has a remarkable effect in enhancing the sensations of touch, smell, hearing, and sight. After strychnine small differences of colour or illumination are more easily discriminated and the field of vision is increased.

Strychnine also acts on the alimentary canal. It has a bitter taste and therefore increases the appetite. It has a peripheral stimulant action on intestinal muscle, which is probably due to an action on Auerbach's plexus and the drug has been used in the treatment of constipation.

Strychnine Poisoning

In spite of its bitter taste, strychnine has proved popular as the drug of choice amongst murderers. After a high dose the subject will become restless and small sensory stimuli will cause jerking of the limbs and this quickly leads to generalized convulsions. The trunk and limbs become rigidly extended and the face distorts. Each convulsion lasts a few minutes, is very painful, and is followed by a period of exhaustion. After five or six convulsions the respiration fails to return and he dies of asphyxia.

Strychnine is one of the very few poisons whose effects can be counteracted after absorption. It is important to stop the convulsions and to achieve this sensory stimuli must be reduced to a minimum and a general anaesthetic can be administered. Treatment with one of the barbiturates or with mephenesin is often an effective antidote.

Picrotoxin

The active principle in picrotoxin is picrotoxinin and it is a powerful stimulant which affects all parts of the nervous system to some extent. It is extremely effective in restoring respiration that has been depressed by barbiturates or by morphine. The stimulant action of picrotoxin potentiates the excitatory actions of morphine on the CNS.

The difference between a therapeutic and a toxic dose of picrotoxin is small and convulsions are easily produced so that it is rarely used today. Picrotoxin is known to act in the spinal cord by blocking presynaptic inhibition. This may occur by directly depressing the synapses or by competing with the natural transmitter whose identity is not yet established.

Leptazol (Pentylenetetrazol)

Leptazol stimulates the brain and, to a lesser extent, the spinal cord. It is particularly effective in stimulating the medulla which has been depressed by drugs and it is therefore a useful analeptic but it is less effective than picrotoxin. The use of leptazol in place of insulin or electroconvulsive therapy has not proved successful. Leptazol is sometimes used in the diagnosis of epileptic conditions. It is injected intravenously in subconvulsive doses while the electroencephalogram is recorded and this will often reveal potential epileptic foci. It seems unlikely that leptazol blocks either pre- or postsynaptic inhibition, nor does it seem to excite motoneurones by causing depolarization.

Nikethamide

Nikethamide is a weak analeptic and, in high doses, produces convulsions similar to those obtained with leptazol. The myocardium may be depressed but stimulation of the vasomotor centre will cause vasoconstriction and a rise in blood pressure. Nikethamide is used as a stimulant when respiration is depressed by barbiturates. It has been used in the past as a cardiovascular stimulant but it is not now used for this purpose because of its action on the myocardium.

Bicuculline

Bicuculline is a phthalide-isoquinoline alkaloid isolated from corydalis species and is as potent a convulsant as strychnine. It is known to be a specific and reversible antagonist of the inhibitory action of GABA on some central neurones and its site of action is likely to be in those regions of the brain where GABA is a major transmitter. Considerable evidence has accumulated to make it very likely that GABA is an inhibitory transmitter in the brain. This evidence includes the identical nature of natural IPSP and a GABA-induced hyperpolarization, the regional and subcellular distribution of GABA, its uptake by nerve tissue, and its release during central inhibition. The action of GABA is not antagonized by strychnine or picrotoxin but the specific antagonism of bicuculline to GABA hyperpolarization and natural IPSPs confirms GABA as a transmitter in those regions of the brain so far studied, namely the cerebral cortex, Purkinje cell neurones, mitral and thalamic cells.

Bemegride

Bemegride resembles leptazol in its stimulant action on the CNS. It has been used as an antidote to barbiturate poisoning but it is rarely used for this purpose now. Like leptazol it may be used for the diagnosis of epilepsy.

Amiphenazole

Amiphenazole is a central stimulant which was originally thought to be a specific antagonist of certain depressant actions of morphine without affecting analgesia. It now seems that it is a straightforward analeptic. Large doses will produce convulsions.

It has been used as a respiratory stimulant during respiratory insufficiency but its effectiveness is in doubt.

Lobeline

Lobeline is a powerful alkaloid obtained from *Lobelia* and has general actions like nicotine. Its most marked action is to stimulate respiration via the carotid sinus receptors, and it has been used to revive patients who have had an overdose of a narcotic. It causes stimulation and then depression of autonomic ganglia, the adrenal medulla, and the neuromuscular junction.

It is not now normally used as a respiratory stimulant because its action is rather unpredictable and it may have unpleasant and dangerous side-effects.

Ethamivan

Ethamivan is a vanillic acid derivative with a structural resemblance to nikethamide. It is a respiratory stimulant and is usually preferred to nikethamide to treat cases of barbiturate poisoning. Ethamivan has proved particularly useful, when given by mouth, in the treatment of respiratory distress in the new-born.

HALLUCINOGENS

Compounds which act on the CNS to produce hallucinations can be loosely classified as stimulants although their mode of action is completely unknown and their effects are certainly not always of a stimulating nature.

Many hallucinogenic compounds are known and they have always proved attractive to those who hope to enrich and widen their perception and who seek novel experiences. Although these compounds have become rather widely used in some sectors of society, their use is like the use of any powerful and poorly understood drug and is fraught with danger.

The effects of these compounds are hard to predict from one individual to another and may cause permanent or semi-permanent psychological damage in some people. In addition to this danger there are reports of genetic effects associated with these compounds and the possibility of the development of serious dependence.

Because these drugs are subject to strict controls they can normally only be obtained from illegal sources and this always raises the possibility that they are contaminated by other more harmful compounds.

Animals appear to be remarkably resistant to LSD and although many species have been subjected to tests with the drug, only primates show any response in doses up to ten times those effective in man.

The effect of LSD in man has been claimed to resemble, in some aspects, the symptoms of schizophrenia and as little is known of the mechanism of action of the drug as is known of the causes of schizophrenia.

It is well known that LSD antagonizes the action of 5-HT *in vitro* and since 5-HT may be a control neurotransmitter it has been suggested that this may form the basis of action of LSD. This hypothesis became less tenable when it was found that powerful 5-HT antagonists, such as bromo-lysergic acid diethylamide, had no hallucinogenic activity. It is also now known that LSD and 5-HT act in a similar way at central synapses, for instance in the lateral geniculate nucleus, apparently to compete with action of the natural neurotransmitter.

With high doses of LSD there are signs of sympathetic stimulation and an amphetamine-like desynchronization of the electroencephalogram occurs so the basis of action of LSD may be associated with central noradrenergic mechanisms.

Many of the effects of LSD can be relieved with chlorpromazine. Tolerance to the behavioural effects of LSD develops quickly and there is cross-tolerance between LSD and mescaline. LSD is used in psychotherapy but its usefulness in this field is not yet proven. On the other hand it has been widely used as a research tool in the study of central synaptic transmission and, because of its high potency and specificity, it is likely to continue to be used in the study of sensory transmission processes.

Cannabis (Marihuana)

Hallucinations are only caused by large doses of cannabis but it is the most widely used drug of this type.

The drug is obtained from the hemp plant (*Cannabis sativa*) and has been in use longer than almost any other drug. It may be taken in the form of a cigarette ('reefer') but can be taken orally.

The active principle is tetrahydrocannabinol and many synthetic derivatives of this compound have been produced and many are more potent than the parent compound.

In small amounts cannabis produces euphoria and elation and there is often a loss of appreciation of time and space.

The mode of action is unknown although it does appear that changes in the catecholamine content of the brain occur.

The dangers associated with the use of cannabis are controversial but there is evidence that some dependence and psychological damage can occur. Perhaps the greatest danger is that the drug may be adulterated with more habit-forming compounds or that the consumer will be persuaded or will desire to proceed to the use of more dangerous drugs.

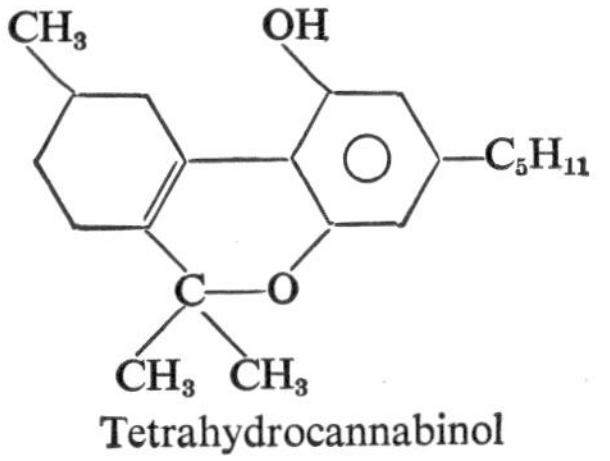

Tetrahydrocannabinol

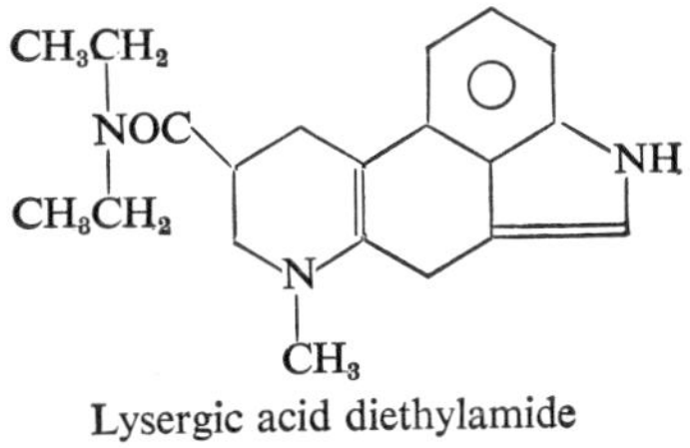

Lysergic acid diethylamide

FIG. 4.6. The structures of hallucinogenic compounds.

Lysergic Acid Diethylamide (LSD)

Powerful hallucinogenic drugs such as mescaline, which were isolated in 1896 from the peyoti cactus, have been used for various reasons, often involving religious rites, from the early nineteenth century. In 1943 the psychological effects of a much more powerful synthetic hallucinogen, lysergic acid diethylamide, were discovered accidentally by Hofmann. This compound will produce hallucinations in man in doses as low as 20 μg. taken orally but has few actions outside the CNS at this or at higher dose levels.

FURTHER READING

CURTIS, D. R. (1963) The pharmacology of central inhibition, *Pharmacol. Rev.*, **15**, 333.

FELDBERG, W. (1963) *A Pharmacological Approach to the Brain from its Inner and Outer Surface*, London.

HAHN, F. (1960) Analeptics, *Pharmacol. Rev.*, **12**, 447.

HOLTZ, P., and WESTERMANN, E. (1965) Psychic energizers and antidepressant drugs, in *Physiological Pharmacology*, ed. ROOT, W. S., and HOFMANN, F. G., Vol. 2, New York.

KRNJEVIĆ, K. (1967) Chemical transmission and cortical arousal, *Anesthesiology*, **27**, 100.

5

LOCAL ANAESTHETICS

MECHANISM OF ACTION

LOCAL anaesthetics prevent the generation and conduction of nerve impulses and, while this is a property of a great number of drugs, only those which have this as a predominant characteristic when in low concentrations are classed as local anaesthetic agents. Their site of action is the cell membrane and the block they produce is the result of interference with changes in membrane permeability to potassium and sodium ions. These permeability changes are responsible for the rising and falling phases of the action potential and they follow depolarization of the membrane. In the presence of a local anaesthetic the electrical excitability of the tissue gradually decreases until, eventually, complete block ensues.

How local anaesthetics affect the transient changes in ionic permeability is unknown but the potency of these compounds is matched by their ability to increase the surface pressure of monomolecular lipid films. It has been suggested that the anaesthetic 'squeezes' the lipid molecules closer together. In the lipid membrane layers of nerves this could have the effect of closing membrane 'pores' so reducing ionic permeability; this would have the effect of stabilizing the membrane and reducing its excitability.

DIFFERENTIAL SENSITIVITY OF NERVE FIBRES

Not all nerve fibres are equally vulnerable to the actions of local anaesthetics. As a general rule, small diameter fibres are more easily blocked than large ones and if cocaine is applied to a mixed nerve trunk it is found that the small diameter γ fibres block first and the large α fibres last. The sensitivity of nerve fibres is not, however, entirely determined by their diameter, because some small myelinated fibres block more easily than even the small diameter C fibres.

It is now known that there is no difference in the vulnerability of motor and sensory fibres of the same diameter.

After administration of a local anaesthetic the various sensations are not lost simultaneously, probably because they are mediated by nerves of different diameters. The order of sensation loss is rather variable but usually pain is abolished first, followed by the sensations of cold, warmth, touch, and deep pressure in that order.

THE EFFECT OF pH

The most useful local anaesthetics are secondary or tertiary amines and they can exist as uncharged or positively charged molecules, depending on the pH of the solution and on the pK_a of the compound.

Procaine, for instance, is a weakly basic tertiary amine and in solution may exist as a mixture of the uncharged compound [B in FIG. 5.1] and the cationic form (BH$^+$). The amount of each form present in a given solution will depend on the pH of the solution according to the equation $\log {}^B/_{BH^+} = pH - pK$.

Since the pK_a of procaine at 20° C. is 8·7, at pH 7, 2 per cent. of the drug will be in the uncharged form and at pH 9, 67 per cent. of the procaine will be in the uncharged form.

The penetration of a local anaesthetic to its site of action depends on its ability to cross lipid barriers and the uncharged form has a high oil/water distribution coefficient and can therefore penetrate into lipid layers with ease. The cationic form is hydrophilic and therefore

$$B + H_3^+O \rightleftharpoons BH^+ + H_2O$$

$$NH_2\text{—}Ph\text{—}COOCH_2CH_2N(C_2H_5)_2 \xrightarrow{H_3^+O} NH_2\text{—}Ph\text{—}COOCH_2CH_2N^+\begin{matrix}C_2H_5\\H\\C_2H_5\end{matrix}$$

FIG. 5.1. The ionization of procaine.

penetrates lipid layers very slowly. It would be expected, therefore, that procaine would be more effective at the higher pH because of the much larger fraction of the uncharged form that is present in solution. This is not, however, the whole story, because once the drug has penetrated the lipid barriers and reached its site of action it appears that the charged, rather than the uncharged, form is most effective in producing an anaesthetic effect. This suggestion has been confirmed by Ritchie and his co-workers who showed convincingly that alkaline anaesthetic solutions were more effective in nerves with their outer sheathing intact but that neutral solutions were more effective in desheathed nerves, the cation being the active form of the anaesthetic and the uncharged molecule being important only for penetration.

PHARMACOLOGICAL ACTIONS

In addition to their action in blocking conduction in nervous tissue, the local anaesthetics interfere with the function of all organs in which the transmission of electrical impulses occurs. The most important effects are on the CNS and heart.

Central Nervous System. Most local anaesthetics stimulate the CNS and overdoses may lead to tremors, restlessness, and convulsions. Central depression may occur later and death may result from respiratory depression. The stimulant action may be the result of a block in vulnerable central inhibitory pathways. Although all local anaesthetics cause stimulation, cocaine is unique in having a powerful effect on the cerebral cortex and it may be this which makes cocaine addictive. Synthetic local anaesthetics have less stimulant actions on higher centres and do not cause addiction.

Cardiovascular System. If given systemically, local anaesthetics have a quinidine-like action on the myocardium and reduce its excitability and force of contraction; they also prolong the refractory period and slow conduction. These effects cannot easily be taken advantage of because the drugs are rapidly destroyed and their CNS effects usually predominate.

All local anaesthetics except lignocaine and cocaine produce vasodilatation by a direct action on arterioles.

FATE AND METABOLISM OF LOCAL ANAESTHETICS

All local anaesthetics are broken down in the liver to non-toxic products and procaine is also inactivated in the plasma by circulating cholinesterase.

CHEMISTRY OF LOCAL ANAESTHETICS

The very large number of local anaesthetics available have many actions in common and their chemical structures show many similarities. They are all water-soluble salts of lipid-soluble alkaloids and consist basically of three parts, an amino group, a connecting group which is an ester or amide, and an amino alcohol residue in which the amino group

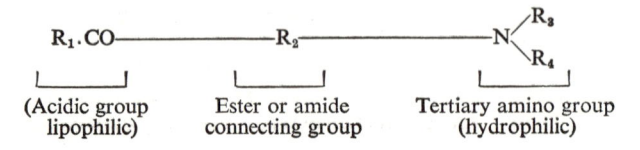

$$R_1.CO\text{——————}R_2\text{——————}N\begin{matrix}R_3\\R_4\end{matrix}$$

(Acidic group lipophilic) | Ester or amide connecting group | Tertiary amino group (hydrophilic)

FIG. 5.2. The basic structure of local anaesthetics.

may be substituted by alkyl groups or form part of an alicyclic ring. Alterations in all three parts of the molecule give compounds of varying potency and toxicity. Local anaesthetics may be divided into three main groups: (1) cocaine, a naturally occurring alkaloid and the first local anaesthetic to be used; (2) para-aminobenzoic acid derivatives (procaine, amethocaine, etc.); (3) agents including lignocaine, cinchocaine, benzocaine, many of which chemically resemble the para-aminobenzoic acid drugs.

THE ADMINISTRATION OF LOCAL ANAESTHETICS

Local anaesthetics may be administered in a number of ways. (1) As a cream, ointment, spray, solution, or powder to mucous membranes or to damaged skin around wounds. (2) By infiltration. The drugs may be injected locally into subcutaneous tissue to block sensation for the performance of minor, superficial surgery. (3) By injection into the subarachnoid space of the spinal cord to procure block of motor and sensory roots and autonomic fibres. This is known as spinal anaesthesia and will block the sensation of pain from the regions of body innervated by the affected segments of the cord. (4) By injection near major nerve trunks to block sensation from the innervated region of the body, e.g. brachial plexus block.

Amethocaine (Tetracaine)

This compound is suitable both for injection and application to mucous membranes. It is the most powerful local anaesthetic after cinchocaine and is used for infiltration anaesthesia, spinal and extradural block. It is often mixed with procaine or lignocaine to combine the rapid action of these compounds with its own more prolonged effect.

Like most other local anaesthetics, amethocaine is usually administered with adrenaline in order to constrict blood vessels and thus reduce absorption and thereby confine the area of anaesthetic effect and increase the duration of action.

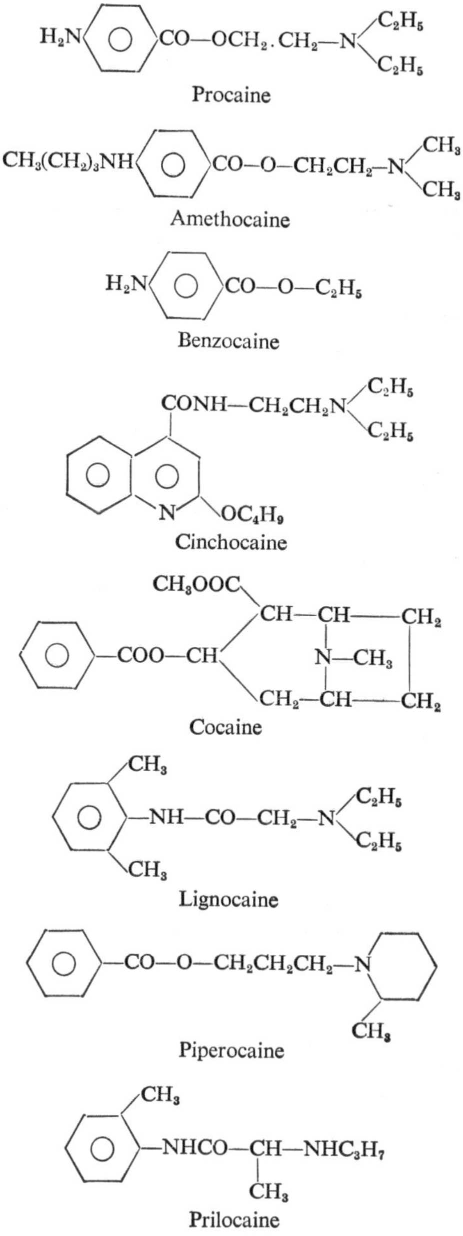

FIG. 5.3. The structures of some local anaesthetics.

Cinchocaine (Dibucaine)

Cinchocaine is a powerful local anaesthetic with an onset of action slower than procaine but with a longer duration. It is absorbed from mucous membranes and is 2–5 times more toxic than cocaine but, because it is more active, it can be used in lower concentrations. It sometimes produces inflammation at the site of injection. It is still widely used for spinal anaesthesia.

Cocaine

Cocaine is obtained from the leaves of *Erythroxylon coca*, a tree found in South America.

It has pharmacological actions on the nervous and cardiovascular systems similar to those of other local anaesthetics.

In some respects it differs from other local anaesthetics because it has its own adrenergic action and blocks the uptake of catecholamines into adrenergic nerve terminals and so enhances the action of adrenaline, noradrenaline, and sympathetic nerve stimulation [CHAPTER 7].

It produces marked stimulation of the higher centres in the brain which results in restlessness and euphoria. This stimulation will give way to depression, paralysis of medullary centres, and death.

Cocaine potentiates the excitatory and inhibitory responses of sympathetically innervated tissues to the action of noradrenaline and adrenaline and to stimulation of sympathetic nerves. This effect is produced because cocaine prevents the reuptake of noradrenaline into nerve terminals and thus produces a build-up of the neurotransmitter. The increased concentration of neurotransmitter at the receptors causes a type of supersensitivity to develop. Probably the most important result of this action is possible occurrence of ventricular fibrillation. It is a potent surface anaesthetic and produces intense vasoconstriction. Because of its toxic actions in the body its use is mainly limited to surface anaesthesia.

Cocaine is a drug of addiction and the results of its persistent administration are unpleasant and the victims, who become tolerant to the drug and therefore increase their intake, lose all self-control. They develop tremors, hallucinations, and eventually become melancholic and insane. Treatment for cocaine addiction consists in withdrawal of the drug, which does not cause serious symptoms like those following the withdrawal of morphine, but relapses are common.

Poisoning by Cocaine. The early symptoms of poisoning are due to actions on the CNS. There is excitement, restlessness, and mental confusion with giddiness, fainting, and vomiting. Due to stimulation of the sympathetic nervous system the skin is pale, the pupils dilated, and the temperature raised. Large doses cause convulsions followed by central paralysis and death from failure of respiration.

Lignocaine (Lidocaine)

Lignocaine acts rapidly and has a strong anaesthetic action on mucous membranes. It has no action on blood vessels and produces long-lasting general analgesia when given intravenously. It is used for local anaesthesia by infiltration, nerve, epidural, and caudal block. It is not used widely for spinal anaesthesia.

Lignocaine is also used to produce general analgesia and toxic side-effects are rare except when high doses are administered intravenously.

Prilocaine

Prilocaine closely resembles lignocaine in structure. It is as effective as lignocaine as an anaesthetic but it is less toxic and lasts longer. It is also active topically and on mucous membranes. There is not yet full clinical data on this local anaesthetic but it appears to be safe and free of serious side-effects.

Procaine

Procaine is a safe and effective local anaesthetic. It is used for infiltration anaesthesia and all types of regional, spinal, and extradural block. Its duration of action may be prolonged by combination with amethocaine. It is also used for the relief of post-operative pain by producing general analgesia, to prevent cardiac arrhythmias during cyclopropane and trichlorethylene anaesthesia, and as a supplement to nitrous oxide and oxygen anaesthesia.

Procaine has a vasodilator action so it is rapidly absorbed after local injection and this action is used to produce vasodilatation in peripheral vascular disease, acute arterial spasm, and in venous spasm.

Procaine antagonizes the actions of sulphonamides and anticholinesterase drugs inhibit its hydrolysis and therefore its removal. It is normally rapidly hydrolysed by pseudocholinesterase in the plasma to give para-aminobenzoic acid and diethylaminoethanol, the former being excreted in the urine and the latter being largely metabolized in the liver.

FURTHER READING

ADRIANI, J. (1960) The clinical pharmacology of anaesthetics, *Clin. Pharmacol. Ther.*, **1**, 645.

DE JONG, R. H., and WAGMAN, I. H. (1963) Physiological mechanisms of peripheral nerve block by local anesthetics, *Anesthesiology*, **24**, 684.

DOUGLAS, W. W., and RITCHIE, J. M. (1962) Mammalian non-myelinated nerve fibres, *Physiol. Rev.*, **42**, 297.

MATTHEWS, P. B. C., and RUSHWORTH, G. (1957) The relative sensitivity of muscle nerve fibres to procaine, *J. Physiol. (Lond.)*, **135**, 263.

RITCHIE, J. M., and GREENGARD, P. (1966) On the mode of action of local anaesthetics, *Rev. Pharmacol.*, **6**, 405.

SKOU, J. C. (1961) The effect of drugs on cell membranes with special reference to local anaesthetics, *J. Pharm. Pharmacol.*, **13**, 204.

WIEDLING, S. (1963) Local anaesthetics, *Progr. Med. Chem.*, **3**, 332.

6

CHOLINERGIC SYSTEM

There is now sufficient evidence to be sure that acetylcholine is liberated from motor nerve terminals and that it transmits the nerve impulse across a synaptic gap to the end-plate region on skeletal muscle cells. There is also good evidence that acetylcholine acts as a neurotransmitter at Renshaw cells in the spinal cord and at autonomic ganglia. It seems likely that a similar mechanism of transmission occurs at some motor terminals on smooth muscles and there is growing evidence that cholinergic synapses are present in the brain.

Since acetylcholine has important actions at so many sites in the body it is not surprising that its effects, and the effects of acetylcholine-like drugs and their antagonists, are varied and often complex.

A convenient division of the actions of cholinergic drugs exists because it has long been recognized that they act on two main types of membrane receptor. These receptors are called 'muscarinic' and 'nicotinic' receptors because muscarine and nicotine were found to stimulate them selectively before other, even more specific, drugs were discovered.

The effects of acetylcholine-like drugs on nicotinic receptors are blocked by curare and muscarinic actions are blocked by atropine.

Although it is now becoming clear that the differences between these two types of receptors may not be as clear-cut as was previously thought, they still form a useful way of classifying the action of acetylcholine.

This chapter is divided in the following way:

1. Methods of studying the cholinergic system.
2. Nicotinic receptors—drugs acting at the skeletal neuromuscular junction.
   Nicotinic receptors—drugs acting at the autonomic ganglion.
3. Muscarinic receptors—drugs acting at parasympathetic, postganglionic nerve junctions.
4. Mixed receptor sites—the spinal cord and brain.
5. Individual cholinergic drugs and their antagonists.

METHODS OF STUDYING THE CHOLINERGIC SYSTEM

DRUGS WHICH ACT AT NICOTINIC RECEPTORS

The action of drugs on nicotinic receptors can best be studied by their effect on neuromuscular transmission. This can be most easily investigated by recording muscle contractions evoked by the direct application of drugs or by maximal stimulation of the motor nerve in the presence of drugs. The drugs may be applied over the whole muscle or injected into the blood vessels entering the muscle. The latter method of drug application has been more widely used, the injection being made into an artery as near as possible to the insertion of the nerve. This is known as a close arterial injection and ensures a high concentration of drug at the neuromuscular junction. Acetylcholine delivered in this way will produce a twitch of voluntary muscle.

Maximal stimulation of the motor nerve produces contraction of the muscle and the effect of drugs on neuromuscular transmission may be tested by recording changes in the extent of the contraction.

Among the muscle preparations commonly used are the cat tibialis anterior, the frog gastrocnemius, and the rat diaphragm. The first preparation is used *in situ* but the other two are conveniently used as isolated preparations. They are illustrated in FIGURE 6.1.

Information about acetylcholine-like drugs may also be obtained from muscles containing multiply-innervated fibres. These fibres are especially sensitive to the action of acetylcholine-like compounds and respond with a prolonged, non-propagated contracture rather than a twitch. Examples of this type of preparation are the frog rectus and the dorsal muscle of the leech. Because of their sensitivity, these techniques are useful for assaying very small amounts of acetylcholine.

Since microelectrophoretic techniques were introduced, many advances have been made in understanding the mechanism of neuromuscular transmission, and the pharmacology of drugs which affect nicotinic receptors. The basic techniques for recording membrane potentials and applying drugs are described on pp. 15–16. Variations of this technique are now used almost exclusively for the detailed study of pharmacological events at the neuromuscular junction, and other cholinergic receptor sites.

TESTS FOR MUSCARINIC ACTIVITY

The muscarinic activity of a drug may be conveniently tested on the isolated guinea-pig ileum preparation [FIG. 1.1]. It should be remembered that when a drug like acetylcholine is being tested for its muscarinic activity it is essential to eliminate any interference due to its action on nicotinic receptors. With the guinea-pig ileum preparation it is impossible to separate the muscle receptors from the autonomic ganglia which are nicotinic, but effects on the latter may be blocked by the use of a ganglion blocking drug such as hexamethonium.

The muscarinic activity of a drug may be estimated by its ability to lower blood pressure [FIG. 6.9] and it can be tested on the rate and force of contraction of the isolated perfused heart. If the drug is acting on muscarinic receptors its action should always be abolished by atropine.

Another convenient, but less quantitative test of muscarinic activity, is on the diameter of the pupil of the eye and on the blood vessels of the perfused rabbit ear or the perfused rat hind quarters.

THE BIOLOGICAL ASSAY OF ACETYLCHOLINE

One of the most sensitive assay preparations for acetylcholine is the dorsal muscle of the leech treated with an anticholinesterase. This tissue contracts in a concentration of about 1×10^{-9} g./ml. of acetylcholine.

The frog rectus preparation, which is easier to use, is about ten times less sensitive than leech muscle. The heart of the clam (*Venus mercenaria*) is extremely sensitive but lacks the specificity to choline esters that is shown by the leech and frog rectus preparations. Other useful preparations are the cat blood pressure, the frog heart, and the rabbit auricle. All these methods involve a comparison of the activity of the unknown solution with a solution containing a known amount of acetylcholine [see CHAPTER 19]. If two or more tests on different preparations agree quantitatively in terms of acetylcholine it is good evidence that the test solution contains acetylcholine or a very similar choline ester. The presence of acetylcholine in the test solution can only be confirmed by the use of further tests including: (1) the abolition of activity on the frog rectus and leech preparations by the addition of D-tubocurarine; (2) the blocking of a depressor response in blood pressure preparations by the addition of atropine-like compounds; (3) loss of activity in the test solution following alkali hydrolysis; (4) loss of activity in the test solution following incubation with acetylcholinesterase; and (5) chromatographic analysis of the active principle and a comparison of its Rf characteristics with those of acetylcholine and similar choline esters.

Cholinergic System

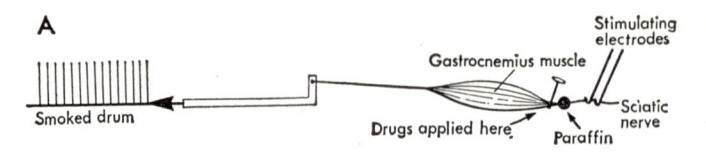

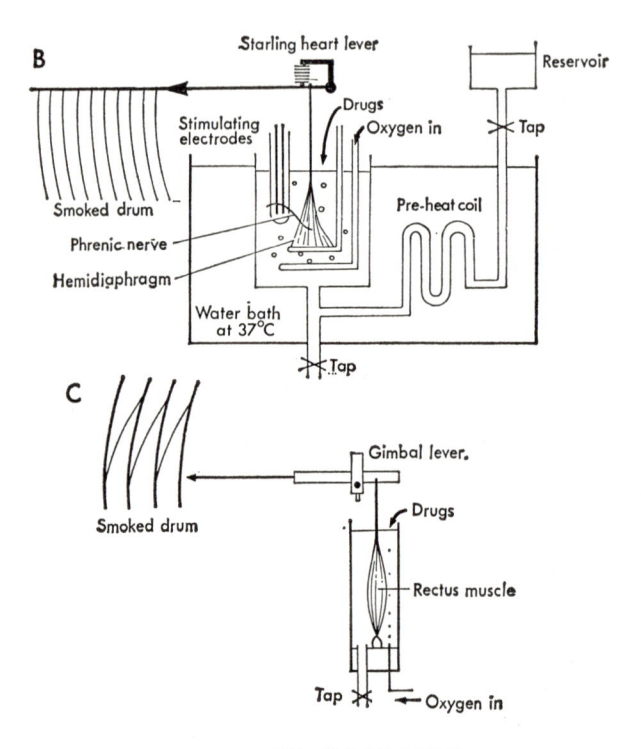

FIG. 6.1. Schematic illustrations of three simple, isolated preparations, which can be used to study the action of drugs on the neuromuscular junction.
  A. The frog sciatic-gastrocnemius preparation. Notice use of paraffin to prevent short-circuit of stimulating electrodes by drug solutions.
  B. Isolated rat phrenic nerve-diaphragm preparation.
  C. Frog rectus preparation.

NICOTINIC RECEPTORS

Peripheral nicotinic receptors are located on the postsynaptic membrane of the neuromuscular junction and on autonomic ganglion cells. A considerable amount is now known about the actions of agonist and antagonist drugs at these sites and they will be considered in the following section.

THE NEUROMUSCULAR JUNCTION

Detailed accounts of the histology and general properties of the neuromuscular junction and the electrical changes which occur during the transmission of an impulse may be found in most textbooks of physiology.

As shown in FIGURE 6.2, the myelinated motor nerve fibre loses its myelin sheath near the tip and the axon spreads under the sarcolemma where it is separated by a cleft of about 300 Å from the folded structure of the muscle end-plate (the postsynaptic membrane). Although the nerve terminal and the postsynaptic membrane lie close together there is no continuity between them and it is this gap

Fig. 6.2. A. Diagram of frog neuromuscular junction. B. End-plate region of frog neuromuscular junction magnified ×19,000.

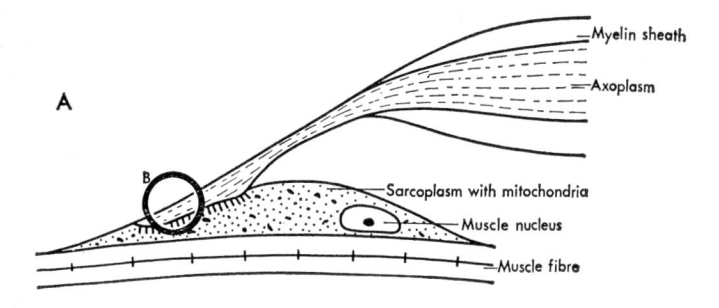

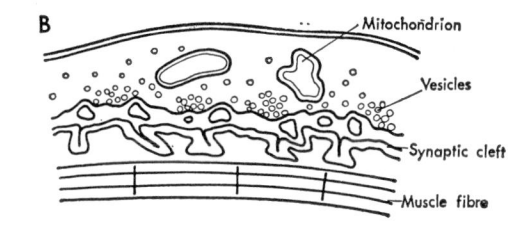

which acetylcholine bridges to generate an electrical potential at the end-plate.

The sequence of events which results in a muscle contraction may be summarized as follows:

1. An action potential travels down the motor nerve fibre and invades the fine, unmyelinated terminal.
2. Depolarization of the terminal causes the release of about 100 'quanta' of acetylcholine each containing roughly 10^6 molecules. Each quantum is thought to be the contents of one synaptic vesicle. The vesicles are concentrated in the motor nerve terminal, close to the presynaptic membrane.
3. The liberated acetylcholine quickly diffuses across the synaptic gap and interacts with receptors on the end-plate of a muscle fibre. The receptors can be shown to be on the outer surface of the muscle fibre membrane, because when acetylcholine is injected intracellularly it is ineffective.
4. The action of acetylcholine on the receptor results in a massive increase in the ionic permeability of the end-plate region allowing Na^+ and K^+ ions to flow down their concentration gradients and so reduce the membrane potential from above -70 mV to near zero. The acetylcholine is then rapidly hydrolysed by cholinesterase.
5. If the evoked end-plate potential is sufficiently large, it will trigger off a further sequence of events resulting in the generation of a propagated muscle action potential which in turn activates the contractile processes of the muscle fibre. When no action potentials are passing down the motor nerve there is a continuous, spontaneous release of acetylcholine quanta from the nerve ending which produces miniature end-plate potentials (mepps). These potentials are not large enough by themselves to produce muscle spikes and are thought to be the result of the random bursting of single vesicles.

Cholinergic System

Hemicholinium (HC-3)

Triethylcholine (T.E.C.)

FIG. 6.3. Drugs which interfere with the synthesis of acetylcholine.

The synthesis of acetylcholine occurs in the motor nerve terminals and requires glucose, oxygen, sodium ions, choline, and the enzyme choline acetyltransferase, for its maintenance. If synthesis is blocked then transmission fails and this happens rapidly at high rates of stimulation of the motor nerve.

One way of stopping synthesis is by interfering with the uptake of choline by the nerve terminal. This can be achieved with **hemicholinium** (HC–3) which has some structural similarities to choline and appears to compete for a choline carrier in the nerve membrane. The transmission block which occurs can be overcome with excess choline. A striking demonstration that HC-3 reduces acetylcholine synthesis and hence the content of each vesicle was provided by the demonstration that the size of mepps, but not the frequency, was reduced after the drug. A compound with an effect similar to that of HC-3 is **triethylcholine** [FIG. 6.3].

Myasthenia gravis, a disease characterized by muscular weakness, is likely to be due to a defect in acetylcholine synthesis because the amplitude of the mepps is reduced.

Little is known of the way in which acetylcholine is released from the motor nerve terminal but it is known that a reduction in extracellular calcium or an increase in magnesium reduces spontaneous acetylcholine release and that local anaesthetics, acting on the fine terminals of the nerve, stabilize the membrane and so block release.

Botulinum toxin causes muscular fatigue and paralysis due to the abolition of acetylcholine release. This is well illustrated by the reduced frequency but unimpaired amplitude of mepps which follows botulinum poisoning.

Black widow spider venom produces paralysis of skeletal muscle and it does so by causing the explosive release of all the acetylcholine stores in motor nerve terminals. The use of this venom experimentally has shown that the synaptic vesicles disappear from the motor nerve terminal when the acetylcholine is lost, thus adding support to the idea that they contain the transmitter.

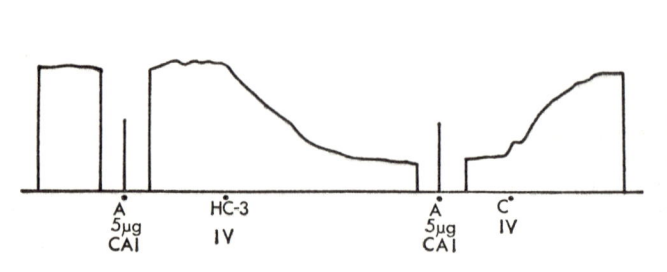

FIG. 6.4. The effect of HC-3 on neuromuscular transmission. Maximal twitches of the cat tibialis anterior muscle elicited by stimulating the motor nerve at a frequency of 1/sec.

In this, and in all subsequent diagrams of the effect of drugs on muscle twitches, the individual records of twitches are not shown. Instead they are enclosed in a common envelope, the top edge of which indicates the height of the twitches.

A, acetylcholine; C, choline; CAI, close arterial injection.

FIG. 6.5. A depolarizing block of neuromuscular transmission by acetylcholine. Cat tibialis anterior muscle. Stimulus frequency, 0·1/sec. A, acetylcholine; N, neostigmine. Note the potentiating effect of intravenously injected neostigmine on the maximal twitches and on the effect of injected acetylcholine. When neostigmine is injected arterially it reaches the end-plates in a high concentration and a depolarizing block occurs as the acetylcholine accumulates. A further injection of acetylcholine makes the block worse.

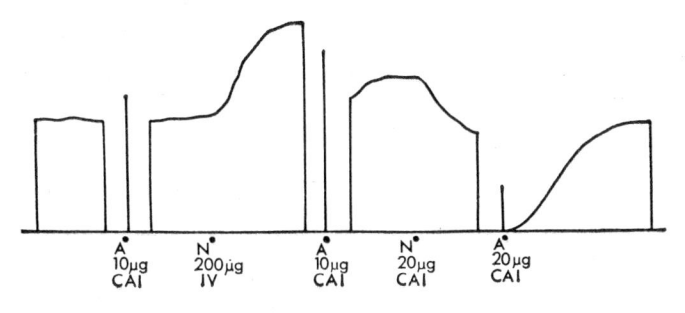

There is some evidence that cholinergic receptors exist on the presynaptic motor nerve terminal and these may be affected by acetylcholine if anticholinesterase drugs are present. The result of this will be increased depolarization of the terminal and a consequent increase in acetylcholine release, leading to enhanced muscle activity.

Most drugs which affect neuromuscular transmission do so by an action at the postsynaptic membrane. Acetylcholine has important effects at this site and, although its action is too brief to make it of clinical importance, its mode of action is relevant to the action of many other drugs which are clinically useful.

The close arterial injection of acetylcholine to a skeletal muscle causes a twitch, and if an anticholinesterase is present to prevent enzymic destruction of acetylcholine, there may be prolonged fasciculations. The twitch and fasciculations are the result of the depolarizing action of acetylcholine on the end-plate region. If a large amount of acetylcholine is injected, and if there is abundant anticholinesterase present, the stage of excitation may develop into a stage of block known as a depolarizing block.

This depolarizing action of acetylcholine is an effect on nicotinic receptors and is antagonized by curare-like compounds which act as antagonists to acetylcholine by competing

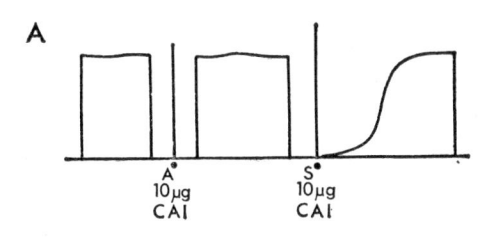

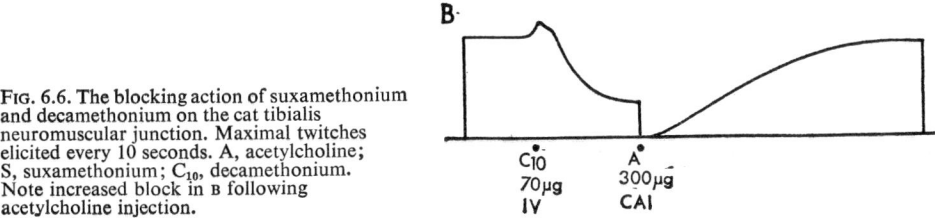

FIG. 6.6. The blocking action of suxamethonium and decamethonium on the cat tibialis neuromuscular junction. Maximal twitches elicited every 10 seconds. A, acetylcholine; S, suxamethonium; C_{10}, decamethonium. Note increased block in B following acetylcholine injection.

for the receptors and thereby preventing depolarization.

An acetylcholine block is made worse by tetanic stimulation of the motor nerve and by the addition of drugs which depolarize the membrane.

There are other important drugs, notably the methonium compounds, which depolarize the end-plate and thereby block neuromuscular transmission.

Suxamethonium, which resembles two molecules of acetylcholine laid end to end, has this property and so does **decamethonium.** The former drug is hydrolysed by pseudocholinesterase but has a sufficiently prolonged action to make it clinically useful. Decamethonium is not hydrolysed and so it has a longer action. Both these compounds may cause an initial facilitation of transmission in the period before a block develops.

It is interesting that both these compounds which activate the nicotinic receptor are long, slender molecules having a pair of charged groups separated by a carbon chain. It is known that the neuromuscular blocking activity in methonium compounds is greatest when the charged nitrogen groups are separated by ten to twelve carbon atoms. Any alteration in this chain length reduces blocking activity, presumably because the drug molecule fits less well on to the receptor. Methonium compounds also block transmission across autonomic ganglia but, in this case, the optimum number of carbon atoms in the chain is five or six, a strong suggestion that the nicotinic receptors at this site and at the neuromuscular junction are not identical [see Fig. 6.7].

The depolarizing block and paralysis produced by the methonium compounds at the neuromuscular junction are the result of prolonged depolarization. This might be expected to produce a sustained tetanic spasm limited only by the refractory period of the membrane, but, in fact, this only occurs in slow-contracting multiply-innervated muscles.

The flaccid paralysis that occurs has been studied in the cat gracilis muscle and it is found that depolarization by decamethonium extends slightly beyond the region of muscle from

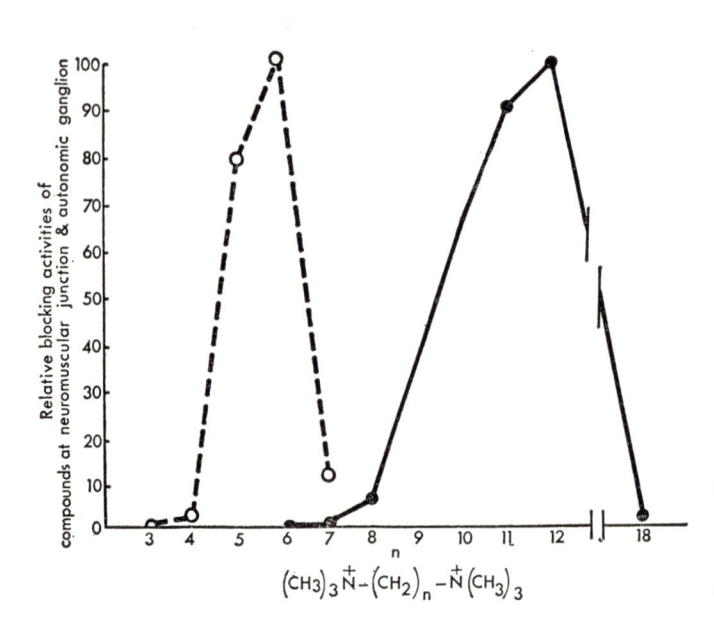

Fig. 6.7. The effect of altering the length of the methylene chain in methonium compounds on their ability to block transmission at the neuromuscular junction and at the autonomic ganglion. ●———●, neuromuscular junction (cat tibialis). ○-- --○, autonomic ganglion (cat superior cervical ganglion). (From data of Paton and Zaimis (1949 and 1951) *Brit. J. Pharmacol.*, **4**, 381, and **6**, 155.)

which the end-plate potentials can be recorded. After applying decamethonium there is a brief increase in end-plate sensitivity but it then becomes less sensitive as does the region around the end-plate.

This loss of excitability may be due to inactivation of the sodium carrier in the membrane leading to the development of a 'zone of inexcitability' round the end-plate. A muscle action potential evoked at one end of the muscle fibre cannot then propagate across this zone. The block is very similar to that obtained with persistent cathodal stimulation.

A second important class of neuromuscular blocking drugs act in a very different way. They do not depolarize the postsynaptic membrane and they have no direct effect on the membrane potential, but they do prevent the action of depolarizing drugs.

Their blocking action may often be overcome by any procedure which increases the amount of transmitter in the vicinity of the end-plates. Tetanization of the motor nerve and the addition of an anticholinesterase will achieve this.

An example of this type of non-depolarizing blocking drug is **curare**, which is a South American arrow poison prepared from various species of plant. There are three varieties, known as pot-curare, tube-curare, and calabash-curare, named after the vessels in which they are kept. Tubocurarine is the dextroisomer of a pure alkaloid, obtained from tubecurare and from plant extracts.

Tubocurarine is not absorbed when taken orally and must be injected, but once in the plasma it disappears rapidly, so that the concentration is reduced by half every 13 minutes. About one-third of the dose is excreted in the urine, while the remainder is inactivated in the body in a few hours. The rapid rate at which the drug disappears ensures that its action lasts only a few minutes and that it is relatively ineffective when slowly absorbed.

The rat phrenic nerve–diaphragm preparation [p. 56] is a convenient method for the assay of tubocurarine.

The nerve is stimulated every 5–10 seconds and the resulting contractions remain constant for hours unless a drug is added to the bath.

The effect of curare is reversible; doses can be applied every 10 minutes, and standard and unknown solutions compared with one another.

Tubocurarine is still one of the most widely used neuromuscular blocking drugs and has played a part in balanced anaesthesia for many years. It is also used in the management of tetanus and has, in the past, been used in the diagnosis of myasthenia gravis.

Other neuromuscular blocking agents include **gallamine, dihydro-β-erythroidine,** and **benzoquinonium**; these are described on pages 71–2.

DRUGS WHICH PRESERVE ACETYLCHOLINE

Drugs which inhibit or inactivate cholinesterase are called **anticholinesterases** and their action prevents the destruction of acetylcholine and so potentiates its effect. These drugs have a variety of uses as insecticides, as 'nerve gases', and as therapeutic agents.

They may be divided into two major groups, the reversible anticholinesterase drugs and the organophosphorus compounds which permanently inactivate cholinesterase. Both classes of drug react with cholinesterase in much the same way as does the natural substrate. If acetylcholine is the substrate then the molecule is bound to an active unit of the enzyme at an anionic and an esteratic site. From this choline is split off leaving an acyl group attached to the enzyme. The latter reacts with water to produce acetic acid and the regeneration of the enzyme.

This reaction is theoretically reversible but in practice moves rapidly to the state where acetylcholine is hydrolysed.

A weak anticholinesterase such as **edrophonium** produces a reversible inhibition of the enzyme by combining with it only at the anionic site thus blocking the attachment and subsequent destruction of acetylcholine.

More potent anticholinesterases like **physostigmine** and **neostigmine** form attachments at both sites and they are then hydrolysed in the same way as acetylcholine. The difference between this reaction and that with acetylcholine is that hydrolysis of the acyl enzyme is about a million times slower than the hydrolysis of the acetyl enzyme. These compounds therefore act as anticholinesterases because they form alternative substrates for the enzyme and are hydrolysed extremely slowly.

The organophosphorus anticholinesterases such as **diisopropylfluorophosphonate** (D.F.P.) only bind with the enzyme at the esteratic site but the reaction then proceeds as it does with other anticholinesterases. In this case, however, the resultant phosphorylated enzyme is extremely stable and if isopropyl groups are involved virtually no hydrolysis or regeneration of the enzyme occurs. Cholinesterase activity will then only return as new enzyme is synthesized.

The negligible reactivation of phosphorylated forms of cholinesterase can be greatly speeded up if oximes are used to react with the enzyme instead of water. The best example of these compounds is **P-2-AM** (pralidoxime, PAM). The rate of combination of this type of compound is greatly helped by electrostatic forces between the quaternary nitrogen and the anionic site on the enzyme.

This type of enzyme reactivator will protect against otherwise lethal doses of anticholinesterases but phosphorylated cholinesterase 'ages' rapidly and, in a matter of minutes or hours, may become completely resistant to reactivators. The process of 'ageing' is likely to be due to the splitting off of an alkyl group leaving a more stable mono-alkyl phosphorylated compound.

The pharmacological effects of the anticholinesterases are largely due to the accumulation of acetylcholine that they cause at all cholinergic synapses in the body.

Some of the anticholinesterase agents, particularly the quaternary ammonium compounds like neostigmine, have their own direct action on cholinoceptive sites. Neostigmine has a direct depolarizing action on the neuromuscular junction, an effect which is not surprising in view of the fact that it reacts efficiently with the same enzyme as acetylcholine.

The actions of anticholinesterases at autonomic effector cells, and to some extent in the CNS, are antagonized by atropine and at the neuromuscular junction and autonomic ganglia some antagonism may be effected by curare-like drugs and hexamethonium respectively.

The therapeutic uses of the anticholinesterases are limited to effects on the pupil and the intestine, and to the treatment of myasthenia gravis.

When applied locally to the eye the anticholinesterases cause pupil constriction and spasm of accommodation. Intraocular pressure falls because the miosis allows the reabsorption of aqueous humour.

Anticholinesterases, particularly neostigmine, increase motor activity in the small and large bowel and this action can be used to overcome atonic conditions.

THE AUTONOMIC GANGLION

Transmission at autonomic ganglia is not unlike that at the neuromuscular junction, acetylcholine is the transmitting chemical at both parasympathetic and sympathetic ganglia and the main receptors are nicotinic. There is some evidence to suggest that muscarinic-type receptors exist on the postganglionic membrane but their physiological function is not yet clear.

Small spontaneous potentials, similar to mepps at the neuromuscular junction, can be recorded from the postsynaptic ganglionic neurones and it is likely that when a large number of them occur simultaneously, a full ganglion spike potential will be generated.

The site which has been most fully studied is the cat superior cervical ganglion, because it can easily be perfused through its artery or studied *in vitro*. It contains no interneurones and transmission across the synapses can be measured by recording electrically from the

FIG. 6.8. The effects of nicotine on a sympathetic ganglion. The tracing shows contractions of the nictitating membrane of a cat. The superior cervical ganglion was perfused with Locke's solution. A–D show the stimulant action of small doses of nicotine injected in the perfusion fluid; E and G show the effect of stimulating the cervical sympathetic. The injection of a large dose of nicotine (0·05 mg.) at F caused a contraction followed by paralysis of the ganglion. (From Feldberg and Vartiainen (1934) *J. Physiol. (Lond.)*, **83**, 120.)

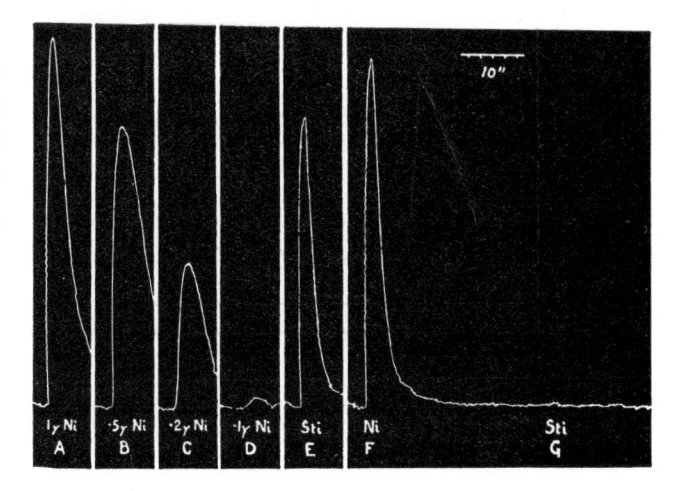

postganglionic fibres or by measuring contractures of the nictitating membrane which it innervates. The stimulant and paralysing actions of nicotine on the ganglion and the effect on the nictitating membrane are illustrated in FIGURE 6.8.

The evidence for cholinergic transmission at the ganglion is good. Choline acetyltransferase is present, cholinesterase is present, applied acetylcholine depolarizes the postsynaptic membrane, and acetylcholine is released from the stimulated preganglionic terminals.

The synthesis and turnover of acetylcholine in the preganglionic terminal have been studied in some detail and, as at the neuromuscular junction, choline and glucose are essential for synthesis. As might be expected, hemicholinium, triethylcholine, calcium and magnesium ions, and botulinum toxin all affect the synthesis and release of acetylcholine in apparently the same way as at the neuromuscular junction.

The effect of stimulating transmission through autonomic ganglia is best considered in relation to nicotine, acetylcholine, and T.M.A., which all work by depolarizing the postganglionic cell bodies.

Nicotine is readily absorbed from all mucous membranes, and more slowly on subcutaneous injection, or through intact skin. It causes excitation followed by inhibition at all sympathetic and parasympathetic ganglia. The first phase is the result of depolarization of the postganglionic membrane and the second phase results from the persistent depolarization of the membrane, probably by inactivation of the sodium carrier mechanism.

The peripheral responses to nicotine are complicated, because not only are there the excitatory and depressant effects, but also sympathetic and parasympathetic ganglia are equally affected. It imitates the effects of muscarine by stimulating the ganglia from which cholinergic nerves arise. It also imitates the actions of catecholamines by stimulating sympathetic ganglia and by causing a release of adrenaline from the adrenal medulla.

Nicotine is the most important pharmacological constituent of tobacco and the smoke from an average-sized cigarette may contain 6–8 mg. of nicotine. Attention has been focused in recent years on the hazards of tobacco smoking and a strong association between the incidence of carcinoma of the lung and tobacco smoking has been established. This is not the only hazard, however, because there is evidence that the action of nicotine, particularly on the cardiovascular system,

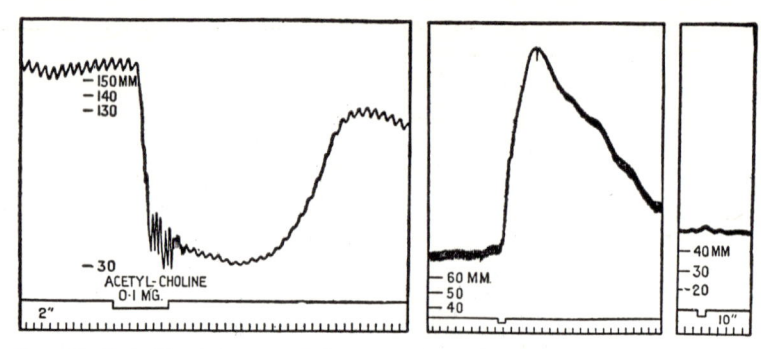

Fig. 6.9. Cat's blood pressure. Left—muscarine action of acetylcholine (0·1 mg.). Vasodilatation and slowing of heart. Middle—nicotine action of acetylcholine (5 mg.) after 1 mg. of atropine, which antagonizes muscarine actions. The rise of blood pressure is partly due to the liberation of adrenaline and partly due to the stimulation of sympathetic ganglia. Right—after 30 mg. of nicotine, the nicotine action of 5 mg. of acetylcholine disappears. (From Dale (1914) *J. Pharmacol.*, **6**, 152.)

can be deleterious when taken over long periods. The effects of cigarette smoking may include peripheral vasoconstriction, a rise in systolic and diastolic blood pressures, the occasional initiation of premature systoles, and attacks of atrial tachycardia. Smoking also causes bronchial irritation and the long-term addict can usually be recogized by his wheezing and dyspnoea. He is often subject to upper respiratory infections and may suffer chest pains. Most of these symptoms disappear if smoking is discontinued.

Despite the unpleasant and sometimes fatal side-effects of smoking which are now recognized and publicized, the use of tobacco shows only slight signs of declining. This is likely to be partly due to the addictive nature of the whole smoking ritual and to the pleasant central effects that nicotine has for many individuals.

Other effects of nicotine include the stimulation of respiration, vomiting by an action on central and peripheral receptors, antidiuresis by stimulating the release of ADH, and an increase in tone and motor activity of the bowel due to parasympathetic stimulation.

The ganglion-stimulant action of nicotine, acetylcholine, and related compounds may be clearly illustrated in the whole animal by the effect of acetylcholine on the blood pressure of the cat [FIG. 6.9].

A small dose of acetylcholine produces a dramatic fall in the blood pressure because the muscarinic effects of acetylcholine [see p. 65] slow the heart and cause peripheral vasodilatation. If atropine is now given to block this action and a higher dose of acetylcholine is injected, the nicotinic actions are unmasked and revealed as a rise in blood pressure. This is the result of ganglion stimulation causing activity in postganglionic vasoconstrictor fibres and the release of adrenaline from the adrenal medulla. The former effect may be abolished by giving a ganglion blocking compound.

Tetramethylammonium (T.M.A.), like acetylcholine and nicotine, stimulates all autonomic ganglia and causes a rise in the cat blood pressure after atropine because the effect of stimulating the sympathetic ganglia then predominates. It has only very weak muscarinic activity and it excites the ganglia in much lower concentrations than it does the neuromuscular junction.

Other drugs with ganglion stimulating actions include **lobeline** [p. 46] and **dimethyl-4-phenylpiperazium** (D.M.P.P.).

The stimulant action of nicotine, choline esters, and related compounds is often followed by a block of transmission due to persistent depolarization but there are other drugs which block ganglionic transmission by a non-depolarizing antagonism. These drugs, like curare at the muscle end-plate, do not alter the ganglion cell potentials nor do they interfere with the release of acetylcholine. They paralyse all autonomic ganglia and so have a variety of effects in all parts of the body. The paralysis of sympathetic ganglia dilates blood vessels and so a general fall in blood pressure occurs. This effect has been made use of clinically in cases of hypertension but because all ganglia are affected, there are numerous side-effects associated with this treatment. In addition, cardiovascular reflexes will be abolished and this may result in postural hypotension.

Paralysis of parasympathetic ganglia reduces gastric secretion, causes a dry mouth, paralysis of the iris and ciliary muscles, paralytic ileus, retention of urine, etc. These side-effects limit the clinical usefulness of the compounds.

Tetraethylammonium (T.E.A.) was the first drug to be used clinically to block ganglia but it is not very active or specific and has now been replaced by other compounds.

It is interesting that T.M.A. stimulates the ganglion by depolarization but substitution of the methyl groups by ethyl groups produces a compound which blocks transmission by a non-depolarizing action.

Although the ammonium salt T.E.A. has ganglion blocking activity, it was only with the development of the bisonium compounds that the sustained and specific action necessary for extensive clinical use could be obtained.

The bisonium compound **hexamethonium** has a highly specific action on ganglia, but, like most antagonists, in very large doses it will have other actions; these include atropine-like and curare-like effects.

It was employed in the treatment of hypertension but is now replaced by drugs with fewer side-effects that can be given orally. It is still used to produce hypotension during anaesthesia.

Other compounds which block transmission at autonomic ganglia include **pentolinium, pentamethonium,** and the orally active hypotensive agents, **pempidine** and **mecamylamine** [FIG. 6.16].

MUSCARINIC RECEPTORS

The action of acetylcholine and acetylcholine-like drugs on 'muscarinic' receptors resembles the effect of stimulating the parasympathetic nervous system. These muscarinic actions are postganglionic and are exerted on the heart, the exocrine glands, and smooth muscle. They include:

1. Heart—slowing.
2. Eye—constriction of the pupil, contraction of the ciliary muscle (for near vision).
3. Blood vessels—most blood vessels have muscarinic receptors and acetylcholine will produce vasodilatation.
4. Exocrine glands—stimulation of secretion from sweat glands, salivary glands (watery secretion), mucous glands, lacrimal glands. Gastric, intestinal, and pancreatic secretions are also increased.
5. Stomach and intestine—increase in motility and tone, relaxation of sphincters.
6. Gall-bladder and ducts—contraction.
7. Bladder—contraction of detrusor and relaxation of sphincter.

Drugs which produce these effects include **acetylcholine, carbachol, pilocarpine, muscarine, arecoline, methacholine,** and the **anticholinesterases.**

All the muscarinic actions of these drugs are abolished or reduced by atropine and atropine-like compounds.

The postganglionic fibres of the parasympathetic nervous system innervate smooth muscle effector cells, and release acetylcholine on to muscarinic receptors. Very much less is known about these neuromuscular junctions than about skeletal muscle junctions because the nerve terminals are not so easy to define and the muscle cells are small and hard to pierce with electrodes. There is, however, good evidence to suggest that acetylcholine is the only excitatory transmitter released when these nerves are stimulated.

The arrangement of nerve and muscle fibres is quite different from that existing in skeletal muscle; there is no organized end-plate and the nerves ramify widely over the muscle fibres. The action of acetylcholine, whether produced by stimulation of the nerves or by local application, is slow, and the tension developed by the muscle is graded continuously up to a maximum.

The electrical events associated with smooth muscle cells have been investigated with intra- and extracellular electrodes and the resting potential, which is rather variable, has been found to be lower than in skeletal muscle, about -50 mV, and to be altered by changes in the tension applied to the muscle. The state of membrane polarization determines the rate of muscle action potential discharge and therefore the activity of the contractile mechanism. When acetylcholine and other drugs interact with the muscarinic membrane receptors a state of membrane depolarization is produced with a consequent increase in spike frequency and muscle tension.

As with the end-plate on skeletal muscle, the action of acetylcholine on the post-junctional membrane appears to be associated with changes in membrane permeability to sodium and potassium ions.

The muscarinic receptors on smooth muscle are specifically stimulated by muscarine and this action is antagonized by atropine and by atropine-like compounds which compete for the receptor sites.

A rather different situation exists at the junction between postganglionic vagal parasympathetic fibres and the heart. As at smooth muscle parasympathetic junctions the transmitter is acetylcholine but it acts as an inhibitory transmitter and the effect of its release is primarily to produce a slowing of the heart rate. The acetylcholine acts on muscarinic receptors and its action is abolished by atropine, but unlike all other peripheral cholinergic sites in the body, except those of the secretory glands, the response to acetylcholine is a hyperpolarization of the membrane with a consequent reduction in membrane excitability.

In 1953 it was shown that the resting potential of the cat auricle fibres was increased (hyperpolarization) in the presence of acetylcholine and parasympathetic drugs. This effect was greatest when the diastolic membrane potential was furthest from the equilibrium potential for potassium ions (-90 mV) and it was suggested that the effect was mediated by a large selective increase in membrane permeability to potassium, this ion passing out of the cell.

When the inhibitory action of acetylcholine on the heart is compared with its excitatory action at the neuromuscular junction it may be seen that both effects are essentially the same. They both involve a fall in membrane resistance, the difference being in the species of ions whose movement is facilitated. At the neuromuscular junction there is a non-selective increase in cation permeability while at cardiac muscle the increase is largely restricted to potassium ions [FIG. 6.10].

Drugs which act as agonists at muscarinic receptor sites have the actions described on page 65. If the drug also has nicotinic activity then these effects will be superimposed on the muscarinic action. The individual compounds with muscarinic stimulating activity are described on pages 74–5.

Drugs which antagonize the action of cholinergic drugs at muscarinic receptors are known as antimuscarinic or **atropine-like compounds.** Except in high doses, their action is specific and clinically their main use has been for premedication before operations in order to prevent excessive salivary and bronchial secretions.

The drugs in this group have many pharmacological properties in common and these are well illustrated by considering the characteristics of atropine.

Various plants, including deadly nightshade

FIG. 6.10. Intracellular recording from a fibre of the sinus venosus of the frog heart. At S the vagus was stimulated at 20/sec. and the dotted line shows the effect of the liberated acetylcholine on the membrane potential. The continuous line shows the membrane potential in the unstimulated sinus venosus.

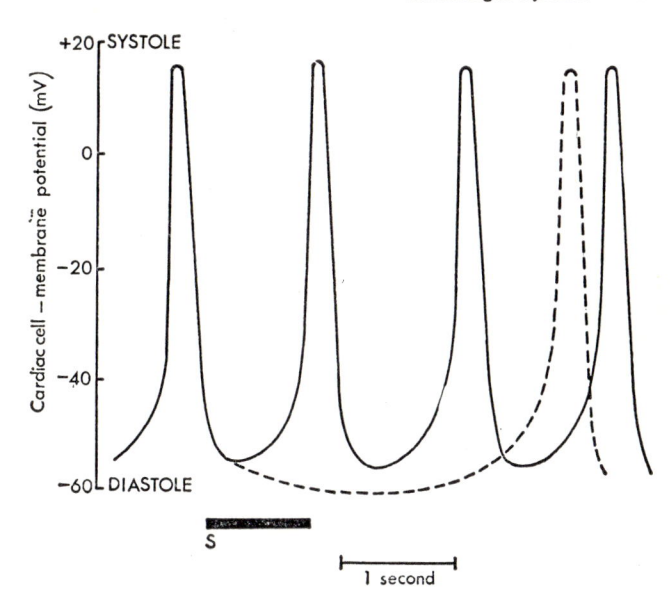

(*Atropa belladonna*), contain the alkaloids **l-hyoscyamine** and **l-hyoscine**. Racemization occurs easily and the racemic dl-hyoscyamine is known as **atropine**. These compounds all have some actions on the CNS [p. 21] but their most important actions are concerned with their antagonism at peripheral muscarinic receptors.

Most of the actions of atropine can be deduced from a knowledge of the effect of muscarine-like drugs. It stops secretion, including tears, sweat, and saliva, and the secretions of the pancreas and mucous glands in the alimentary canal and respiratory passages but has no effect on the secretion of bile, milk, or urine. It abolishes vagal action, dilates the bronchi, and inhibits the emptying of the bladder. It dilates the pupil and paralyses accommodation so that the eye is focused for distant objects.

Atropine is a reversible antagonist of muscarine-like drugs and its effect can usually be overcome if the agonist concentration is made sufficiently high.

Atropine is used to reduce salivary and bronchial secretions during anaesthesia, to protect the heart from vagal inhibition, and to reduce the muscarinic actions of any anticholinesterases that may be given. It is sometimes given to reduce the pain of renal and intestinal colic. It is used locally in the eye when a prolonged mydriatic effect is required.

A person poisoned by atropine has a dry mouth and finds it difficult to swallow or speak; he has a dry skin, a rash like that of scarlet fever, and a high temperature; his pupils are dilated and owing to the action on the CNS he may be restless and even have convulsions followed by paralysis. The convulsions can be controlled by a general anaesthetic and the subsequent paralysis by central stimulants and warmth. The peripheral effects of atropine are comparatively harmless.

A large number of other atropine-like compounds have been discovered or synthesized. Some of these are described on page 75 and include **hyoscine, homatropine, dibutoline, methantheline, propantheline,** the longer-acting drug **lachesine,** and the irreversible antagonist **benzilylcholine mustard** [FIG. 6.17].

MIXED RECEPTOR SITES

THE SPINAL CORD

The synapses between collateral fibres from the motor axon and Renshaw cells in the spinal cord are of particular interest because it is at these sites in the CNS that evidence for the identity of the transmitting chemical is most complete. The transmitter is almost certainly acetylcholine and much of the evidence for this has been obtained by the microelectrophoretic application of cholinergic agonists and antagonists to the Renshaw cell. When the blood–brain barrier is circumvented, as it is with the electrophoretic technique, there are no anomalous features in the response of Renshaw cells to these compounds [FIG. 6.11].

In addition, acetylcholine has been shown to be released by the motor axon collaterals when they are stimulated just as it is from the other terminal of the same axon, the motor nerve terminal.

The Renshaw cells appear to have both nicotinic and muscarinic-type receptors. They are excited by the application of acetylcholine and related choline esters, by nicotine, and by tetramethylammonium and they are weakly excited by muscarinic agents such as muscarine and acetyl-β-methylcholine. Transmission across the synapse is blocked by dihydro-β-erythroidine, tetraethylammonium, hexamethonium, and weakly by d-tubocurarine, and the actions of acetylcholine are potentiated by anticholinesterases. Although muscarinic agents excite only weakly, their action is resistant to block by nicotinic antagonists but is blocked by atropine, thus indicating the presence of muscarinic-type receptors.

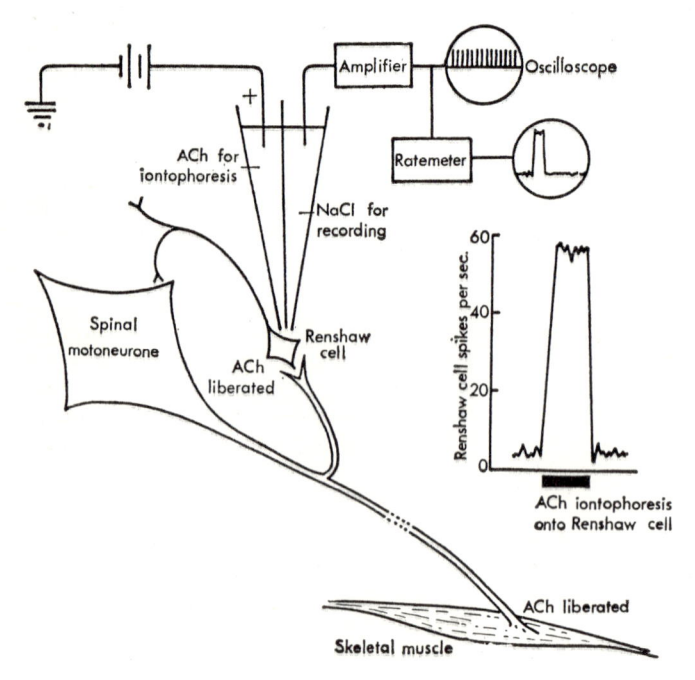

FIG. 6.11. Block diagram of the method used to investigate the action of iontophoretically applied drugs on Renshaw cells.

Many attempts to find cholinergic synapses elsewhere in the spinal cord have failed.

THE BRAIN

When it was realized that acetylcholine was a transmitter at peripheral synapses Sir Henry Dale suggested it might also have this role in the CNS. Although there is still no direct evidence for cholinergic synapses in the brain there is abundant indirect evidence to suggest that, at a small proportion of synapses, it does have an important role as a transmitter.

Acetylcholine, choline acetyltransferase, and cholinesterase are all present in the brain and acetylcholine is released from the brain and the rate of this release and also the acetylcholine content are associated with nervous activity and the level of consciousness [see FIG. 6.12]. Microelectrophoretic techniques have located cholinoceptive neurones in many parts of the brain including the cerebral cortex, the cerebellum, thalamus, hippocampus, reticular formation, and medulla. In the cortex the receptors appear to be predominately of a muscarinic type although nicotinic agonists and antagonists sometimes have weak actions. In the thalamus and lower parts of the brain the cholinoceptive cells appear to have a mixture of nicotinic and muscarinic properties, and in the brain stem, for instance, there is evidence that the 'muscarinic' neurones are inhibited by acetylcholine whereas the 'nicotinic' cells are excited.

It seems likely that some of the cholinergic synapses in the brain are associated with major specific and non-specific ascending pathways from the reticular formation and from specific thalamic nuclei and are concerned with the maintenance of consciousness and the level of arousal in the mammalian brain.

From a consideration of all the cholinergic mechanisms discussed it is evident that, at the

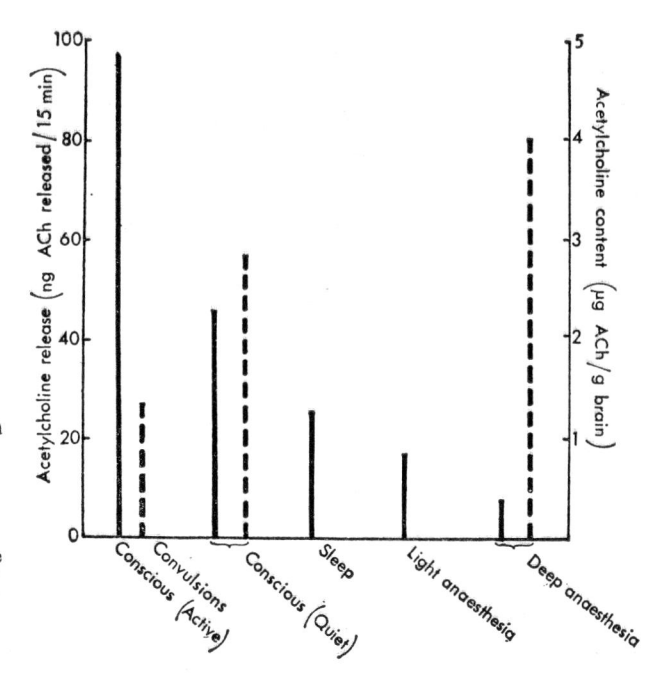

FIG. 6.12. The relationship between nervous activity and central acetylcholine content and release. Acetylcholine content measured in cerebral cortex of rats (dotted lines). Acetylcholine release measured from cerebral cortex of rabbits (full lines). As activity in the brain falls (deep anaesthesia) so the acetylcholine content rises and the release falls. This suggests that less is being liberated from cholinergic nerve terminals in the cortex.

periphery, the receptors are relatively simple and may be clearly divided into those with nicotinic and those with muscarinic characteristics. As one proceeds centrally, so the characteristics of the postsynaptic membranes become more complicated with a variable ratio of muscarinic and nicotinic properties. There is certainly much still to be learnt about these receptor systems and the significance of their distribution and function in the nervous system.

INDIVIDUAL CHOLINERGIC DRUGS AND THEIR ANTAGONISTS

Drugs which block neuromuscular transmission by depolarization:

Nicotine

Like acetylcholine, nicotine depolarizes the neuromuscular junction end-plate but it is not destroyed by cholinesterases, so even in small doses, after an initial twitch, a depolarizing block will appear.

Suxamethonium (Succinylcholine)

Suxamethonium depolarizes the end-plate and is hydrolysed by pseudocholinesterase, but its action is sufficiently prolonged to make it clinically useful as a neuromuscular blocking drug. It is used in short operations where profound muscle relaxation is required for a few minutes. It can be used for longer operations by repeating the dose or by giving infusions.

A few patients suffer prolonged apnoea after the injection of suxamethonium and many of these people have been found to have a reduced level of plasma cholinesterase, usually due to a genetic factor or, more rarely, to hepatic disease or a nutritional deficiency.

Suxamethonium blocks by depolarization but, like acetylcholine, its first effect may be to produce fasciculations which can result in post-operative muscle pains. It has no action on the CNS and unlike acetylcholine it has no muscarinic activity and so does not affect the autonomic nervous system.

When large doses are given, the initial block by depolarization gives way to a non-depolarizing curare-like block, which is relieved by anticholinesterase. This phenomenon is known as 'dual block' and may lead to prolonged muscle paralysis.

Decamethonium (C10)

Decamethonium is not destroyed by cholinesterase so its paralysing action is more prolonged than that of suxamethonium. There is no antidote which may be used safely. The mechanism of its blocking action is similar to that of suxamethonium [above].

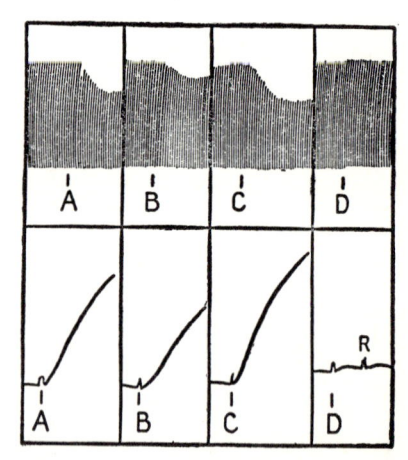

FIG. 6.13. Above—isolated frog's heart (Straub's method). Below—leech muscle sensitized with eserine. A—fluid from perfused sympathetic ganglion collected during stimulation. D—control fluid (no stimulation). B and C—acetylcholine (15 and 30 ng. per ml.). A caused effects between those due to B and C on both preparations. This quantitative agreement between two tests suggests the identification of the active substance in A as acetylcholine. (From Feldberg and Gaddum (1934) *J. Physiol. (Lond.)*, **81**, 314.)

Carbachol

Carbachol is an ester of choline with an action like acetylcholine except that its effect is more prolonged because it is not hydrolysed by cholinesterases. It has both muscarinic and nicotinic actions.

Dihydro-β-Erythroidine (D.H.E.)

This compound contains only one atom of nitrogen in its molecule and is active orally.

It is an effective and highly specific antagonist at nicotinic receptors.

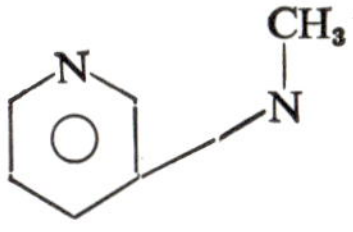
CH3
N
N

Nicotine

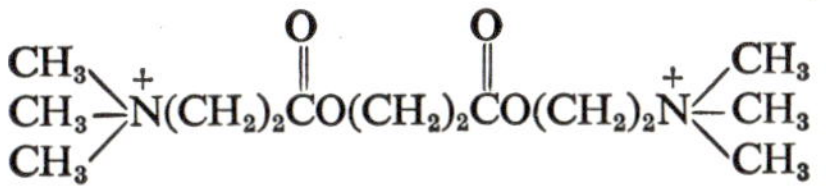
CH3 CH3 CH3 N(CH2)2CO(CH2)2CO(CH2)2N CH3 CH3 CH3

Suxamethonium

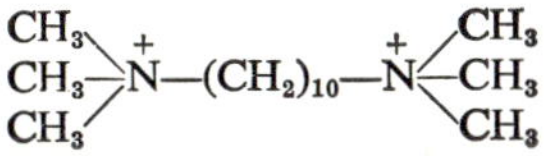
CH3 CH3 CH3 N—(CH2)10—N CH3 CH3 CH3

Decamethonium

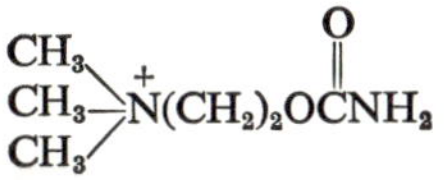
CH3 CH3 CH3 N(CH2)2OCNH2

Carbachol

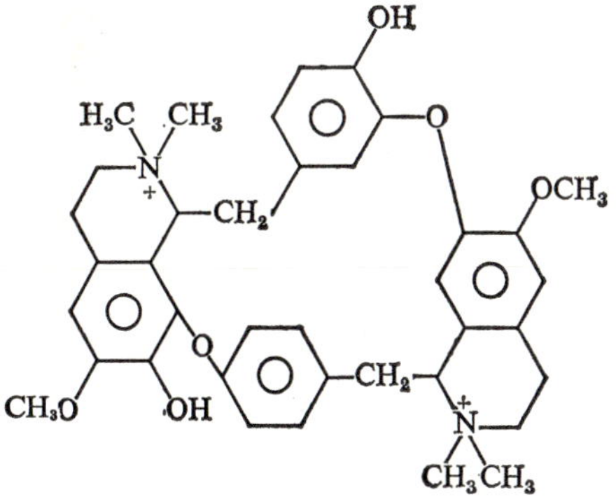
OH
H3C CH3
N
CH2
O
OCH3
O
CH2
N
CH3O
OH
CH3 CH3

d-Tubocurarine

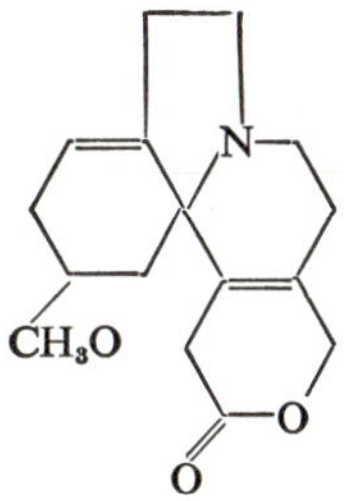
N
CH3O
O
O

Dihydro-β-erythroidine

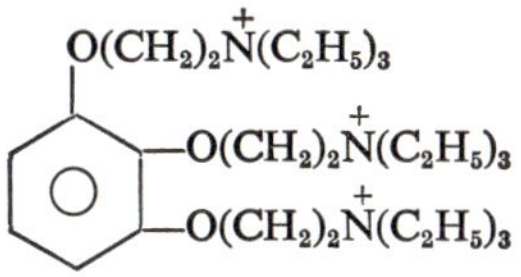
O(CH2)2N(C2H5)3
O(CH2)2N(C2H5)3
O(CH2)2N(C2H5)3

Gallamine

FIG. 6.14. Agonists and antagonists at the neuromuscular junction.

Benzoquinonium (*Mytolon*)

Benzoquinonium is a non-depolarizing blocker but has rather pronounced anticholinesterase properties in mammals, about one-tenth the activity of neostigmine. This may result in bradycardia and increased bronchial and salivary secretions. These are the result of the enhanced action of acetylcholine at muscarinic receptor sites and may all be abolished by atropine.

Because of its anticholinesterase activity it is only weakly antagonized by neostigmine and so it is not considered safe to be used clinically.

Gallamine

Gallamine is a synthetic compound which acts like tubocurarine but is about five times less active. It is widely used clinically to produce muscle relaxation during surgery. It may also be used in small doses to augment the effects of light anaesthesia in minor operations.

ANTICHOLINESTERASES

Edrophonium (*Tensilon*)

Edrophonium has a direct cholinergic action on nicotinic receptors and is a weak cholinesterase inhibitor.

It has a short duration of action and is used to antagonize curare-like drugs, and for the diagnosis of myasthenia gravis. Unlike neostigmine, a large dose of edrophonium produces nicotinic effects with muscle fasciculations leading to paralysis.

Neostigmine (*Prostigmin*)

Neostigmine has similar anticholinesterase properties to physostigmine but like edrophonium it also has a direct action on cholinergic receptors. It is used to antagonize the actions of curare-like drugs and in the treatment of atony of the bladder, myasthenia gravis, glaucoma, and sinus tachycardia. It is usually administered with atropine so that its muscarinic actions are reduced.

Physostigmine (Eserine)

This was the first anticholinesterase to be used clinically. It is absorbed well whether injected or swallowed. Most, if not all, of the actions of eserine are due to the inhibition of cholinesterase. Physostigmine potentiates all the nicotinic and muscarinic actions of acetylcholine and it is a useful drug for increasing the sensitivity of biological assay preparations to acetylcholine and is widely used for this purpose.

Dyflos (Diisopropylfluorophosphonate, D.F.P.)

Dyflos reacts with cholinesterase and loses fluorine. A phosphorylated enzyme is formed which is stable for a week or more. If a choline ester, or a reversible inhibitor such as eserine, is present the active site on the enzyme is occupied and the enzyme is protected from inactivation by organic phosphorus compounds. Dyflos causes a prolonged and powerful constriction of the pupil and is used in glaucoma to reduce intraocular pressure. This last effect is due to contraction of the pupil allowing reopening of the canal of Schlemm in the filtration angle of the eye.

Organo-phosphorus compounds with similar actions to dyflos include the following compounds:

Phospholine	Used to treat glaucoma.
Mipafox	Insecticide and selective inhibitor of pseudocholinesterase.
Sarin	Toxic nerve gas.
Tetraethylpyrophosphate (T.E.P.P.)	Early insecticide. Occasionally used in glaucoma and myasthenia gravis.

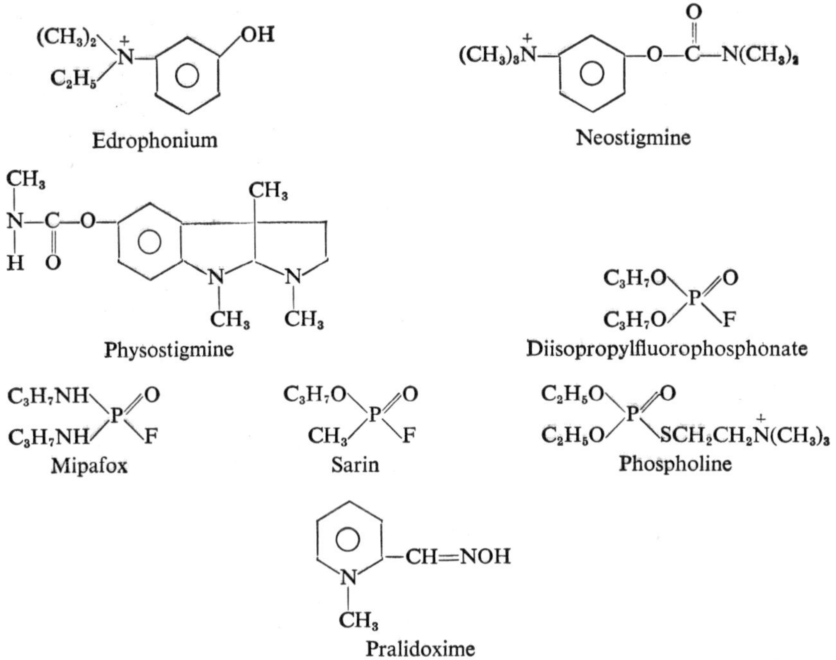

FIG. 6.15. The structures of some anticholinesterases and a cholinesterase reactivator.

DRUGS WHICH BLOCK TRANSMISSION AT AUTONOMIC GANGLIA

Pentamethonium

The actions of pentamethonium are identical to, but slightly less potent than, those of hexamethonium [p. 65]. Pentamethonium is not now used clinically.

Pentolinium

Pentolinium has similar properties to those of hexamethonium but it is more potent.

Mecamylamine

Mecamylamine is a secondary amine and was developed as an orally active hypotensive agent. It has a prolonged action of 8–12 hours and is at least as active as hexamethonium. It suffers from the disadvantage that, unlike quaternary methonium compounds, it enters the CNS with comparative ease and may cause tremor and/or psychoses.

It has side-effects similar to those exhibited by other ganglion blocking drugs.

Pempidine

Pempidine resembles mecamylamine in being absorbed when given orally but has a shorter duration of action. Pempidine is used in the treatment of all types of hypertension but is unsuitable for producing controlled hypotension during anaesthesia because of its prolonged action.

The ganglion blocking activity of mecamylamine and pempidine depends on the presence of a methyl group adjacent to the nitrogen; loss of this methyl group reduces activity.

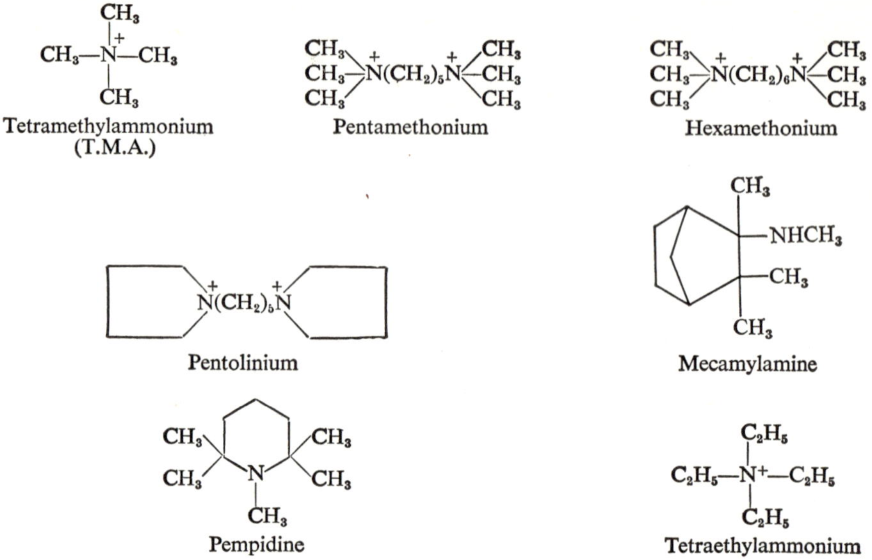

Cholinergic System

Tetramethylammonium (T.M.A.): $(CH_3)_4N^+$

Pentamethonium: $(CH_3)_3N^+(CH_2)_5N^+(CH_3)_3$

Hexamethonium: $(CH_3)_3N^+(CH_2)_6N^+(CH_3)_3$

Pentolinium

Mecamylamine

Pempidine

Tetraethylammonium: $(C_2H_5)_4N^+$

FIG. 6.16. The structures of drugs which act on the autonomic ganglion.

AGONISTS AT MUSCARINIC RECEPTORS

Muscarine

Muscarine was taken as the substance typical of a class of drugs because it was thought to have an action exclusively on pure muscarinic receptors. This is now known not to be entirely true. It is a very stable and active substance and is excreted unchanged in the urine.

Muscarine stimulates the postganglionic parasympathetic receptor and so reproduces the effects of stimulating parasympathetic nerves [see p. 65]. All its actions are antagonized by atropine. It is not used clinically.

Acetylcholine

Acetylcholine produces all the effects which are obtained by stimulation of the parasympathetic nervous system and, in addition, it stimulates nicotinic receptors at the skeletal neuromuscular junction, autonomic ganglion, and the adrenal medulla. Because it is quickly hydrolysed by cholinesterases its action is transient unless anticholinesterases are present.

Small alterations in the acetylcholine molecule produce profound changes in muscarinic activity. The size of the charged cationic head is important for activity, methyl groups being necessary for activity and substitution with more than one ethyl group considerably reduces muscarinic activity.

Replacing the acetyl group by others in the series always leads to a fall in muscarinic activity and homologues higher than butyrylcholine are even found to be acetylcholine antagonists. The changes in nicotinic activity of these substituted compounds do not follow the changes in muscarinic potency [Chapter 1].

If the choline part of the molecule is altered in length, again the muscarinic activity is reduced as in acetylnorcholine which has only weak muscarinic activity.

The introduction of asymmetry into the molecule by the addition of a branched methyl group to the chain also affects activity.

Methacholine, in which the β carbon in acetylcholine has been methylated, has only half the muscarinic activity of acetylcholine and no nicotinic actions.

Methacholine

Methacholine has actions similar to the muscarinic actions of acetylcholine and it is more stable, being hydrolysed by acetylcholinesterase at only one-third the rate of acetylcholine. It is not hydrolysed by pseudocholinesterase. It is a safer drug than carbachol because of its lack of nicotinic effects. Its main actions are to slow the heart and dilate peripheral blood vessels while intestinal tone is raised and salivation and sweating are increased.

Choline

Choline has both nicotinic and muscarinic actions but these are about 1,000 times weaker than those of acetylcholine.

Pilocarpine

Pilocarpine has muscarinic actions but no significant nicotinic activity. It produces marked sweating and the secretion of gastric juices. It is only used clinically to reduce intra-ocular pressure in the treatment of glaucoma.

Arecoline

The pharmacological actions of arecoline resemble those of pilocarpine. Arecoline is the chief alkaloid in betel nuts and has been used by natives of the East Indies from early times to produce euphoria.

Anticholinesterases

These compounds have actions resembling those which result from parasympathetic stimulation because they prevent the destruction of liberated acetylcholine.

The administration of physostigmine produces constriction of the pupil, stimulation of the intestine, and inhibition of the heart. If it is placed in the eye there is constriction of the pupil, spasm of accommodation, and a reduction of intra-ocular pressure [see p. 62].

ANTAGONISTS AT MUSCARINIC RECEPTORS

Hyoscine (Scopolamine)

The peripheral actions of hyoscine resemble those of atropine but it is more effective in stopping secretions.

The central actions of hyoscine differ from those of atropine. They do not produce excitement at any stage but only depression, especially of the motor areas. It is an effective drug against motion-sickness and it is used for this purpose and as a sedative and to prevent secretions during operations.

Homatropine

This is a synthetic derivative closely allied to atropine in chemical structure. It has weaker antimuscarinic actions than atropine and its effect on the eye lasts for only hours instead of for days as with atropine.

Dibutoline

Dibutoline has some structural similarity to carbachol but has antimuscarinic properties. It is less potent than atropine and has ganglion blocking activity in high doses. It has a brief and rapid action and is therefore used for ophthalmic purposes.

Lachesine

Lachesine has obvious structural similarities to acetylcholine but blocking activity is conferred by the presence of the bulky terminal ring structures. The drug is a mydriatic and antispasmodic. Its other pharmacological properties are similar to those of atropine except that, unlike atropine, it produces sedation.

Benzilylcholine Mustard

In 1966 Gill and Rang, in Oxford, discovered an irreversible blocker of muscarinic receptors. It is a β-haloalkylamine which cyclizes in

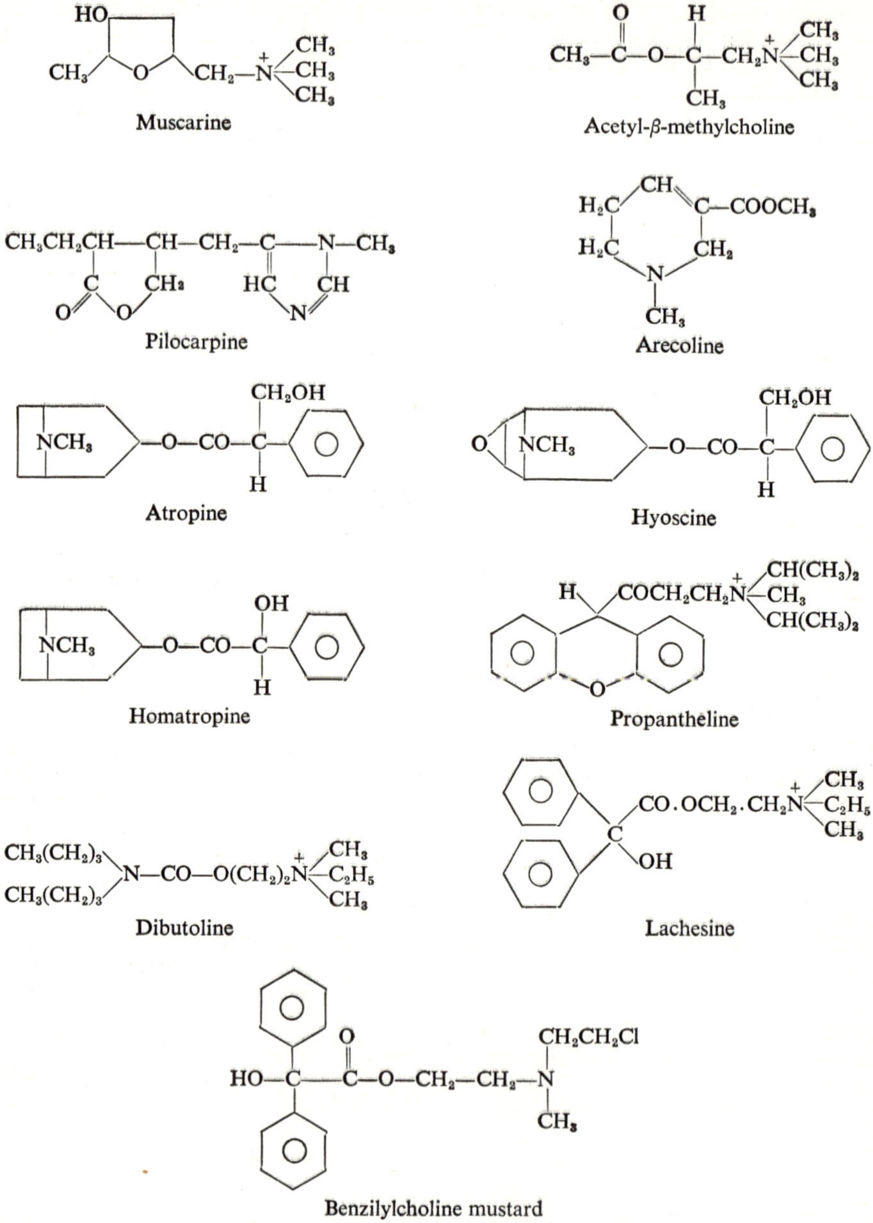

FIG. 6.17. The structures of agonists and antagonists at muscarinic sites.

solution to give an ethyleneiminium derivative. It is a very specific and potent antagonist of muscarinic activity and has no blocking action at the neuromuscular junction or autonomic ganglion.

It produces an irreversible block in a similar way to dibenamine [p. 88] by alkylation of a receptor group with the formation of a very stable, covalent bond. It is found that the degree of irreversible muscarinic block is proportional to the concentration of ethyleneiminium ions present in solution.

Methantheline (*Banthine*)

This is a synthetic quaternary ammonium compound which has a wide clinical use. It differs from atropine in having relatively strong ganglion blocking activity compared to its antimuscarinic activity. The ganglion blocking activity may be apparent even in therapeutic doses.

Propantheline (*Pro-Banthine*)

This is a synthetic compound closely related to methantheline. It is about three times as active as methantheline as an antimuscarinic agent and its ganglion blocking activity is also greater. It was developed in an effort to produce a drug which would inhibit gastric motility and secretion without the undesired side-effects of atropine. Propantheline is used for this purpose either alone or with barbiturates in the treatment of peptic ulcers.

FURTHER READING

BIRKS, R. I., and MACINTOSH, F. C. (1961) Acetylcholine metabolism of a sympathetic ganglion, *Can. J. Biochem.*, **39**, 787.

BOWMAN, W. (1962) Mechanisms of neuromuscular blockade, *Progr. Med. Chem.*, **3**, 88.

BROWN, G. L., DALE, H. H., and FELDBERG, W. (1936) Reactions of the normal mammalian muscle to acetylcholine and eserine, *J. Physiol. (Lond.)*, **87**, 394.

BURNSTOCK, G., and HOLMAN, M. (1966) Effect of drugs on smooth muscle, *Ann. Rev. Pharmacol.*, **6**, 129.

CASTILLO, J. DEL, and KATZ, B. (1957) A study of curare action with an electrical micro-method, *Proc. roy. Soc. B*, **146**, 339.

CHANG, H. C., and GADDUM, J. H. (1933) Choline esters in tissue extracts, *J. Physiol. (Lond.)*, **79**, 255.

COLLIER, B., and MITCHELL, J. F. (1967) The central release of acetylcholine during consciousness, and after brain lesions, *J. Physiol. (Lond.)*, **188**, 83.

CURTIS, D. R. (1966) Synaptic transmission in the central nervous system and its pharmacology, in *Nerve as a Tissue*, ed. Rodahl, K., and Issakutz, B., New York.

DIXON, W. E. (1907) On the mode of action of drugs, *Med. Mag. (Lond.)*, **16**, 454.

KATZ, B. (1967) *Nerve, Muscle and Synapse*, London.

KOELLE, G. B. (ed.) (1963) Cholinesterase and anticholinesterase agents, *Handb. exp. Pharmak.*, Suppl. 15, Berlin.

KRNJEVIĆ, K., and PHILLIS, J. W. (1963) Pharmacological properties of acetylcholine-sensitive cells in the cerebral cortex, *J. Physiol. (Lond.)*, **166**, 328.

McLENNAN, H. (1970) *Synaptic Transmission*, 2nd ed., Philadelphia.

MITCHELL, J. F. (1963) The spontaneous evoked release of acetylcholine from the cerebral cortex, *J. Physiol. (Lond.)*, **165**, 98.

MITCHELL, J. F. (1966) Acetylcholine release from the brain, *Wenner-Gren International Symposium*, Stockholm.

PATON, W. D. M. (1959) The pharmacology of ganglion blocking agents, in *Hypertension*, ed. Moyer, J. H., Philadelphia.

PHILLIS, J. W. (1970) *The Pharmacology of Synapses*, Oxford.

7

ADRENERGIC SYSTEM

THE peripheral sympathetic nervous system is derived from neurones arising in the lateral horns of the grey matter of the spinal cord. These neurones synapse mainly on ganglion cells located in the sympathetic chains which run on either side of the vertebrae, although some ganglion cells are also found in the autonomic nerves going to the peripheral structures innervated, and in some cases also in these tissues. The presynaptic nerves to the adrenal medulla synapse directly upon the medulla cells which are thus homologous to the postsynaptic neurone. The transmitter at these synapses is acetylcholine as it is in the entire cholinergic system. The postsynaptic neurone, on the other hand, contains catecholamines, which can be demonstrated by a brown colour produced by treatment with dichromate, and these cells are therefore called chromaffin cells. The presence of catecholamines can be more selectively demonstrated by a fluorescence technique in which the tissue is treated with formaldehyde vapour and the catecholamines converted to dihydroxydihydroisoquinolines which give a strong green fluorescence [FIG. 7.1]. In the sympathetic neurones this is concentrated in granules collected in little varicosities along the length of the nerve, and it is particularly in these regions that the transmitter, which is noradrenaline (arterenol), is liberated when the nerve is stimulated.

Similar granules are present in very large numbers in the adrenal medulla cells and in this case the transmitter is mainly the N-methyl catecholamine adrenaline (epinephrine). These granules can be isolated by homogenizing the tissue and then separating the granule fraction by centrifuging in a sucrose gradient. The particles contain as much as 7 per cent. catecholamine together with adenine nucleotides, proteins, and lipids. Present evidence suggests that the major part of the catecholamine in the nerve is present in these storage particles and that when catecholamines are liberated in response to nerve stimulation, the nucleotides and protein contained in the granule are liberated too. This suggests that liberation occurs as a result of fusion of the granule membrane with the cytomembrane, and discharge of the contents without their coming into contact with the cell cytoplasm. It is known that, as with acetylcholine transmitter release in response to nerve stimulation, release is dependent on the presence of calcium in the external medium, and it is believed that calcium entry into the nerve is responsible for the granule fusion and discharge.

The reserpine group of alkaloids have a selective action on storage of catecholamines in the granules, probably by increasing the permeability of the lipoprotein envelope of the granule. This causes release of the catecholamine into the neuronal cytoplasm where it is largely metabolized so that pharmacologically inactive degradation products are released into the extraneuronal space. The nerve may become almost wholly depleted of noradrenaline and hence unable to release transmitter on stimulation.

Noradrenaline is synthesized in the neurones from tyrosine which is first hydroxylated in the 3 position by tyrosine hydroxylase to give DOPA (dihydroxyphenylalanine; 3-hydroxytyrosine), which is then decarboxylated by DOPA decarboxylase to give dopamine (3-hydroxytyramine) and finally a β-hydroxyl group is introduced by dopamine β-oxidase to give noradrenaline [FIG. 7.2]. The rate-limiting step in this biosynthetic sequence is the formation of DOPA. In the adrenal medulla a further

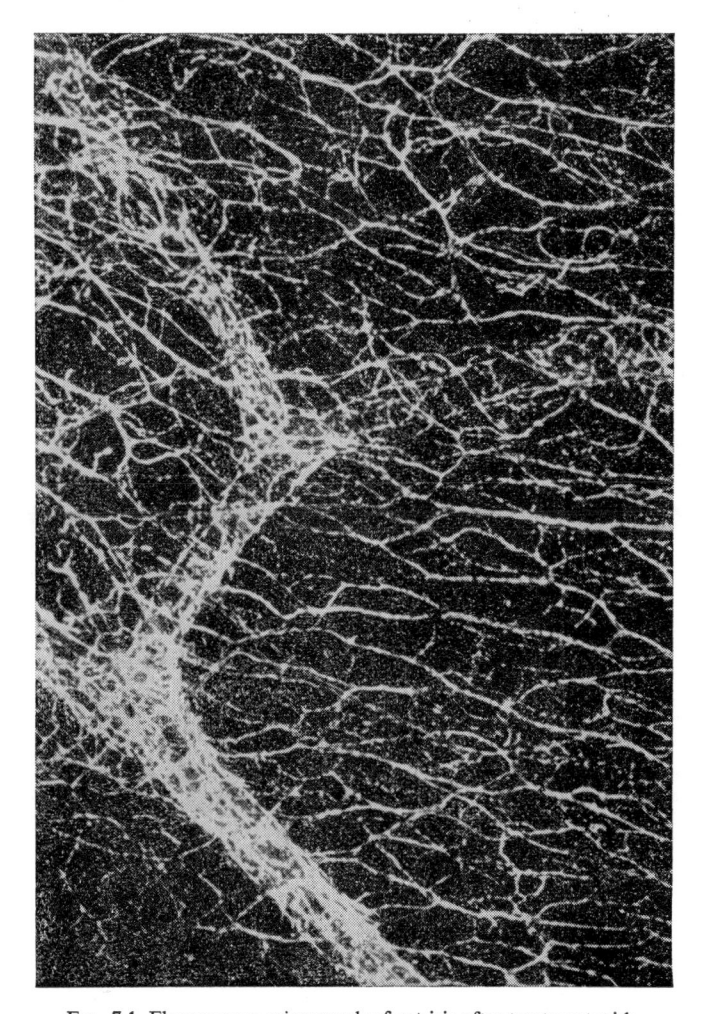

Fig. 7.1. Fluorescence micrograph of rat iris after treatment with formaldehyde. The sympathetic neurones appear as beaded structures with a green fluorescence. The dense mat of sympathetic neurones on the left of the picture surround an arteriole. (Malmfors, T. (1965) *Acta physiol. scand.*, **64**, Suppl. 248.)

step, N-methylation of noradrenaline to give adrenaline, occurs, catalysed by phenylethanolamine-N-methyl transferase. By injecting tyrosine or DOPA labelled with C^{14} or tritium into an animal, the biosynthetic pathway can be studied *in vivo*. Because the conversion of tyrosine to DOPA is rate limiting, higher rates of biosynthesis can be achieved if DOPA is supplied, than with tyrosine.

Adrenergic System

FIG. 7.2. The biosynthesis of noradrenaline and adrenaline.

[Biosynthetic pathway: Tyrosine → (Tyrosine hydroxylase) → DOPA → (Dopa decarboxylase) → Dopamine → (Dopamine β-hydroxylase) → Noradrenaline → (Phenylethanolamine N-methyl transferase) → Adrenaline]

There is some evidence that the level of free noradrenaline in the system is controlled by noradrenaline acting as a feedback controller of tyrosine hydroxylase. Inhibitors for several of these biosynthetic enzymes are known, for instance **α-methyltyrosine** and **3-iodotyrosine** are potent inhibitors of tyrosine hydroxylase and lead to a reduction of the noradrenaline content of the nerves. Inhibitors of DOPA decarboxylase such as **methyldopa** do not appear

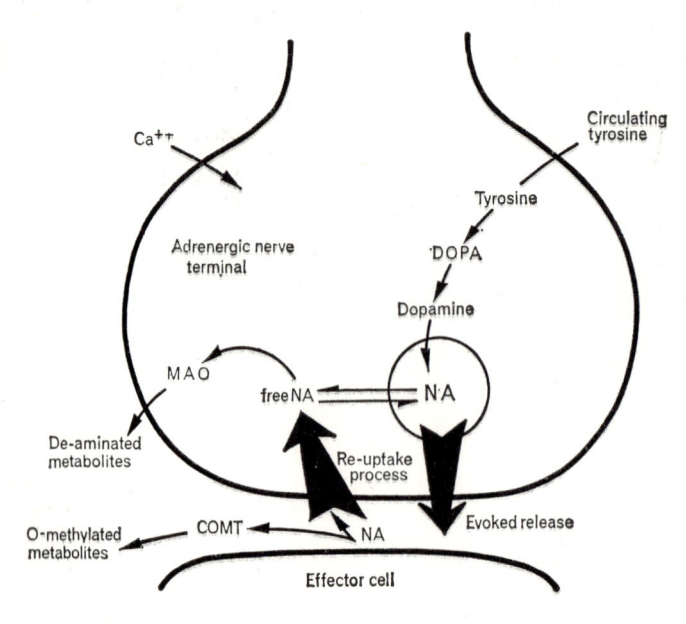

FIG. 7.3. Processes concerned in the synthesis, storage, release, and metabolism of noradrenaline (NA) in sympathetic nerves. MAO, mono-amine oxidase; COMT, catechol-O-methyl transferase.

to reduce noradrenaline synthesis appreciably because the availability of DOPA dominates the rate of over-all biosynthesis. Dopamine-β-hydroxylase is inhibited by the copper chelater **disulfiram** leading to a relative accumulation of dopamine in the nerves. The enzymes in the biosynthetic pathway are not wholly specific and thus methyldopa is a substrate for dopa-decarboxylase and leads to the formation of α-methyldopamine which is β-hydroxylated to α-methylnoradrenaline. This is stored in granules in the same way as noradrenaline and replaces part of the noradrenaline, thus decreasing the content of the latter in the tissue. Similarly tyramine can be β-hydroxylated to **synephrine** (octopamine) which is also stored and replaces noradrenaline [FIG. 7.4].

Two major metabolic pathways exist for the degradation of catecholamines. These are first 3-O-methylation by the enzyme catechol-O-methyl transferase (COMT) which leads to the formation of **normetanephrine** and **metanephrine**. This enzyme appears to be localized exclusively outside the neurone but in close proximity, and is also found in large amounts in the liver and kidneys. The enzyme may be inhibited by the competitive substrates pyrogallol, tropolone, and dopacetamide, none of which are very potent. The second pathway for metabolism is by oxidative deamination by the enzyme monoamine oxidase (MAO) which is found in large amounts in the mitochondria of the sympathetic neurones as well as in the liver, intestine, and elsewhere [FIG. 7.3]. Inside the cell noradrenaline is protected from MAO by segregation in the granules and probably also by other intracytoplasmic membranes. A large number of powerful inhibitors of MAO are known, the most important of which are the hydrazines (e.g. phenelzine). Because of the operation of these two enzymes the main metabolites of catecholamines excreted in the urine are 3-methoxy-4-hydroxy mandelic acid and 3,4-dihydroxymandelic acid [FIG. 7.5].

These metabolic pathways are *not* the major processes dealing either with noradrenaline liberated from sympathetic stimulation or with noradrenaline or adrenaline injected into the circulation. The dominant process is uptake of catecholamine into the sympathetic endings which occurs in two stages: (1) active transfer through the cytomembrane; and (2) storage in the catecholamine granules.

This conclusion has been reached from the following observations:

1. If tritium-labelled noradrenaline is injected intravenously the major portion can be recovered from the tissues as

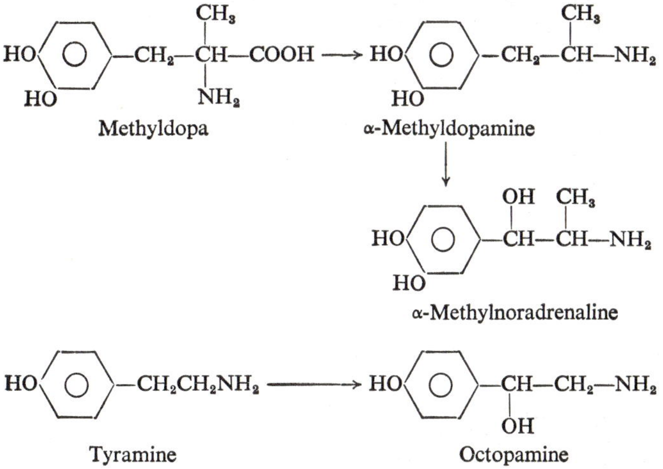

FIG. 7.4. Formation of modified transmitters that can be stored in sympathetic nerves.

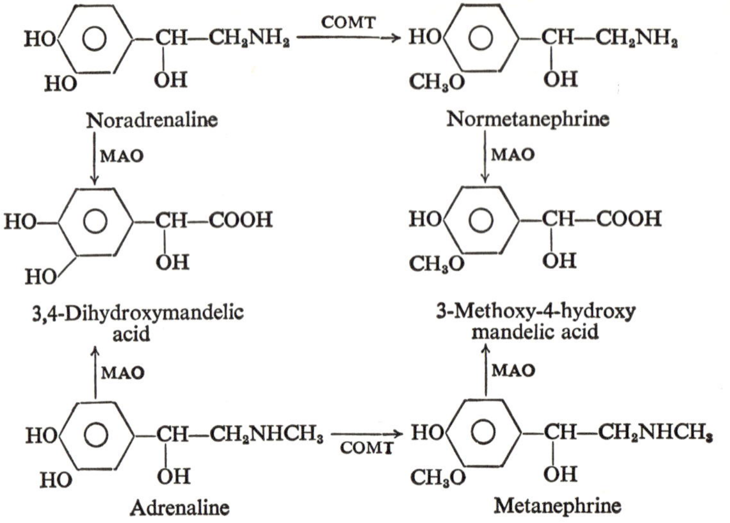

Adrenergic System

FIG. 7.5. The metabolic fate of noradrenaline and adrenaline.

unchanged noradrenaline and a minor part as metabolites.
2. Inhibitors of MAO and COMT *do not* significantly potentiate the actions of injected noradrenaline or of sympathetic stimulation.
3. The uptake process may be inhibited by **cocaine, desipramine,** and **phenoxybenzamine,** and the use of these drugs increases and prolongs the response to sympathetic nerve stimulation and to injected noradrenaline, and also increases the amount of noradrenaline that can be collected in perfused preparations. Present evidence suggests that 80–90 per cent. of the noradrenaline released by nerve stimulation is reaccumulated in the nerve terminals.

This behaviour of the sympathetic transmitter contrasts with the parasympathetic transmitter acetylcholine which is wholly destroyed by hydrolysis by cholinesterase.

The re-uptake mechanism is not very specific and can take up related amines; one of the most interesting of these is 6-hydroxydopamine (3,4,6 trihydroxyphenylethylamine) which is highly toxic to the neurone and causes degeneration. Within a few days the sympathetic nerve endings disappear and with them the tissue noradrenaline. After intraventricular injection 6-hydroxydopamine causes degeneration of most of the noradrenergic nerves in the brain.

Noradrenaline may be released from sympathetic nerves in yet another way. This is by the action of certain sympathomimetic amines such as **tyramine.** When tyramine is injected into an animal it produces effects very much like noradrenaline except that the effects are slightly delayed and more long-lasting and also much larger doses are required.

Certain differences are found on more detailed examination:

1. The effects of repeated doses gradually become less (tachyphylaxis); this does not happen with noradrenaline.
2. The effects are greatly diminished by section of the sympathetic nerves and subsequent degeneration. The effects of noradrenaline, on the other hand, are increased due to denervation hypersensitivity.

3. The effects are also diminished by pre-treatment with doses of reserpine sufficient to deplete the nerves of noradrenaline.
4. The effects of tyramine are also diminished by uptake inhibitors (e.g. cocaine) which, at the same time, potentiate noradrenaline.
5. Successive doses of tyramine cause a progressive depletion of the noradrenaline content of the nerves.
6. In perfused organs noradrenaline can be detected in the perfusate following injection of tyramine.

This evidence is conclusive in showing that the major action of tyramine is to cause release of noradrenaline from the nerves as noradrenaline and not as metabolites (cf. reserpine) and that it is the released noradrenaline that produces the pharmacological effects. It is not certain how the release occurs. There is evidence favouring a displacement of noradrenaline from storage granules with protection from the action of MAO by substrate competition, but also some evidence suggestive of activation of the nerve membrane in a manner comparable to that produced by physiological nerve stimulation. This action is important and sympathomimetic drugs may be divided into *direct acting*, i.e. having actions like noradrenaline, *indirect acting*, i.e. acting through release of noradrenaline, and *mixed acting*, i.e. in which both direct and indirect actions are playing a part.

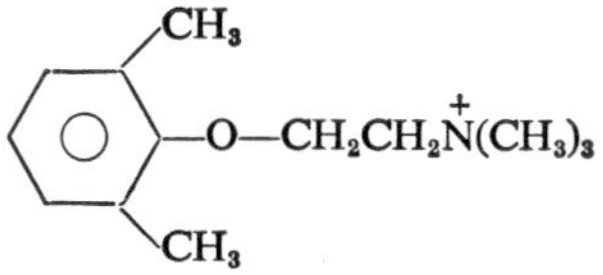

Finally there is a group of drugs that interferes with the release of noradrenaline from sympathetic nerve terminals [FIG. 7.6]. This action was originally found quite unexpectedly in **xylocholine** which produced a selective blockade of the effects of stimulating postganglionic sympathetic nerves without affecting the response to noradrenaline or adrenaline. Xylocholine has some nicotinic actions as might be expected from its structure, but these are absent from β-methylxylocholine. Subsequently high activity was found in other quaternary ammonium compounds of which

Xylocholine (TM 10)

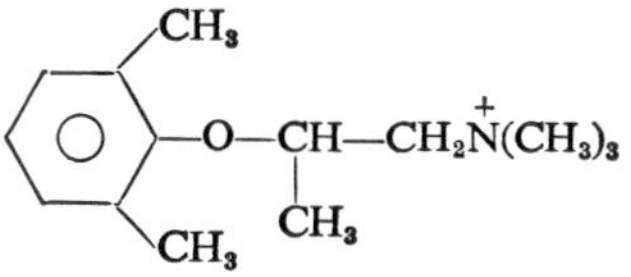

β-Methylxylocholine

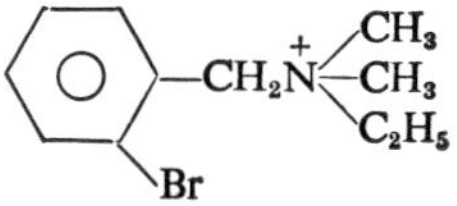

Bretylium

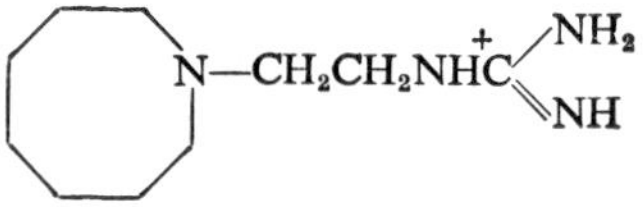

Guanethidine

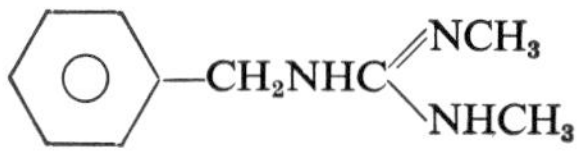

Bethanidine

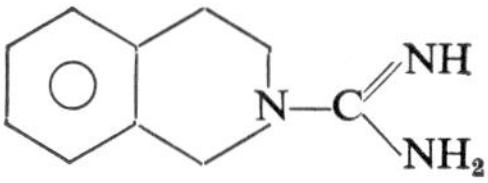

Debrisoquine

FIG. 7.6. The structures of drugs which interfere with the release of noradrenaline.

bretylium is the most active. Bretylium does not deplete the sympathetic neurones of noradrenaline but is itself highly concentrated in these neurones. Since bretylium and related substances are local anaesthetics it has been suggested that they block conduction in the sympathetic nerve filaments, and are selective owing to the specially high concentration in these nerves. Direct evidence that they block

TABLE 7.1 DISTRIBUTION OF ADRENERGIC RECEPTORS

ORGAN	EFFECTS	RECEPTOR TYPE
Heart	Increased heart rate, contractibility, and excitability	β
Coronary arteries	Decreased blood flow	α
	Increased blood flow	β (predominant)
Skeletal muscle arterioles	Increased blood flow	β
Skin arterioles	Decreased blood flow	mainly β
Spleen	Contraction	α
Iris (radial muscle)	Pupil dilated	α
Smooth muscle of gut	Relaxed, rhythmic activity inhibited	β
Bladder	Sphincter contracted	α
	Detrusor relaxed	β
Salivary glands	Secretion	α
Metabolism (liver, fat, heart)	Increased	β

conduction is absent. **Guanethidine** also blocks release of noradrenaline in a similar way to bretylium, but in addition causes depletion of the noradrenaline content. Bethanidine and debrisoquine are related guanidine derivatives.

Burn and Rand have produced a large amount of evidence suggesting that noradrenaline is not directly released by the nerve impulse but that acetylcholine release is the primary event and that this leads secondarily to noradrenaline release. This is referred to as a 'cholinergic link'. Most pharmacologists are unwilling to accept this thesis while admitting that most sympathetic nerves are mixed (i.e. contain cholinergic as well as the predominant adrenergic fibres) and that release of acetylcholine may alter the amount of noradrenaline released.

A substance stimulating the growth of sympathetic neurones has been found in tumours, snake venom, and mouse salivary glands by Levi-Montalcini and her collaborators. It is a protein which, if given to young animals, leads to overgrowth of certain parts of the sympathetic nervous system specifically. It has little or no effect on the adrenal medulla. Antisera against the nerve growth factor can be prepared and, when injected into young animals, cause a selective loss of sympathetic neurones, for instance, in the rat the heart can lose up to 95 per cent. of its noradrenaline content.

THE EFFECTS OF SYMPATHETIC NERVE STIMULATION AND OF NORADRENALINE AND ADRENALINE

When sympathetic nerves are stimulated they cause increase of tone in some varieties of smooth muscle, relaxation in others as well as increasing the rate and force of the heart and stimulation of the secretion of some glands [TABLE 7.1] and also effects on carbohydrate and lipid metabolism.

Qualitatively similar effects are produced by noradrenaline and adrenaline. However, the intensity of the effects produced by these two drugs is not similar, the inhibitory, cardiac, and metabolic effects being greater with adrenaline. Since the chemical difference between adrenaline and noradrenaline is the presence of the N-methyl group in adrenaline, it is interesting that if this group is made larger as in N-ethyl noradrenaline or isoprenaline (N-isopropyl noradrenaline, isoproterenol)

Fig. 7.7. Cyclic AMP.

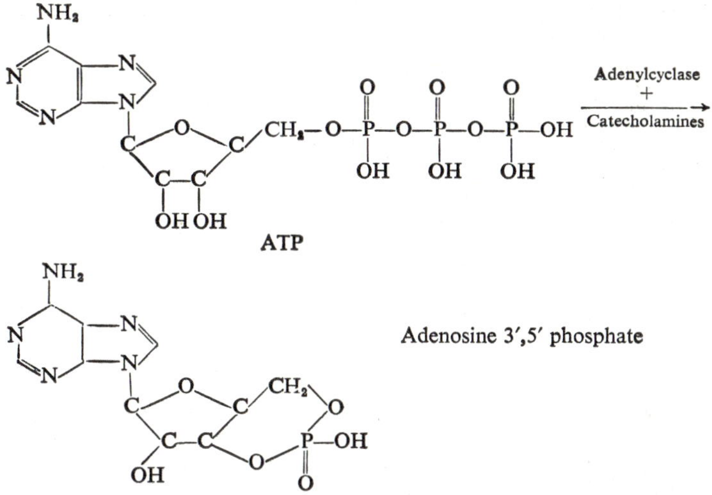

ATP

Adenosine 3′,5′ phosphate

these latter effects are further intensified and the excitor effects on smooth muscle become very weak. The different order of potency, i.e. noradrenaline < adrenaline ≫ isoprenaline for the excitor actions, and noradrenaline < adrenaline ≪ isoprenaline for the inhibitory, cardiac, and metabolic actions is most easily explained if these are mediated by two distinct receptors—this was first pointed out by Ahlquist who named the first type of receptor α and the second β. Strong support for this hypothesis has come from the discovery that antagonists of the catecholamines have a selective action on these two classes of response. The older established antagonists ergotamine, phentolamine, and phenoxybenzamine are selective α-blockers totally without effects on the β-responses. On the other hand, propranolol, iproveratrine, and dichloroisoprenaline block β-responses and have no effect on α-action. It is interesting to note that whereas all the β-blockers so far described are closely related in structure to isoprenaline, the α-blockers bear a less obvious chemical resemblance to the catecholamines. Although the β-actions of noradrenaline are weaker than those of adrenaline it appears that the effects of sympathetic neurones terminating on β-receptor areas are due to the liberation of **noradrenaline**; this is the case for the heart, liver, and intestine to mention just a few areas.

BIOPHYSICAL AND BIOCHEMICAL ACTIONS OF CATECHOLAMINES

On smooth muscle where α-excitation occurs, sympathetic stimulation causes depolarizing junction potentials which, if they are suprathreshold, lead to propagating action potentials. Applied catecholamines similarly lead to depolarization. This is probably produced by an increase in sodium permeability. In the heart, on the other hand, there is little change in either resting or action potential to account for the large positive inotropic action. Under rather abnormal conditions (i.e. raised Mg concentration) catecholamines will increase the magnitude and duration of the action potential probably by increasing entry of both sodium and calcium. In nodal tissues the action of the sympathetic is clearer, depolarizing junctional potentials are produced together with a greater rate of diastolic drift in the resting potential and these are responsible for increasing the rate of impulse discharge. Again the effects are probably mediated by an increase in sodium permeability. Undoubtedly the main part of the positive inotropic effect in the ventricles is unaccounted for by obvious ionic changes and much interest has recently been centred on biochemical changes.

The starting-point of this new approach was the discovery that the amount of the cyclic nucleotide, 3′,5′ adenosine monophosphate (cyclic AMP) in the heart was markedly increased when the heart was stimulated by catecholamines. Further study has shown that this is due to an activation of the enzyme adenylcyclase that forms cyclic AMP from ATP. It was also found that cyclic AMP is destroyed by an intracellular phosphodiesterase which can be inhibited by theophylline; this can also raise the level of cyclic AMP. Since theophylline produces inotropic effects in the heart very similar to those of catecholamines it is interesting that both effects are mediated by a rise in cyclic AMP. Subsequently it was found that adenylcyclase and cyclic AMP are involved in a very wide range of hormone actions, including the lipolytic effects of adrenaline and insulin on fat cells, the action of corticotrophin on the adrenal cortex, the action of catecholamines on cerebellar neurones, the action of parathormone on the kidney, and most interesting, on gene expression in bacteria. It is also the hormone causing colony formation in the free swimming forms of the cellular slime moulds. In nearly every case the action of the initiating hormone can be mimicked in whole or in part by addition of cyclic AMP itself or its more stable, lipid-soluble derivative, dibutyryl cyclic AMP.

The actions of cyclic AMP appear to be due to a general action in which proteins are phosphorylated by the cyclic AMP and thereby change their activity. This class of enzyme is generally referred to as a protein kinase and is responsible for various reactions involving phosphorylation. A well-known example is phosphorylase which catalyses the equilibrium between glycogen and phosphate on the one hand and glucose-l-phosphate on the other. As mentioned earlier theophylline, by inhibiting phosphodiesterase, potentiates actions involving cyclic AMP; other xanthines such as caffeine and 8-chlortheophylline are also active.

THE ACTION OF SYMPATHOMIMETIC SUBSTANCES

The action of sympathomimetic substances depends on their relative activity on α- and β-receptors, the proportion of direct and indirect action, as well as on their metabolic handling.

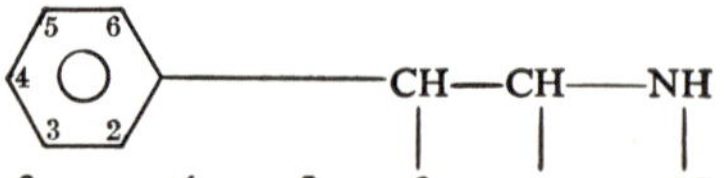

	2	3	4	5	β	α	N
Phenylethylamine	H	H	H	H	H	H	H
Noradrenaline	H	OH	OH	H	OH	H	H
Adrenaline	H	OH	OH	H	OH	H	CH$_3$
Isoprenaline	H	OH	OH	H	OH	H	CH(CH$_3$)$_2$
Methoxamine	OCH$_3$	H	H	OCH$_3$	OH	CH$_3$	H
Methoxyphenamine	OCH$_3$	H	H	H	H	CH$_3$	CH$_3$
Isoxsuprine	H	H	OH	H	OH	CH$_3$	CH(CH$_3$)CH$_2$O⟨O⟩ 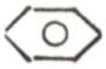
Tyramine	H	H	OH	H	H	H	H
Octopamine	H	H	OH	H	OH	H	H
Metaraminol	H	OH	H	H	OH	CH$_3$	H
Ephedrine	H	H	H	H	OH	CH$_3$	CH$_3$
Amphetamine	H	H	H	H	H	CH$_3$	H
Methamphetamine	H	H	H	H	H	CH$_3$	CH$_3$
Salbutamol	H	CH$_2$OH	OH	H	H	H	C(CH$_3$)

FIG. 7.8. Sympathomimetic amines.

Noradrenaline
Noradrenaline is more active on α-receptors than on β-receptors, but is by no means devoid of β-action. It is rapidly taken up by sympathetic neurones, is a good substrate for COMT but not a particularly good substrate for MAO. Noradrenaline is practically inert when given by mouth because of extensive metabolism in the gut wall and liver.

Adrenaline
Adrenaline is more active on β-receptors than on α-receptors, is less well taken up by neurones and in consequence a higher proportion is metabolized. As with noradrenaline, absorption from the gut is slight.

Isoprenaline
Isoprenaline has a very powerful β-action but is almost devoid of α-actions. Its duration of action is greater than either of the preceding due to its failure to be taken up by neurones and its resistance to MAO. It is active by mouth when given in large doses as is sometimes done in treating Stokes–Adams attacks (intermittent heart block), although it is more usually given by the sublingual route by which absorption is more rapid and complete.

Salbutamol
Salbutamol differs from isoprenaline mainly in having a hydroxymethyl group in the 3-position in place of a hydroxy group; this weakens the action on the heart without affecting the bronchodilator action. Salbutamol may thus be used in asthma with a lower risk of cardiac side-effects. The selective effects of salbutamol and of some β-blockers have led to a subdivision of β-receptors into β_1 receptors on the heart and β_2 receptors on smooth muscle. The hydroxymethyl group also renders salbutamol insensitive to COMT and this gives it a longer duration of action than isoprenaline. Soterenol has a similar pharmacology.

Methoxamine
Methoxamine has nearly pure α-actions, though it has some weak β-blocking action. Being already O-methylated it cannot be inactivated by COMT and like other substances derived from isopropylamine and other secondary amines is not attacked by MAO. For these reasons it has a long duration of action. The chemically related **methoxyphenamine** and **isoxsuprine** are selective β-stimulators.

Tyramine
Tyramine is the archetypic indirectly acting amine. It is low in activity in part because tyramine is an excellent substrate for MAO. Tyramine is found in many foods (notably in mature cheese, broad beans, yeast extract, yoghurt, and wine) but is destroyed by MAO in the gut and liver. However, when MAO inhibitors are administered the tyramine reaches the systemic circulation and causes noradrenaline release which may result in dangerous hypertension and cerebral oedema or haemorrhage. In the presence of MAO inhibitors tyramine is also protected from the intracellular attack of MAO in sympathetic neurones and the preserved tyramine is partially converted to octopamine by dopamine β-oxidase and this leads to partial replacement of noradrenaline by octopamine in the granules.

Metaraminol
Metaraminol is a highly active mixed sympathomimetic agent—it has a strong direct action and is also a noradrenaline releaser. It is taken up and stored in the granules. It is not a substrate for either COMT or MAO and has a long duration of action.

Ephedrine
Ephedrine acts almost wholly indirectly and, as expected from such an action, shows rather a rapid development of tolerance. Because of its resistance to MAO it is active by mouth and is still much used as an orally acting bronchodilator in asthma. Its main disadvantage is a pronounced central action leading to jitteriness and wakefulness.

88 *Adrenergic System*

Amphetamine and Methamphetamine

Amphetamine and methamphetamine have mainly central actions which have a complicated basis. They are directly sympathomimetic, are releasers of noradrenaline and inhibitors of uptake, and are also inhibitors of MAO. Their central actions are discussed in Chapter 4.

These drugs are also used to reduce appetite and hence food intake in the treatment of obesity.

α-BLOCKERS
[FIG. 7.9]

Ergot Alkaloids

These compounds are dealt with in detail in Chapter 8. They are rarely used as pharmacological tools because the strong direct stimulation of smooth muscle complicates their actions. These actions are reduced in the dihydrogenated alkaloids.

Phentolamine and Tolazoline

Phentolamine and tolazoline are substituted imidazolines which are highly selective α-blockers but which also are directly depressant on smooth muscle. They also have some direct sympathomimetic action on the heart. Their action is transient and they are used in the diagnosis and treatment of phaeochromocytoma, a tumour of adrenal medullary cells which secretes noradrenaline and adrenaline often in a paroxysmal fashion.

Piperoxan and Dibozane

These are α-blockers in addition to having direct actions on smooth and cardiac muscle. Toxic effects have made them unsatisfactory for therapeutic use. **Azapetine** is a dibenzazepine with actions rather similar to tolazoline.

Yohimbine

Yohimbine is related to both ergot and reserpine and is another α-blocker with relatively pure action.

-Haloalkylamines

The first of these compounds to be studied was **dibenamine**. This produces a very prolonged block of α-receptors which takes days to recover. The effects develop slowly due to the necessity of forming the intermediate aziridine (ethyleneiminium) which occurs as in the nitrogen mustards [p. 206] by elimination of halogen. The three-membered ring is strained (i.e. bond angles are abnormal so that orbital overlap is imperfect and hence the bonds are weakened) and acts as an alkylator which reacts covalently with some group in the α-receptor. Selectivity is presumably achieved by preliminary non-covalent complex formation determined by the fit of the molecule for the receptor. Recovery from block is dependent on the rate of hydrolysis of the ester bond formed with the group in the receptor.

Phenoxybenzamine

Phenoxybenzamine is both more potent than dibenamine and more selective and has supplanted it in use. Both agents are able to block histamine receptors and muscarinic receptors in higher doses as well as probably having direct actions on cell membranes. Phenoxybenzamine is a very potent irreversible blocker of noradrenaline uptake into neurones and therefore has the property of potentiating β-actions of noradrenaline and of sympathetic stimulation.

The main clinical use of phenoxybenzamine is in controlling hypertensive episodes due to phaeochromocytoma as a preliminary to operation. It has a limited use in traumatic shock as it reduces visceral vasoconstriction provided that perfusion rates are maintained by adequate plasma expansion.

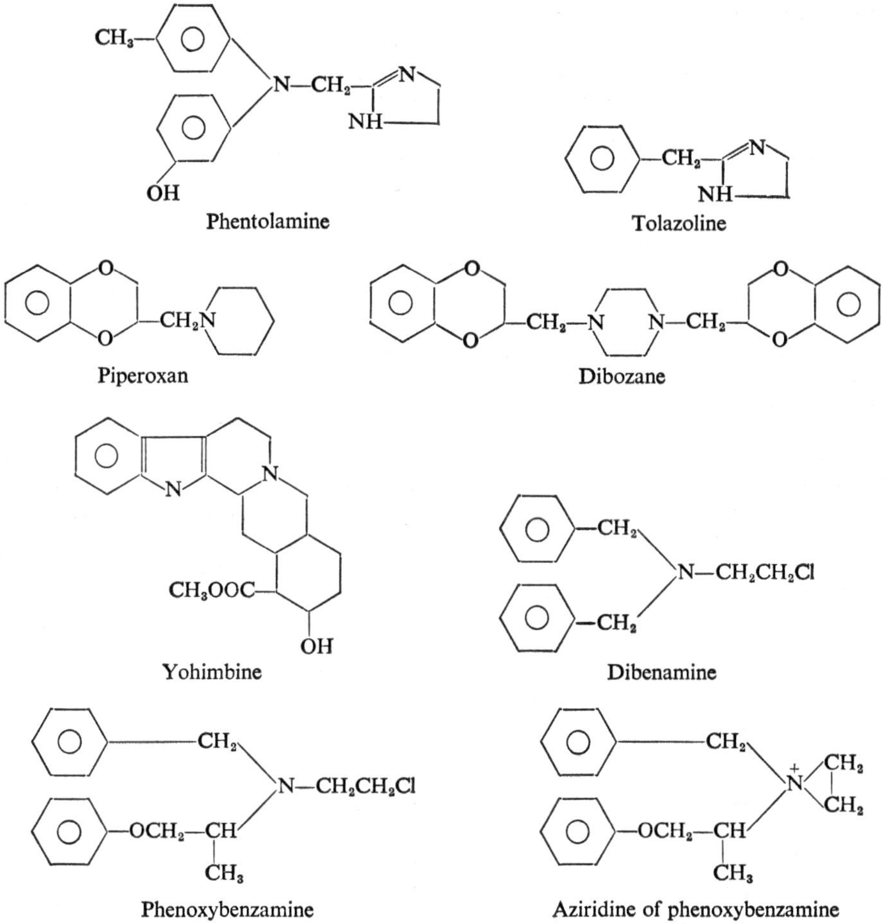

FIG. 7.9. α-blocking drugs.

β-BLOCKERS

[FIG. 7.10]

β-Blockade was first noted with dichloroisoprenaline (DCI). This is really a partial agonist which first stimulates and then blocks β-receptors. Pronethalol is free of the stimulant actions and is more potent. It had two disadvantages: it produced pronounced central nervous side-effects, and also it was found to produce thymic tumours in mice. It has been replaced by the more powerful and specific propranolol and sotalol. As mentioned previously cardiac β-receptors (β_1) differ from other β-receptors and selective blockers are known; of these the most important is practolol. Metabolic actions of catecholamines appear to be mediated through yet another variant of the β-receptor and butoxamine selectively blocks this receptor. It is interesting to note that all the active β-blockers so far discovered can be regarded as derivatives of isoprenaline in which modifications have been made to the aromatic part of the molecule.

β-Blockers have a number of interesting uses. Their effects on the heart are taken advantage of in their use in angina pectoris; by blocking the effects of the increased sympathetic drive in exercise they minimize the increase in cardiac work and hence allow greater exercise before pain develops. However, if the heart is in occult failure and the cardiac output is being maintained by sympathetic drive β-blockers may precipitate overt failure; in a corresponding way they may cause asthma. β-Blockers are potent antiarrhythmics; this is partially due to blocking the excitatory effects of catecholamines, but also due to an anti-arrythmic activity which is analogous to that of quinidine and lignocaine.

One of the most unexpected actions of β-blockers is that they suppress the symptoms of hyperthyroidism in a considerable proportion of patients and are especially useful in thyrotoxic crises. This is very interesting because so many of these symptoms are mimicked by administration of adrenaline. β-Blockers are also of considerable value in combating the effects of excessive catecholamine release from the adrenal medullary tumours (phaeochromocytoma).

DRUGS AFFECTING NORADRENALINE RELEASE

Guanethidine

Guanethidine blocks sympathetic transmission both by depleting the noradrenaline content and by interfering with neurally evoked release. This process does not discriminate between nerve endings in α and β receptive sites. With the usual doses administered therapeutically block develops slowly over several days and also passes off slowly when administration is stopped. Hypersensitivity to noradrenaline develops as it does after surgical denervation. Guanethidine is used almost exclusively as a hypotensive. The major side-effects are diarrhoea, tremors, weakness, mental depression, parotid pain, nasal stuffiness, and failure of ejaculation. **Bethanidine** acts more rapidly and has a shorter duration so that adjustment of dosage is simpler; diarrhoea is also less common. **Guanoxan** and **guanochlor** are related compounds.

Reserpine

Reserpine is a central sedative, acting probably by depleting serotonin and noradrenaline from central neurones; it also depletes peripheral neurones. Effects develop slowly unless very large doses are given. Effects wear off over several days. It has been used both in hypertension and in treating psychoses, but is liable to produce severe depression which may lead to suicide.

Methyldopa

Methyldopa also blocks sympathetic neurones as referred to above, but the mechanism of action is still uncertain. It is likely that its major action is to replace noradrenaline by α-methylnoradrenaline (nordefrin) which is less active on the receptors. It has a number of important, unwanted actions, of which weakness and headache are common, as is the development of hypersensitivity.

The action of MAO inhibitors is considered in Chapter 4.

INHIBITORS OF NORADRENALINE UPTAKE

Noradrenaline uptake is inhibited by **cocaine** but not other local anaesthetics, by **phenoxybenzamine**, and by the antidepressants of the tricyclic group [p. 41] including **imipramine, desipramine, amitriptyline,** and **nortriptyline**.

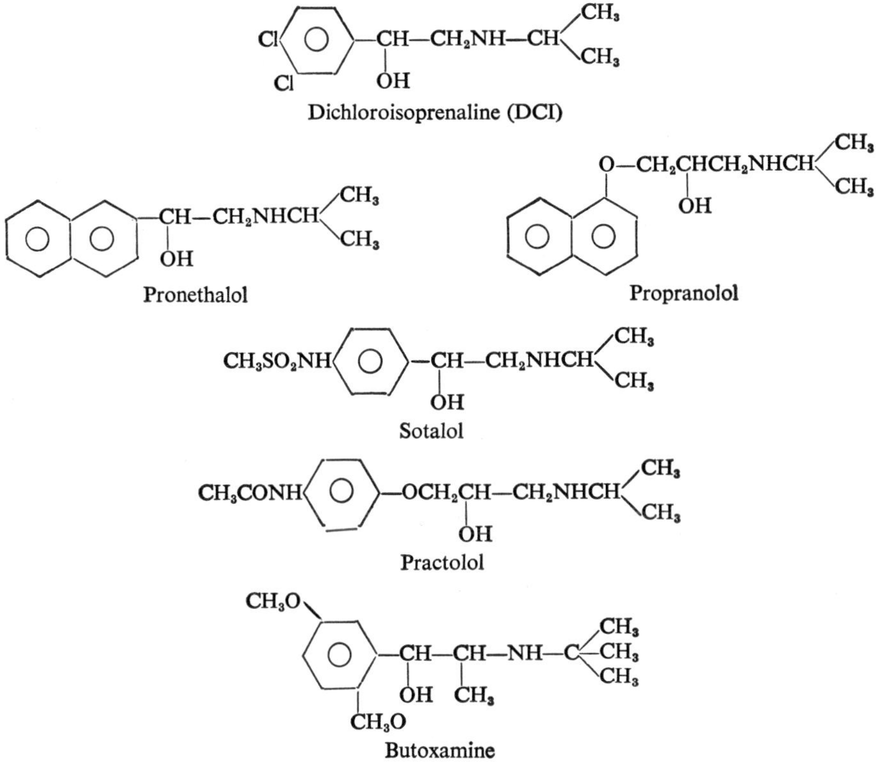

FIG. 7.10. β-blocking drugs.

FURTHER READING

ACHESON, G. H. (1965) Second catecholamine symposium, *Pharmacol. Rev.*, **18**, 1.

ANDEN, N. E., CARLSSON, A., and HÄGGENDAL, J. (1969) Adrenergic mechanisms, *Ann. Rev. Pharmacol.*, **9**, 119.

BOURA, A. L. A., and GREEN, A. F. (1965) Adrenergic neurone blocking agents, *Ann. Rev. Pharmacol.*, **5**, 183.

IVERSEN, L. L. (1967) *The Uptake and Storage of Noradrenaline in Sympathetic Nerves*, Cambridge.

MORAN, N. C. (1967) New adrenergic blocking drugs: their pharmacological, biochemical and clinical actions, *Ann. N.Y. Acad. Sci.*, **139**, 541.

VANE, J. R. (1960) *Adrenergic Mechanisms*, London.

8

SMOOTH MUSCLE

A NUMBER of drugs produce important effects by actions on the smooth muscle of the gastro-intestinal tract, blood vessels, and bronchi. We have already considered drugs acting by the cholinergic and adrenergic systems. In this chapter we will consider other drugs acting on smooth muscle.

Histamine

Histamine like acetylcholine was first isolated from ergot in which it is a contaminant due to bacterial action. Later it was found in animal tissues, being especially concentrated in basophils (mast cells). Histamine is synthesized *in vivo* by enzymatic decarboxylation of histidine by the pyridoxal-requiring enzyme histidine decarboxylase. In mast cells the concentration of histamine may be of the order of several mg./g. and similar concentrations are found in mast cell tissues and in the collections of mast cells in the skin in urticaria pigmentosa.

Histamine is readily released from mast cells by mechanical trauma as shown in the triple response in the skin to a firm stroke, to cold or heat, or ultra-violet radiation. Release is also produced by a variety of chemicals including common drugs such as morphine, atropine, tubocurarine, and stilbamidine. Especially effective is a substance known as 48/80 which is an oligomer of p-methoxyphenylethylmethylamine with formaldehyde. Histamine liberators cause the discharge of granules from mast cells and in larger doses mast cell destruction, with liberation of the histamine (and other substances including heparin, serotonin, and slow reacting substance). Some polymers also cause release of histamine, for instance dextran, and ovomucoid in the rat and polyvinylpyrrolidone in the dog. Mast cell destruction and histamine liberation also result from the immediate type of hypersensitivity reaction. This is seen if an animal is sensitized by giving it an injection of a foreign protein such as ovalbumin and then 10 days later giving a challenging dose of the same protein. The animal has in the meantime developed antibodies and these combine with the ovalbumin in the mast cells and in the presence of plasma factors called complement lead to cell lysis. This phenomenon which is at the basis of immediate sensitivity can be demonstrated both in the whole animal and with isolated tissues such as uterus and bronchi.

Histamine acts on the smooth muscle of the intestine and of the bronchi causing contraction. It has more complicated actions on blood vessels in which there are species variations. In man it relaxes the arterioles and small venules but constricts the larger veins and causes a fall of blood pressure with reflex tachycardia. These effects are visible in man as reddening and increase in temperature in the skin particularly in the blush area of the head and neck. It causes an interesting morphological change in the small venules in which the endothelial cells lining the vessels separate from each other along their edges exposing the underlying basement membrane. As the impermeability of the venule to the plasma proteins depends on the continuity of the endothelial cell barrier the venule now allows protein to escape into the extracellular space and as retention of fluid in the vascular system depends on the colloid osmotic pressure excess in the blood vessels compared with the extracellular space, the loss of this gradient allows fluid to leak out also and oedema results.

When histamine is injected into the skin the triple response of Lewis results, this consists of:

(1) a localized bluish-red area around the injection in the centre of which (2) an area of oedema develops and (3) an irregular area of reddening, called the flare. The site of injection is itchy. The first two responses are due to a direct action on the vessels as described above but the third response is due to stimulation by histamine of sensory nerve fibres, causing impulses to travel up these fibres (to the spinal cord giving the sensation of itch) and also travel down branches and at their terminals liberate a vasodilator substance, whose nature is unknown, which dilates arterioles in the region. The flare no longer occurs after chronic sensory denervation. In the rabbit the predominant change is arteriolar constriction causing a rise of blood pressure, in the cat the pulmonary arterioles are constricted causing a fall of peripheral blood pressure, in the dog the hepatic vein is constricted causing blood to be pooled in the viscera and hence also causing a fall of blood pressure.

Histamine also dilates cerebral vessels and causes a throbbing headache and a rise in intracranial pressure. Histamine contracts the uterus in most species although it relaxes it in the rat and has little effect on the human uterus. It has little effect on the smooth muscle of the bladder or the pupil. Histamine is a strong stimulant of gastric acid secretion [p. 117]. Considerable amounts of histamine are found in the stinging hairs of nettles and are responsible for the wealing and itching produced.

Histamine is rapidly metabolized in the body, by three routes: (1) the primary amine group can be acetylated to give the inactive N-acetylhistamine; (2) the ring is methylated to give 1-methylhistamine; and (3) the side chain is oxidized by diamine oxidase to give imidazole carboxylic acid.

The high concentration of the latter enzyme in the gut wall and liver is responsible for the inactivity of histamine when given by mouth and for the lack of pharmacological effects produced by the rather large amounts of histamine produced in the gut by bacterial histidine decarboxylase.

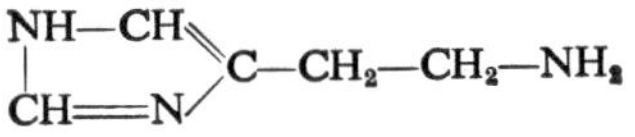

Histamine

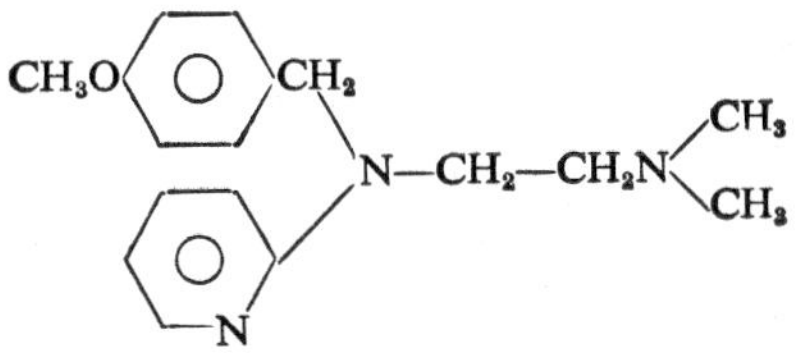

Mepyramine (pyrilamine)

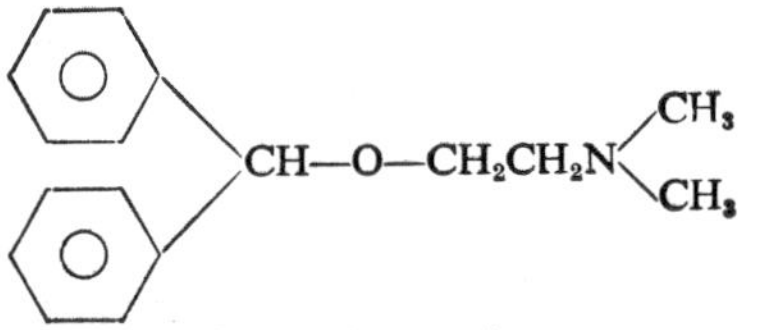

Diphenhydramine

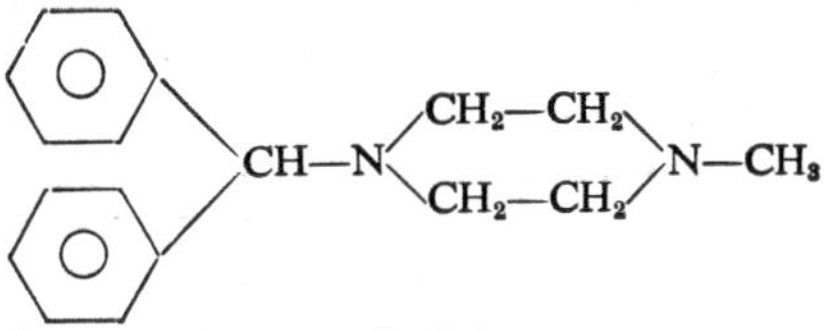

Cyclizine

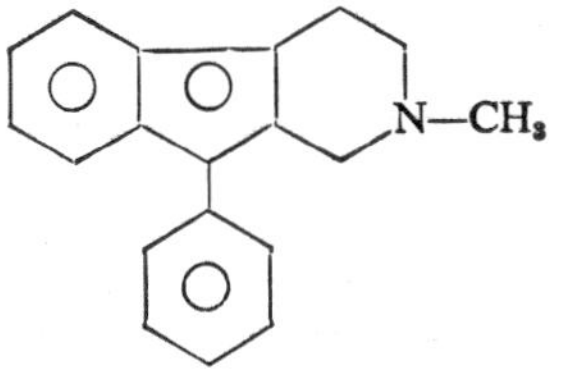

Phenindamine

FIG. 8.1. Antihistamine drugs.

Antihistamines

A large number of highly active antihistamines are known which are basically diaralkylamines. The resemblance to some of the antimuscarines is plain and many of the antihistamines are of low specificity and have also atropine-like actions, a few such as **mepyramine** (pyrilamine) are more specific and almost devoid of atropine-like action.

The antihistamines are highly effective in antagonizing the effects of histamine on smooth muscle and on capillary permeability. They are less active at antagonizing histamine released from mast cells partly because other pharmacologically active substances are released but also because the concentration of histamine released in the neighbourhood of a disintegrating mast cell is so high that very large amounts of antihistamine would be needed to antagonize it. Antihistamines are successful in the therapy of hay fever—an allergic rhinitis due to pollen, and in cutaneous allergies in which they relieve both the urticaria and the itching. None of the antihistamines significantly alter the secretagogue action of histamine on the gastric mucosa. Allergic asthma which is also usually due to airborne allergens is rarely improved by antihistamines and the most likely reason for this is that histamine plays a minor role in the bronchoconstriction. This is thought to be mainly due to SRS (slow reacting substance). Histamine actions on smooth muscle and on permeability can be very effectively annulled by the opposing action of adrenaline and other sympathomimetic substances and this is the basis of the treatment of asthma by these substances. Adrenal corticoids are also used in treating allergic disorders because they reduce the liberation of histamine and the other mediators of the allergic response.

The allergic response and release of histamine can also be interfered with by a new drug, **cromoglycate** (*Intal*), which appears to prevent the cytotoxic effects resulting from the reaction of reagin (monovalent antigens) with a serum antibody (IgE) on the cell surface. Cromoglycate is effective both in hay fever and in asthma. It is not absorbed from the gut and must therefore be given by inhalation into the nose or bronchi.

Apart from their action against histamine, the antihistamines have pronounced central effects causing drowsiness and incoordination, and have some value in treating paralysis agitans (Parkinsonism). Some of them have value against motion sickness, and this seems to be correlated with the possession of atropine-like properties; in general the antihistamines are less effective for this purpose than hyoscine.

Many of the aromatic haloalkylamines are very effective antihistamines.

Serotonin (5-Hydroxytryptamine)

It had been known for a long time that serum (i.e. the fluid part of clotted blood) contained a vasoconstrictor substance. In 1948 this substance was isolated and identified as 5-hydroxytryptamine. Erspamer had previously extracted a substance called enteramine from the gut and in large quantities from the posterior salivary glands of the octopus. This is likewise serotonin. Subsequent evaluation has shown that serotonin is present in large amounts in blood platelets (released in clotting), in the enterochromaffin (argentaffin) cells, and in a small number of neurones in the CNS. In the rat and mouse it is present in mast cells where it largely replaces histamine. Serotonin is also found in plants, notably bananas, pineapples, and nuts as well as in stinging nettles. Serotonin is synthesized in the tissues in a two-stage operation: first tryptophan is hydroxylated by the enzyme tryptophan-5-hydroxylase to give 5-hydroxytryptophan (5-HTP). This is a substrate for both 5-HTP decarboxylase and dopa decarboxylase yielding serotonin. Serotonin is stored in cytoplasmic granules in a manner analogous to that for histamine and catecholamines and like the latter is released by reserpine. Serotonin is metabolized almost wholly by monoamine oxidase to 5-hydroxyindole acetic acid which is excreted in the urine.

Serotonin acts by stimulation of smooth muscle directly and also by stimulation of nerve fibres and these effects are often difficult to separate. In the cardiovascular system direct vasoconstriction is produced in most vascular beds and is especially intense in the renal vessels. In skeletal muscle vasodilatation is usually produced, but the over-all effect is an increase in the peripheral resistance. In man a dusky red flush is produced in the skin show-

FIG. 8.2. Serotonin and serotonin antagonists.

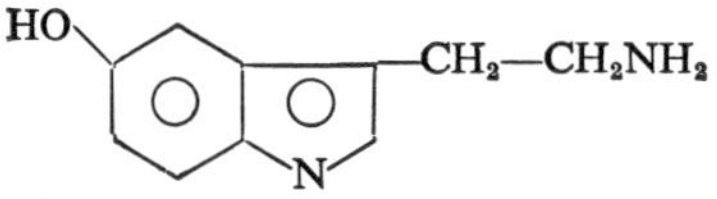

Serotonin

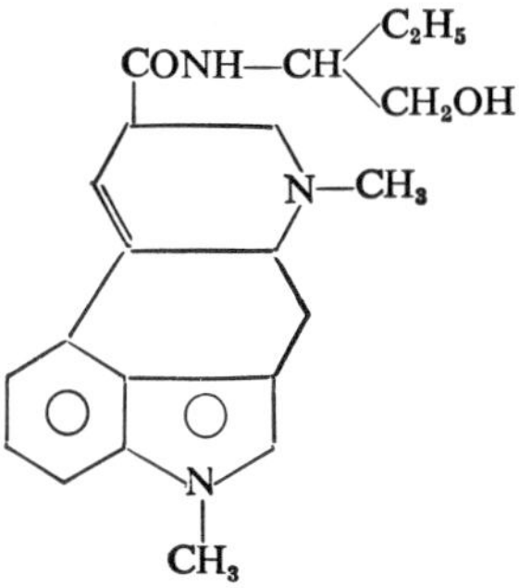

Methysergide

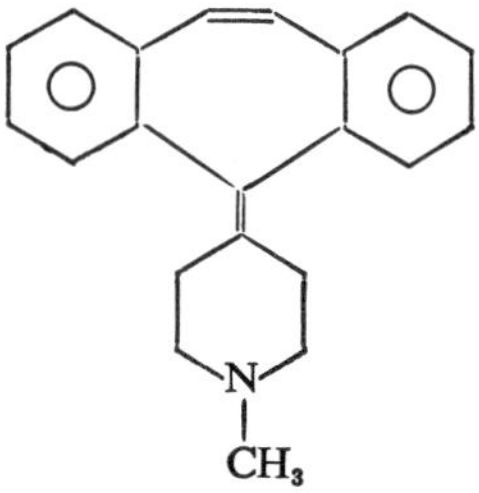

Cyproheptadine

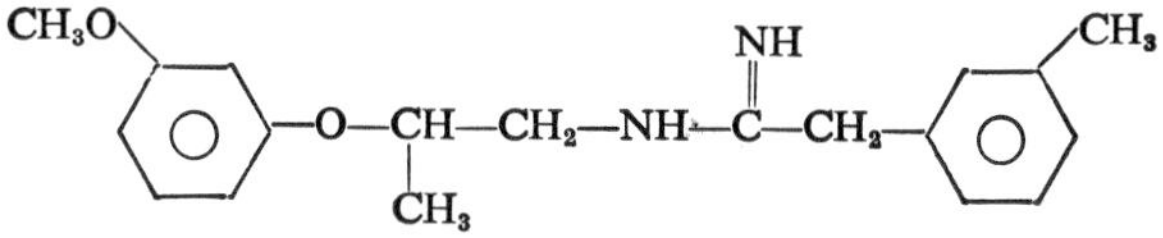

BW 545 C64

ing that dilatation of some small vessels, possibly venules, is occurring. In rats and mice serotonin produces small vessel permeability changes similar to those caused by histamine and this is consistent with the alternative release of serotonin from the mast cells of these species. In man permeability changes are minimal. Direct effects on the heart are not prominent and the over-all effects on the circulation are affected by stimulation of ventricular afferent nerves (Bezold reflex) and the carotid and aortic chemoreceptors and baroceptors. The effect of serotonin on blood pressure is commonly triphasic, the initial fall in pressure being due mainly to ventricular afferent stimulation, followed by a rise due to the direct vasoconstrictor effects and chemoreceptor stimulation. The final depressor phase is due mainly to the muscle vasodilatation.

The motility of the gastro-intestinal tract is increased by serotonin. In part this is a direct effect on the smooth muscle but in large measure it appears to be due to stimulation of ganglion cells in the myenteric plexus and to sensitization of the afferent stretch endings that initiate local peristaltic action. It has been suggested that serotonin produced by the enterochromaffin cells has an important role in regulating intestinal mobility.

Serotonin also causes constriction of the bronchioles, and contraction of the ureter and uterus. In pregnant rodents large doses of serotonin cause resorption of foetuses, probably due to an intense constriction of the umbilical vessels.

Serotonin has no direct effects on the CNS probably because it cannot penetrate the blood–brain barrier. On the other hand, 5-hydroxytryptophan penetrates into the brain and is there decarboxylated to serotonin which may produce behavioural changes. Serotonin injected directly into the ventricular system produces a catatonic state and a sleep-like state. In view of this evidence and the correlation of behavioural changes with serotonin content of the brain after administration of reserpine or monamine oxidase inhibitors, there is a disposition to assign an important role to serotonergic neurones in the control of mood and behaviour.

Serotonin Antagonists

The actions of serotonin are countered by two different groups of antagonists. The neuronal effects are antagonized by **morphine,** the direct effects on smooth muscle by phenoxybenzamine, by ergot derivatives of which **methysergide** and **bromo-lysergic acid diethylamide (BOL)** are the most useful, and by the tricyclic compound **cyproheptadine** which is also a powerful antihistamine. A new class of antagonists are substituted amidines (BW 545 C64).

Angiotensin

Saline extracts of kidney when injected intravenously cause a hypertension that develops rather slowly and is sustained. The activity of the kidney extract is destroyed by heating. On the other hand, if the kidney extract is first allowed to stand with plasma for a few minutes and the mixture injected an immediate pressor action is produced. This action is not destroyed by heating the kidney extract–plasma mixture. The action in the second case has been shown to be due to a decapeptide angiotensin I. This substance is itself inactive but through the action of an enzyme ('converting enzyme') the C-terminal dipeptide is removed to give the active octapeptide angiotensin II [Fig. 8.3]. This enzyme is present in many tissues especially the lungs. Angiotensin I is split off from a precursor, plasma protein angiotensinogen, by the selective protease in the kidney extract which is called renin.

Asp–Arg–Val–Tyr–Ileu–His–Pro–Phe–His–Leu
Angiotensin I

Asp–Arg–Val–Tyr–Ileu–His–Pro–Phe
Angiotensin II

Lys–Arg–Pro–Pro–Gly–Phe–Ser–Pro–Phe–Arg
Kallidin

Arg–Pro–Pro–Gly–Phe–Ser–Pro–Phe–Arg
Bradykinin

Fig. 8.3. Vasoactive peptides formed by enzymatic action on plasma protein precursors.

Angiotensin is a powerful smooth muscle stimulant particularly on arterioles, but also on gut and uterus. It is relatively persistent, the recovery depending on the removal of amino acid residues by tissue peptidases.

Angiotensin also has a powerful action on the adrenal cortex causing the release of the mineralocorticoid, aldosterone, and its physiological function is believed to be in the control of aldosterone secretion. No effective antagonists for angiotensin are known.

Bradykinin

In an analogous way to the discovery of angiotensin the injection of an extract of pancreas causes a fall of blood pressure on injection and this has been shown to be due to the release of two peptides bradykinin and kallidin from a protein precursor due to the action of another proteolytic enzyme, kallikrein. Kallikrein is widely distributed, and is found particularly in parenchymal tissues and in plasma—it is usually held inactive by inhibitors or by segregation within cells.

Bradykinin is a very potent vasodilator having an especially strong action on skin vessels and causes hypotension by dilatation of all the small vessels. On local injection vascular permeability is increased and a local flush is produced but a flare does not normally occur. Bradykinin is a powerful stimulant of pain endings in the skin. The actions of bradykinin are antagonized by aspirin and related antipyretic-analgesics and the formation of bradykinin can be reduced by the kallikrein inhibitor **trasylol**, a peptide extracted from ox parotid glands.

It is believed that activation of kallikrein and the formation of bradykinin play a key role in the local phenomena of inflammation, particularly the vasodilatation, oedema, and pain.

In the malignant carcinoid tumour, there is evidence that while serotonin is released in excess the major symptoms are produced by release of a kallikrein.

Oxytocin and Vasopressin [Fig. 8.4]

These are two related cyclic peptides produced in the hypothalamus and posterior lobe of the pituitary gland. They both have actions on smooth muscle and an antidiuretic action but differ in the relative intensity of these actions. For instance oxytocin has about 1 per cent. of the activity of vasopressin on the kidney whereas vasopressin has about 10 per cent. of the activity of oxytocin on the pregnant uterus.

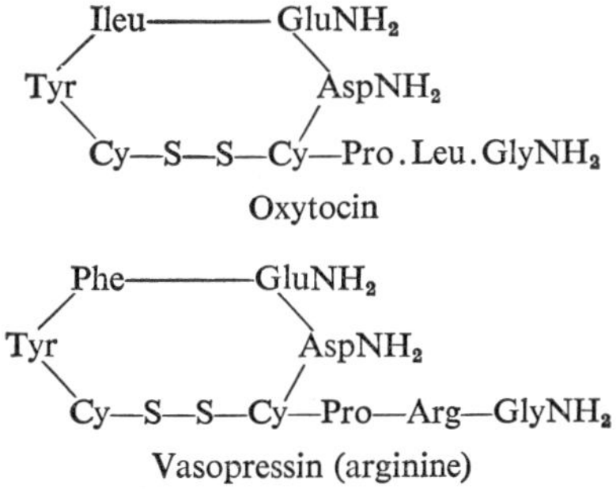

Vasopressin contracts vascular smooth muscle and so raises the blood pressure but with excessive doses the pressure falls because the constriction of the coronary vessels leads to anoxic hypodynamism of the myocardium. The doses needed to produce a rise in blood pressure are much greater than those required to produce an antidiuresis.

Both peptides contract the non-pregnant uterus. Sensitivity of the immature uterus is low and can be markedly increased by prior treatment with an oestrogen; the activity of vasopressin is a little greater than oxytocin. During pregnancy the sensitivity of the uterus increases particularly to oxytocin and this becomes very prominent at the time of parturition. In small doses oxytocin will initiate

$$
\begin{array}{c}
\text{Ileu} \longrightarrow \text{GluNH}_2 \\
\text{Tyr} \qquad \text{AspNH}_2 \\
\text{Cy—S—S—Cy—Pro.Leu.GlyNH}_2 \\
\text{Oxytocin} \\
\\
\text{Phe} \longrightarrow \text{GluNH}_2 \\
\text{Tyr} \qquad \text{AspNH}_2 \\
\text{Cy—S—S—Cy—Pro—Arg—GlyNH}_2 \\
\text{Vasopressin (arginine)}
\end{array}
$$

Fig. 8.4

contraction or increase the force and frequency of a pre-existing rhythm, in larger doses it causes a maintained increase in tone.

Oxytocin is not commonly used to initiate labour but it is frequently used in the second stage when the cervix is well dilated to stimulate a flagging uterus and is also used in the third stage to cause expulsion of the placenta and blood and to contract the uterus down to stop post-partum bleeding. For these purposes oxytocin is usually administered by a continuous intravenous infusion. Oxytocin acts on the smooth muscle in the trabeculae of the mammary gland and will cause expulsion of milk; this is known as milk let-down in animals. Oxytocin is sometimes used to aid milk ejection.

Ergot [Fig. 8.5]

Ergot is a fungus (*Claviceps purpurea*) which grows on rye so that the infected ears turn dark. Ergot contains many interesting substances but we are concerned here only with the characteristic alkaloids which are all amides of lysergic acid. We have previously referred to methysergide, the N-methyl lysergic butanolamide. Ergometrine (ergonovine) is the closely related lysergic propanolamide. Ergometrine stimulates smooth muscle in blood vessels and hence causes a rise of blood pressure with reflex bradycardia, contracts smooth muscle of the gut, ureter, biliary tract, and the uterus. It is the action on the latter that provides the main use for ergot.

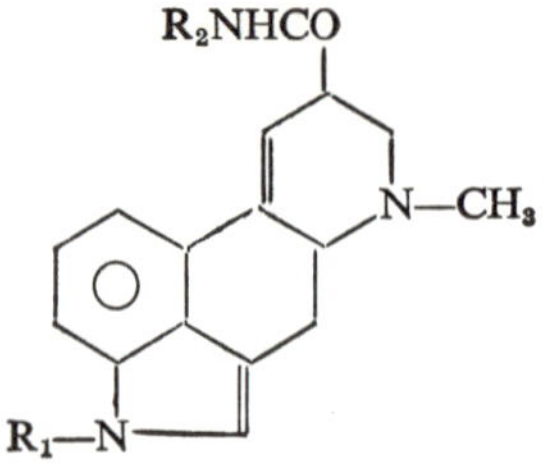

Smooth Muscle

Fig. 8.5. Ergot alkaloids.

	R₁	R₂
Ergometrine (ergonovine)	H	—CH(CH₃)CH₂OH
Methysergide	CH₃	—CH(C₂H₅)CH₂OH
Lysergic diethylamide (LSD)	H	(C₂H₅)₂

Ergometrine will contract the uterus even when not oestrogen-primed, but the sensitivity of the uterus is greatly increased in the latter stages of pregnancy. Ergot produces a great increase in the rhythmic activity rather than of tone. It is given routinely by most obstetricians at the beginning of the third stage of labour to aid the expulsion of the placenta and blood clots. It has a long duration of action.

Ergot alkaloids are also used in the treatment of migraine which is a paroxysmal dilatation of vessels related to the internal and external carotid arteries leading to severe throbbing headache, and often visual disturbances. Ergot alkaloids are effective by virtue of their vasoconstrictor actions. Ergometrine and methysergide are most frequently used.

The main toxic effect of the alkaloids is due to their powerful and prolonged effect on arteries, which may lead to peripheral gangrene partieularly of fingers or toes. It was this action which was recognized in the Middle Ages as St. Anthony's Fire after the shrine where peopie sought a cure. Other toxic effects include nausea, vomiting, diarrhoea, dizziness, and confusion. The side-effects unfortunately frequently make it impossible to give adequate doses to migraine sufferers.

Prostaglandins

Extracts of seminal fluid and of the vesicular gland cause a fall of blood pressure when injected intravenously. The active substance was named prostaglandin by Von Euler and he showed it was a lipid acid. Elucidation of the structure of prostaglandin showed that it was not a single substance but a large family of related substances based on a hydrocarbon skeleton called prostenoic acid. This consists of a cyclopentane ring with adjacent attached hydrocarbon chains, one of which terminates in a carboxyl group. The two most important groups are the E and F series which differ in their ring substituents; in the F series they are both hydroxyl, whereas in the E series there is one hydroxyl and one ketone [Fig. 8.6]. The prostaglandins can be made biosynthetically by incubating a homogenate of sheep vesicular glands with polyunsaturated fatty acids such

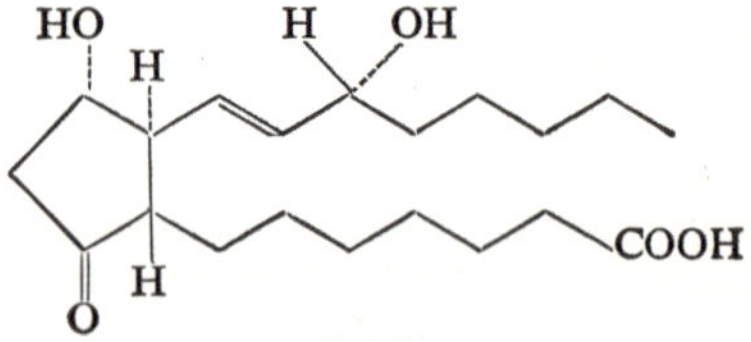

PGE₁

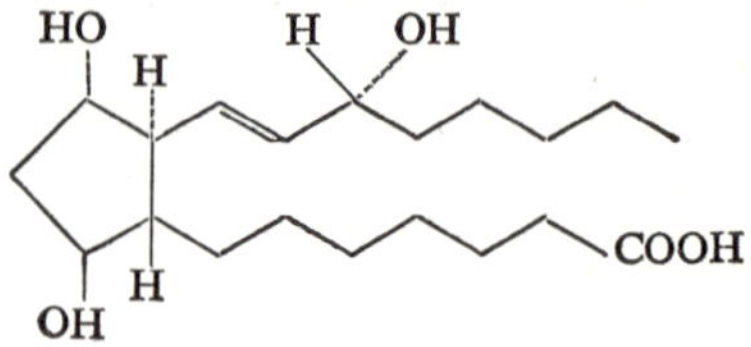

PGF₁α

Fig. 8.6. Prostaglandins.

as arachidonic acid and this leads to ring closure giving the cyclopentane ring, and thus to prostaglandins. The type of prostaglandin formed depends on the exact structure of the substrate fatty acid. Similar enzyme systems are found in other tissues. There is evidence to suggest that free unsaturated fatty acids in the tissues are rapidly converted into prostaglandins, so that the rate limiting step is the release of the fatty acids from their combined state in lipids such as phospholipids. Phospholipase A may therefore be an important controller of prostaglandin formation. Prostaglandins when released are rapidly metabolized by saturation of the side chain double bond and oxidation of the side chain hydroxyl to ketone; the products are pharmacologically inert.

The pharmacology of prostaglandins is very complex. They are active on most preparations of smooth muscle and in general the E series are more active than the F series. They contract the small and large intestine and the uterus. The latter action may be used to induce labour at term or abortion in early pregnancy. They relax the bronchi and are under trial as possible therapy in asthma; they also lower the blood pressure by relaxing arterioles and venules.

It was shown some years ago that injection of PGE_1 into the cerebral ventricles produces sedation and stupor; the most clear-cut central action so far described is that of PGE_1 which blocks the inhibitory action of noradrenaline on the Purkinje cells of the cerebellum. Prostaglandins are powerful inhibitors of lipolysis, reducing the lipolytic effects of adrenaline, corticotrophin, and other hormones. They inhibit the action of antidiuretic hormone on the kidney and toad bladder, and they can also inhibit gastric and other secretion. On the other hand, on the thyroid, adrenal, and corpus luteum, the effects of PGE and PGF mimic those of the hormones TSH, ACTH, and LH. A further interesting action is in preventing the aggregation of platelets.

The difference between the various prostaglandins is mainly in potency and selectivity, but in some cases it is also a difference in sign—for instance, PGF tends to be bronchoconstrictor whereas PGE is bronchodilator. There are also marked species differences. Many of the actions of prostaglandins can be attributed to actions on adenylcyclase and thus on cyclic AMP [see p. 86]. It seems not impossible that prostaglandins act on cell membranes and thus influence membrane-bound enzymes. Recently it has been shown that acetylsalicylic acid and other anti-inflammatory drugs are potent inhibitors of PG release from tissues; this may be related to their anti-inflammatory action and to their analgesic action.

The prostaglandins are among the most interesting agents discovered for many years. Their therapeutic action is limited by the broad range of actions and evanescent activity. If analogues can be found that are metabolically more stable they may form the basis for a new range of drugs.

Slow Reacting Substance and Related Compounds

Slow reacting substance (called for short SRS-A) is released from sensitized tissues in many species when challenged with antigen. It is responsible for most of the activity released from sensitized tissues other than histamine. The chemical nature of the substance is obscure. It may either be a lipid, glycolipid, or perhaps carbohydrate material and is rather unstable. The release is slower than that of histamine and responses on tissues are also slower. Its effects are much more specific than the agents previously discussed. It contracts bronchial and ileal muscle but is without effect on the blood pressure or uterus. The importance of SRS-A is that it probably accounts for the ineffectiveness of antihistamine in bronchial asthma. No antagonists to SRS-A are known.

A number of other pharmacologically active lipids have been extracted from tissues; these include **darmstoff**, a mixture of phosphatidic acid and other acidic phospholipids, and **irin**, an unsaturated hydroxy fatty acid.

Xanthines

Theobromine, theophylline, and **caffeine** are respectively di- and tri-methyl xanthines [Chapter 4]. These substances are the most important ingredients of coffee, tea, cocoa, and colas. The most important of the three for actions on smooth muscle and cardiac muscle is theophylline. In general this substance relaxes smooth muscle, notably on the bronchi, intestine, and biliary tract. It also dilates blood vessels and tends to decrease peripheral resistance by a direct action while at the same time the central actions increase sympathetic activity and hence cause an increase in peripheral resistance. Theophylline stimulates cardiac contractility in a manner similar to that of adrenaline and leads to an increase in stroke output. The over-all effect on the circulation is an increase in minute output, with some increase in blood pressure and little change in heart rate.

The present evidence suggests that the xanthines produce their effects by inhibiting phosphodiesterase, the enzyme that inactivates cyclic 3',5' adenylic acid. There is considerable evidence that glycogenolysis is controlled by the level of 3',5' AMP, so that if phosphodiesterase is inhibited the level of 3',5' AMP rises, glycogen is broken down, and hence the level of carbohydrate intermediates for cell metabolic usage rises.

Theophylline itself has a low solubility in water so that it is used as a salt either with ethylene diamine (**aminophylline**) or with choline (**oxtriphylline**) which may be given intravenously, orally, or by rectum.

Aminophylline finds its most valuable use in severe cases of asthma where status asthmaticus may be relieved by intravenous administration, and in cardiac failure, particularly left ventricular failure with paroxysmal dyspnoea.

Aminophylline must be given with some care and may cause dizziness, headaches, nausea and vomiting, palpitations, and precordial pain.

FURTHER READING

BERGSTRÖM, S., CARLSON, L. A., and WEEKS, J. R. (1968) The prostaglandins, *Pharmacol. Rev.*, **20**, 1.

CALDEYRO-BARCIA, R., and HELLER, H. (1961) *Oxytocin*, Oxford.

DALE, H. H., and LAIDLOW, P. P. (1910) The physiological action of β-iminazolyl-ethylamine, *J. Physiol. (Lond.)*, **41**, 318.

ERSPAMER, V. (1966) *5-Hydroxytryptamine and Related Indolealkylamines*, Berlin.

GARATTINI, S., and VALZELLI, L. (1965) *Serotonin*, Amsterdam.

KEELE, C. A., and ARMSTRONG, D. (1964) *Substances Producing Pain and Itch*, London.

LEWIS, T., and GRANT, R. T. (1924) Vascular reactions of the skin to injury, *Heart*, **11**, 209.

PATON, W. D. M. (1957) Histamine release by compounds of simple chemical structure, *Pharmacol. Rev.*, **9**, 269.

PICKLES, V. R., and FITZPATRICK, R. J. (1966) *Endogenous Substances Affecting the Myometrium*, Cambridge.

RAMWELL, P., and SHAW, J. E. (1971) Prostaglandins, *Ann. N.Y. Acad. Sci.*, **180**, 1.

ROCHA E SILVA, M. (1966) Histamine and antihistamines, *Handb. exp. Pharmakologie*, Vol. xviii/i, Berlin.

SAWYER, W. H. (1961) Neurohypophyseal hormones, *Pharmacol. Rev.*, **13**, 225.

SCHACHTER, M. (1960) *Polypeptides which Affect Smooth Muscle and Blood Vessels*, Oxford.

Symposium on Pharmacologically Active Lipids (1963) *Biochem. Pharmacol.*, **12**, 401.

WOLSTENHOLME, G. E. W., and O'CONNOR, C. M. (1956) *Histamine*, London.

9

CIRCULATION

DRUGS acting on the circulation may produce their primary effects on the heart or the vessels or more frequently on both but, because of the complex integration of the circulation, the final effects of drugs may be greatly modified by the homeostatic processes involved. For this reason, before we attempt to analyse drug actions, we will briefly describe the main circulatory control mechanisms.

The stroke output of the ventricles is primarily dependent on the filling pressure at the end of diastole, in that the more the ventricular muscle is stretched the greater is the stroke ejection. However, if the pressure is increased far enough the stroke output reaches a maximum and no longer responds to changes in filling pressure. The range over which there is a proportionality between filling pressure and stroke output is often referred to as the operating range. This is a very important regulator that has the effect of increasing the stroke output in response to the venous return and is the means by which the output from the two sides of the heart is balanced. The output curve is not invariant and can be modified, for instance, if the ventricular muscle is damaged or is anoxic the curve will be depressed and displaced so that to achieve the same stroke output the filling pressure must be increased or alternatively if the filling pressure remains unchanged the output is reduced and the emptying of the ventricles in systole is reduced.

The characteristic curve can be elevated by sympathetic stimulation or by catecholamines and certain other drugs and in these circumstances for any specified filling pressure the stoke output is increased and the ventricle more completely emptied in systole, or alternatively to maintain a specified stroke output a reduced filling pressure is needed. The effect of the sympathetic in speeding up the heart results in an even greater increase in minute output with respect to any reference filling pressure. This action of the sympathetic is of great importance in the regulation of heart action and its influence is seen in emotional excitement, in exercise, after blood loss, and, as a compensatory effect, in hypodynamism of the ventricular muscle in disease.

It has been emphasized that stroke output depends most directly on the diastolic filling pressure and this in turn depends on certain characteristics of the venous system. A part of the arterial blood pressure is transmitted through the capillaries to the small venules and it is the pressure difference between these vessels and that in the right atrium that drives blood back to the heart. However, the mean pressure within the venous system depends also upon the volume of blood contained in the venules and veins and the tone of the walls of these vessels; the veins are not merely passive vessels but are under tonic control of sympathetic nerves and are also susceptible to the effects of drugs. Thus if the venous tone is decreased the blood becomes pooled in the venous system, the pressure in the right atrium decreases and the stroke output diminishes, and on the contrary, if the venous tone increases the pressure gradient diminishes and the pressure in the right atrium will increase provided that venous tone does not increase so much that the resistance to flow in the veins, which is usually slight, becomes a limiting factor. It is clear that the venular pressure will also depend on the state of tone of the arterioles —if these dilate the venular pressure will rise and the venous return will increase. Finally the arterial blood pressure will depend both on

102   Circulation

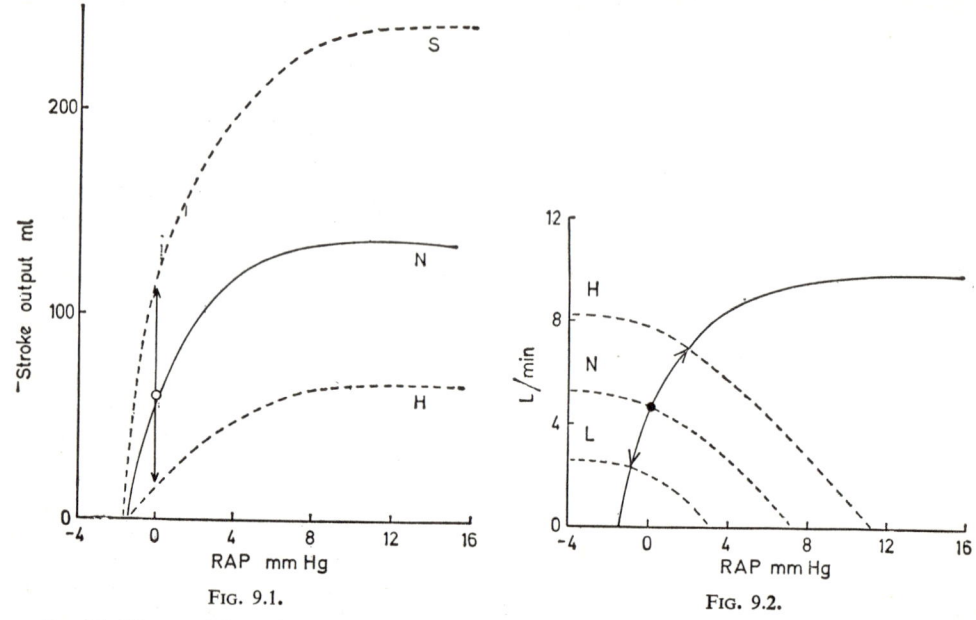

Fig. 9.1.

Fig. 9.2.

Fig. 9.1. Characteristic stroke output curve of the right ventricle.
  N shows the relationship of stroke output of the normal ventricle at different values of right atrial pressure.
  H those of the hypodynamic (i.e. depressed ventricle).
  S those of the ventricle stimulated by sympathetic stimulation.

Fig. 9.2. The effect of venous return on minute output of the right ventricle.
  N is the normal venous return curve—the operating point of the ventricle is at the intersection of this curve with output curve.
  H high venous return (e.g. in exercise).
  L low venous return (e.g. peripheral venous pooling).

the output of the left ventricle and the ease with which blood can leave the great arteries and pass through the capillary bed. This peripheral resistance is mainly controlled by the calibre of the arterioles which are affected both by local conditions, notably oxygen and carbon dioxide partial pressures and the release of vasodilating metabolites, as well as a general control by sympathetic nerves and catecholamine release from the adrenal medulla. The latter causes vasoconstriction in the skin and viscera and dilatation in skeletal muscle and the coronary bed. These opposing effects may be regarded as a special adaptation of the requirements of exercise.

Set over the haemodynamic mechanisms we have described are various regulating systems of which the dominant is normally that exerted through the carotid-aortic pressor receptors. These structures are in the aortic arch and carotid artery and are sensitive both to the mean pressure within them and also to the dynamic pressure variation during the course of a cardiac cycle. A rise in pressure or an increase in pressure swing causes an increased rate of firing in the sino-aortic sensory nerves and this alters the state of activity of cells in the CNS, notably in the medulla, and leads to a decreased sympathetic discharge to the heart and peripheral vessels as well as an increase in the vagal discharge to the heart. The over-all effect is to reduce both the stroke output of the heart and the peripheral resistance and hence to lower the blood pressure, thus minimizing the alteration in blood pressure which would have occurred if this compensation were inoperative. Other modifications of cardiovascular tone are produced through peripheral chemoreceptors and by alterations in central nervous activity.

Much has been learned of the way drugs act on the cardiovascular system by using simplified preparations, such as the heart perfused through the coronary vessels, perfused peripheral beds, isolated artery and vein strips, and heart–lung preparations and these remain invaluable objects for the study of drugs, but major advances in the understanding of how cardiovascular drugs act has come in recent years from new methods, particularly those that can be used in unanaesthetized animals and man, and include cardiac catheterization for measurement of pressures, Fick and dye methods for measurement of cardiac output, and the attachment of radiopaque markers to the ventricles for the measurement of ventricular contraction.

We will now consider the action of some major groups of drugs on the cardiovascular system.

NORADRENALINE AND RELATED COMPOUNDS

Noradrenaline [CHAPTER 7] is a catecholamine acting predominantly on the sympathetic α-receptors and has in most species a relatively weak β-action. It produces a considerable increase in blood pressure and slowing of the heart with cutaneous vasoconstriction. The primary effects are to increase the stroke output (the positive inotropic action) and to increase the heart rate, and also to constrict arterioles in the skin and viscera while having little effect on the vessels in skeletal muscle. It is also venoconstrictor and hence raises left atrial pressure further augmenting the increase in stroke output. These effects are modified by the baroreceptors which in compensation increase vagal tone and so slow the heart but the vagus has little inotropic effect (there are few vagal fibres ending on the ventricular myocardium). There will also be a reduction in sympathetic tone to the vessels. The slowing of the heart tends to counteract the direct effects of noradrenaline tending to increase the minute output, so that over all the cardiac output may not be much changed.

Methoxamine which seems to be completely devoid of β-actions is without any direct effect on the heart but increases the blood pressure purely by its effect on peripheral resistance. A secondary bradycardia is produced through the baroreceptors.

The actions of **isoprenaline (isoproterenol)** are exerted almost entirely on the β-receptors. There will, therefore, be strong positive inotropic and chronotropic actions on the heart, but there will be no vasoconstriction in the skin and viscera, and marked vasodilatation in muscle, and some venodilatation too. The effects on the mean arterial blood pressure will therefore depend on the balance between the direct effects on the heart increasing stroke and minute output, and hence tending to raise the pressure, and the decrease in peripheral resistance and increase in venous capacity tending to reduce pressure. The balance of effects differs in different animals. In man the mean pressure is not much changed. In other animals there may be a precipitous fall in pressure or a modest rise. In all cases there is a tachycardia and an increase in pulse pressure. The chronotropic action of isoprenaline is made use of in intermittent heart block (Stokes–Adams syndrome) where the increase in excitability of the conducting tissue restarts impulse production.

The action of **adrenaline (epinephrine)** is intermediate between those of noradrenaline and isoprenaline. It acts effectively on both α- and β-receptors. This means that it has a strong cardiac inotropic and chronotropic action, but it has a mixed peripheral action. It constricts skin and visceral vessels, dilates muscle vessels, and constricts most veins. The over-all effect on the peripheral resistance is a modest reduction. The net effect on the blood pressure is a small rise and since the direct cardiac effects are strong and the stimulus to the baroreceptors rather slight, the direct positive chronotropic effect is not annulled by increased vagal tone.

The contrast between noradrenaline and adrenaline is an interesting one and has some relevance to the use of these agents in raising blood pressure in hypotension. Noradrenaline is the more reliable drug for this purpose and also causes a smaller increase in cardiac work for a given rise in blood pressure, because the cardiac output is lower. Both agents have the serious disadvantage of raising blood pressure at the cost of vasoconstriction in the viscera which may cause dangerous ischaemia. **Metaraminol** is sometimes used for the same purpose and has the advantage of a more prolonged action.

HYPOTENSIVE DRUGS

A wide variety of drugs can lower the blood pressure and we will deal here only with some of the more interesting ones.

Ganglion Blockers

Ganglion blockers such as **hexamethonium**, **pempidine**, or **mecamylamine** [CHAPTER 6] cause a rapid and marked fall in arterial pressure with a moderate increase in heart rate. The fall in arterial pressure is mainly due to block of ganglia in the sympathetic vasoconstrictor path, with reduction in vasomotor tone and hence a fall in peripheral resistance.

This would increase the pressure in the small venules, but because of the simultaneous block of sympathetic tone in the veins, the venous capacity is also increased and the right atrial pressure falls, hence the cardiac output falls. This occurs despite the tachycardia due to block of vagal ganglia, which would otherwise tend to increase the minute output. The ganglion blocking drugs were the first drugs to be used in the treatment of hypertension but they are now little used owing to certain undesirable complications. One of these is the large fall in blood pressure that usually occurs in changing position from recumbency to standing. This is due mainly to pooling in the veins and the absence of any baroreceptor reflex consequent on the blocking of all the efferent paths of the autonomic system. The drugs retain a limited usefulness in treating acute hypertensive attacks and sometimes in malignant hypertension. The other unpleasant side-effects are due to the fact that these drugs block all autonomic ganglia including those in the gut causing constipation, in the eye affecting accommodation, and in the bladder causing difficulty with micturition, and in the salivary and lacrimal glands causing dryness of the mouth and eyes.

Sympathetic Block

A more selective effect can be produced by blocking the sympathetic system alone. Direct α-blockade has proved rather ineffective in hypertension largely because although the peripheral resistance is decreased the cardiac sympathetic effects are not blocked so that an increase in heart rate and cardiac output occur. Curiously β-blockers, such as propranolol, do lower the blood pressure by reducing cardiac output and have a place in the treatment of mild hypertension. The details of this action will be described later.

Selective block of sympathetic action is, however, best produced by the agents interfering with noradrenaline biosynthesis and release, namely **guanethidine** and **bethanidine** and **methyldopa**. Because these drugs interfere with the sympathetic neurone rather than with the sympathetic receptor they are effective in blocking both α and β types of effect. They therefore reduce blood pressure by effects both on peripheral vessels and on the heart. Because they leave the vagal effects intact orthostatic hypotension is less marked due to this route of compensation being still available, and indeed there remains available a reduced but significant tachycardia in exercise. These three drugs are the most satisfactory ones available for the treatment of hypertension and are relatively free of side actions, except for rather frequent development of hypersensitivity to methyldopa.

Reserpine produces hypotension in part by its action on peripheral sympathetic neurones, interfering with the storage of noradrenaline, but since the drug is also a sedative it is quite likely that part of the hypotensive effect is due to a depression of the vasomotor centre.

Veratrin Alkaloids

The ester alkaloids from Veratrum species, of which **veratridine** may be taken as typical, have a complicated pharmacology. Their major action is to affect excitable structures, decreasing the threshold for discharge and often causing single impulses to be converted into bursts. Repetitive firing is associated with a large increase in the negative after-potential of the spike which acts as a source of depolarization for excitation. The ionic mechanism of this change is apparently by an interference with the mechanism which shuts off sodium permeability after an action potential. The effects of veratrin can be reversed by lowering the external sodium concentration.

When veratridine is injected intravenously there is pronounced bradycardia and a fall of blood pressure. The bradycardia is vagal in origin and is abolished by atropine, which, however, does not affect the hypotension. The cardiovascular response is totally abolished by bilateral vagal section. This suggested that veratridine caused stimulation of vagal afferents. These have been localized by the demonstration that very small doses of veratridine injected into the coronary arteries or applied to the visceral pericardium produce the same cardiovascular effects as much larger amounts injected intravenously. The afferent fibres concerned originate mainly in the left ventricle and its overlying pericardium and the effect of veratridine on such fibres may be demonstrated by isolating single fibres from the vagal fibres coming from the heart. Some fibres show phasic activity, firing in systole and being silent during the rest of the cardiac cycle; after administration of veratridine, firing is continuous and at a high rate.

The cardiovascular response to veratrin was first described by Bezold in 1867 and the receptors in the heart are therefore usually called Bezold receptors. This type of action is not confined to veratrin but is also found with a variety of phenylguanides and amidines and with serotonin. Veratrin is not used much therapeutically because of the small margin between the therapeutic and the side-effects, the most consistent of which is nausea and vomiting.

Hydralazine

Hydralazine produces general vasodilatation accompanied by tachycardia. Its mode of action is far from settled but appears to be in large measure due to a direct reduction of tone in arterioles, with some depression of vasomotor centre activity. The drug has been extensively used in hypertension but has been dropped mainly because of a wide range of serious side actions including jaundice, pancytopenia, polyneuritis, and a syndrome resembling chronic lupus erythematosus.

Nitrites and Nitrates

Inorganic nitrites have a general relaxant effect on smooth muscle, and this applies to all elements of the peripheral vascular system. However, the veins and venules are particularly affected. The effect on the circulation is to cause a marked fall of blood pressure with tachycardia, cutaneous vasodilatation especially noticeable in the blush area where the skin temperature rises, arterial pulsation becomes marked, and a throbbing headache develops. The blood pressure and heart rate changes are accentuated in the upright posture and fainting may ensue. These changes follow mainly from the decrease in tone in the venules and veins increasing the capacity of this system, and hence causing peripheral blood pooling. Thus despite the arteriolar dilatation and hence greater transmission of arterial pressure to the veins the venous return to the heart is not increased in the supine position and is reduced in the upright position. The change in cardiac output follows the change in venous return. Because the peripheral resistance is reduced the cardiac work is also reduced.

The mechanism of action of the nitrite ion is uncertain, thus in common with cyanide and azide it reacts with cytochrome oxidase and it is of interest that these agents are also powerful vasodilators, and it may be that the interference with oxygen transfer in the cell is responsible for the pharmacological action. However, other factors must be involved as nitrites have a much smaller effect on general oxygen utilization otherwise they would not have their relative freedom from toxicity. Indeed, the main toxic effect of nitrites is due to oxidation of haemoglobins to methaemoglobin.

Qualitatively identical actions to those of inorganic nitrites are produced by aliphatic nitrites such as **amyl nitrite**. This is a volatile substance (b.p. 130° C.) which can be inhaled and is rapidly absorbed from the lungs thus producing effects in a very short time. Other aliphatic nitrates such as **glyceryl trinitrate**, **pentaerythritol tetranitrate**, and **triethanolamine nitrate** have similar actions and are much more potent than inorganic nitrite. It was formerly believed that these substances must first be reduced to nitrites (by the enzyme, polynitrate reductase) before acting. Doubt is thrown on this both by the high activity and rapid action of the ester nitrates and the lack of correlation between the amount of nitrite produced and the intensity of action. There remains the possibility that the ester nitrates owe their high activity to rapid penetration into the target cells with local reduction to nitrites.

The ester nitrates have a prolonged duration of action, whereas sodium nitrite produces effects for less than 1 hour, the effects of pentaerythritol tetranitrate and triethanolamine nitrate (trolnitrate) last for about 6 hours.

Nitrites are a group of drugs to which marked tolerance develops in a few days and becomes maximal after a few weeks, but sensitivity is restored on withdrawal.

ANGINA PECTORIS

Angina pectoris follows the structural narrowing of one or more coronary arteries. In its milder form it is an angina of effort in that the pain develops when an extra task is carried out and ceases rapidly if rest is taken. In severe cases the effort that can be undertaken is very restricted. The pain is due to anoxia in the ventricles affecting directly or indirectly pain afferents in the myocardium. During exercise cardiac work is increased and if the myocardial blood flow cannot be increased in proportion to the oxygen utilization the oxygen tension will fall. Vasodilator drugs like the nitrites enable a patient to undertake more severe exercise before pain develops. Since nitrites can readily be shown to increase coronary flow in isolated perfused hearts it was assumed for many years that nitrites must be increasing exercise tolerance in angina by coronary dilatation. However, since it has been shown in intact animals and in man that it is more common to see a small fall in coronary flow rather than any sustained rise when nitrites are administered, it is very doubtful if this is true. Furthermore, the pathological changes in the coronary artery system affected by atheroma lead to rigidity of the larger vessels which will not be dilatable by any drugs. The remaining possibility is further dilatation of very small vessels and of collaterals. It is possible that these vessels may be dilated more by nitrites than by direct effects of anoxia and myocardial metabolites but the changes are probably marginal. If nitrites do not increase exercise tolerance by dilating the coronary vessels what alternative have we? We noted above that by the combination of action on peripheral venules and arterioles nitrites reduced peripheral resistance without normally increasing cardiac output, resulting in a diminution in cardiac work and hence in cardiac oxygen requirements. It seems likely therefore that nitrites act more by reducing the demand for oxygen by the myocardium than by increasing the supply.

Because of the brief duration of angina of effort there is little value in treating an attack with nitrites which therefore have their main use in prophylaxis, i.e. in enabling individuals to do more than they could otherwise. For this purpose tablets of **glyceryl trinitrate** are chewed, allowing rapid and efficient absorption from the buccal mucosa. By contrast, if the tablets are swallowed absorption is slower and much more irregular. The longer-acting nitrates (pentaerythritol tetranitrate and triethanolamine nitrate) are swallowed rather than chewed.

Recently it has been found that the β-adrenergic blocking agent **propranolol** is effective in angina. The mode of action of this drug is interesting; it does not dilate the coronaries, indeed there are suggestions that it may even reduce coronary flow, nor does it reduce peripheral resistance, but the increase in cardiac work in exercise is in large part mediated by the cardiac sympathetic nerves which increase heart rate, and contractility. By enabling exercise to proceed with a reduced increase in cardiac work propranolol increases exercise tolerance. Since the effects of nitrites are different these drugs are complementary and may be used with profit in combination. A third drug with some value in angina is **dipyridamole**. The present evidence suggests that this drug acts by potentiating the effects of normal metabolic products such as purine nucleotides which are natural coronary dilators.

THE CARDIAC GLYCOSIDES

The rational use of digitalis (foxglove) leaf in cardiac conditions is due to William Withering. He was struck by cases of dropsy (oedema) that had been improved by herbal remedies and came to the conclusion that the active ingredient was foxglove. He then systematically explored the use of the drug, the preparation and standardization of extracts, described many of the toxic effects, and recognized that the improvement of the patient was associated with an improvement in the pulse. He published his results in 1785 in a book entitled *An Account of the Foxglove, and some of its Medical Uses*. The main active principle of purple foxglove is digitoxin, a glycoside of a sterol lactone, digitoxigenin, which is known as the aglycone. Similar substances with actions on the heart are found not only in Digitalis species, but in a number of Strophanthus species, in lilies and in hellebore, and most curious of all, secretions of the skin of toads. The latter is the basis of a traditional Chinese remedy Ch'an su.

A large number of active glycosides have been isolated which differ in the substituent groups and position of unsaturated groups in the sterol, in the structure of the lactone, and in the sugar residues. The sterol skeleton is a peculiar one differing from that in adrenal steroids. In adrenal steroids the A and C and B and D rings are coplanar whereas in the cardiac glycosides the A and D rings are coplanar giving an over-all structure that is much less planar.

The actions of digitalis on the heart may be divided into ones on contractility (inotropic) and on rate and rhythm (chronotropic). The inotropic effect is readily shown under conditions in which the ventricular muscle is hypodynamic, i.e. producing less tension than usual. This can be seen in the ordinary Langendorff preparation in which the coronary arteries are perfused with Krebs salt solution, or when isolated papillary muscles from man or other animals are stimulated *in vitro*. With relatively large doses of ouabain the effects are well developed in a few minutes, but with smaller doses the effects take rather longer to appear. The counterpart of this effect is seen in the intact animal or man when the ventricular contractility is low because of anoxia or muscle damage. The cardiac glycosides shift the filling curve up in the same way that adrenaline does, so that the stroke output and work rise for a given diastolic filling pressure, and also the maximum stroke work is increased. The alternative way of looking at this is to say that to maintain the same stroke output, a lower filling pressure is needed, and hence the pressure in the venous system falls and if oedema is present it will be removed. A more subtle effect on contractility is a consistent increase in the rate of development of tension in the ventricle and this is seen in the normodynamic as well as the hypodynamic myocardium.

The heart rate is slowed in the isolated beating heart, but the slowing is greater *in vivo* and this additional slowing is attributable to an increased rate of discharge of the vagal efferents to the heart, due to a direct action of digitalis on the vagal nucleus; a bradycardia develops when cardiac glycosides are applied directly to the floor of the fourth ventricle in the neighbourhood of the vagal nuclei. In addition to these effects the glycosides potentiate the effects of peripheral vagus stimulation. The vagal slowing of the heart by the glycosides can be removed by atropine administration but the direct effect remains. When digitalis is given in heart failure in therapeutic doses these effects on cardiac rate are not of significance as factors leading to improvement of cardiac function. Indeed, the slowing of the heart that is usually seen as heart failure improves is secondary to the improved function, with a consequent reduction in the sympathetic drive to the heart. However, with increased dosage chronotropic effects become important and these may evolve into partial and finally complete atrioventricular dissocation due to depression of the excitability of the nodal tissue of the atrioventricular bundle. In addition extra systoles arising from the ventricular muscle may occur, a characteristic form being bigemy or coupled beats in which a normally conducted beat is followed at a short interval by an extra systole. With lethal doses the ventricle may fibrillate or be arrested in systole.

It was noticed by Mackenzie that digitalis was particularly effective in heart failure in which the atria were fibrillating and the ventricle was beating excessively fast. A marked slowing of the ventricular rate is produced due to a direct effect on the excitability of the bundle tissue reducing the passage of impulses arising in the subnormal phase of excitability; the direct effect on the atrium is usually to increase the rate of fibrillation.

The cellular mechanism of action of the cardiac glycosides is complex and still incompletely known. However, it is likely that all the actions will eventually be found to stem from the highly specific action of the glycosides on membrane bound ATPase. Membrane bound ATPase is an enzyme found in cell membranes which is activated by sodium and potassium ions; in intact cells enzyme activity depends on the sodium concentration inside the cell and the potassium concentration outside the cell, the enzyme is able to split phosphate from adenosine triphosphate although it is likely that its function in the cell is to transfer a group from ATP to some membrane component. This enzyme is inhibited by cardiac glycosides in the same range of concentrations required to produce the inotropic effect. Furthermore, there is a striking parallelism between the potency of the drugs as inhibitors of the enzyme and as positive inotropic agents. The cardiac glycosides also inhibit the active transport of sodium by cell membranes and it is therefore likely that these two actions are related either because the operation of the ATPase supplies the energy for the sodium pump or because it combines both functions. The most obvious consequence of inhibiting the sodium pump is that the intracellular concentration of sodium rises and that of potassium falls. This may explain the small decrease in resting potential and decreased velocity of contraction, but it is hard to see how it could cause an increase in contractile response directly. On the other hand, it has been established that cardiac glycosides increase the rate of calcium entry with each beat and since there is good evidence that contractile force is dependent on intracellular calcium release, a plausible theory is that the rise in intracellular sodium secondarily facilitates calcium entry which is responsible for the inotropic effect. In fact, cardiac glycosides are known to depress a number of membrane processes which transport substances into cells and these processes are all dependent on extracellular sodium for activity. It should be noted that the effects of digitalis on ionic movements are not restricted to the heart but are exerted on all

FIG. 9.3

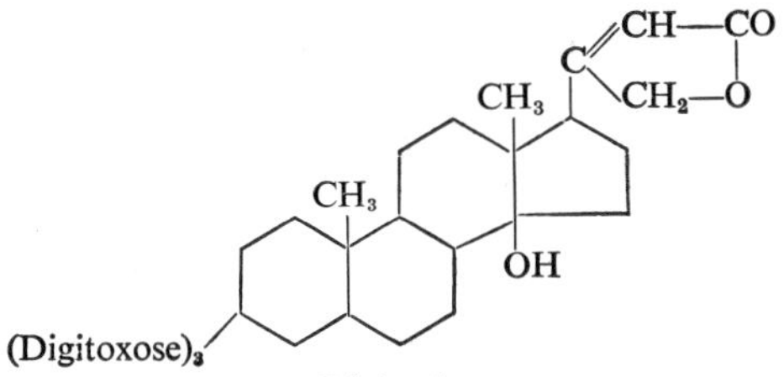

Digitoxin (with (Digitoxose)₃)

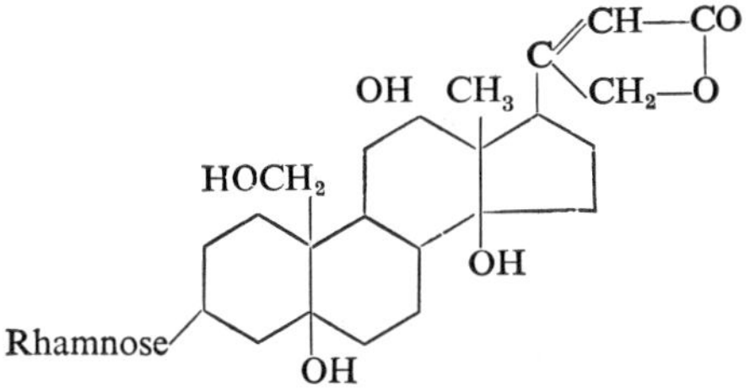

Ouabain (Strophanthin G) (with Rhamnose)

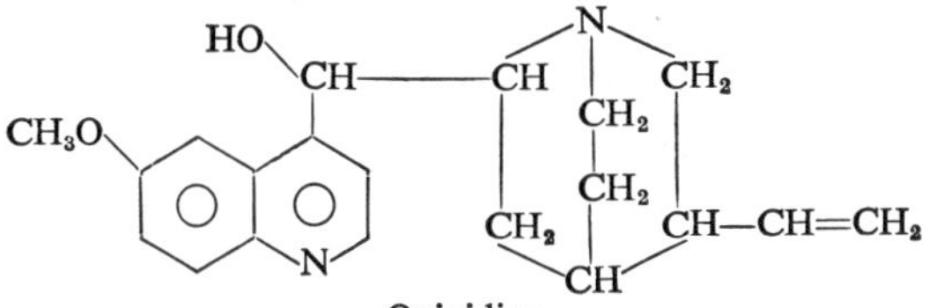

Quinidine

tissues. However, their effect on the physiological state of the tissue will be related to the turnover of ions in the tissue.

The glycosides that are in common use are **digoxin** and **lanatoside C** from *Digitalis lanata*, **digitoxin** from *Digitalis purpurea*, and **ouabain** (strophanthin G) from *Strophanthus gratus*. They have very similar actions in very similar dosage and differ mainly in the rapidity with which effects come on and how long they last; in order of speed and shortness of action they range from ouabain, the fastest, through digoxin and lanatoside C to digitoxin which has effects lasting for about 2 weeks.

In therapeutic use the effects are produced by a loading dose given either by mouth or by injection followed by a daily maintenance dose which in the case of digoxin is about one-quarter of the loading dose.

It has been said that every patient who is on chronic administration of cardiac glycosides suffers from toxic effects at some time or another; this situation exists because the toxic effects of digitalis are those of overdose rather than hypersensitivity or cytotoxicity and in heart failure there is a natural tendency to obtain as much improvement in cardiac function as the drug is capable of giving. Nausea and vomiting are common and are mainly due to stimulation of the chemoreceptor trigger zone in the medulla; as mentioned above arrhythmias may occur and bigeminy is a sign of overdosage as is excessive slowing of the rate. Digitalis toxicity depends on the levels of potassium and calcium in the plasma, and thus toxic effects may be precipitated by a diuretic such as chlorothiazide which causes hypokalaemia; contrariwise the toxic effects may be antagonized by the cautious use of potassium salts. Propranolol has proved a useful agent in dealing with digitalis arrhythmias.

ANTIARRHYTHMIC DRUGS

Arrhythmias are due to the development of new pacemakers in the myocardium distinct from the normal pacemakers in the nodal tissue. In nodal tissue the membrane potential is not constant during diastole but gradually falls ('the diastolic drift') and at a critical potential level a regenerative response develops with the initiation of an action potential. In non-nodal tissue the diastolic drift is absent and no intrinsic rhythmicity is present. However, in injured myocardial tissue pacemaker activity may develop in non-nodal tissue and this may lead to a very high rate of discharge as in atrial or ventricular fibrillation, a lower rate as in flutter or paroxysmal tachycardia or isolated extrasystoles. These effects can be counteracted by agents which:
(1) raise the threshold for excitation; and
(2) prolong the refractory period.

The first effect means that a greater diastolic drift is needed for excitation, the second that the possibility of re-excitation from adjoining active areas of membrane is reduced. The agents that produce these effects are local anaesthetics and the effects are due mainly to a reduced sensitivity of the membrane sodium carrier to depolarization and a reduced ability to reload the sodium carrier. The effects of antiarrhythmic drugs are always accompanied by a reduced contractility. The first agent to be used for this purpose was quinine but it was subsequently found that the stereoisomer **quinidine** was more effective and less toxic. **Procaine** was later found to be effective but suffered from the disadvantage of a very brief action and excessive central nervous actions. Replacement of the ester linkage in procaine by an amide grouping gave the stable substance **procainamide** with reduced central side-actions. **Lignocaine** administered by intravenous infusion is the most effective antiarrhythmic of all, and is particularly of use after cardiac surgery and myocardial infarction. More recently the β-blocking drug **propranolol** has been found to be a very effective antiarrhythmic agent. There does not appear to be any necessary connexion with β-blocking action as some β-blockers are devoid of antiarrhythmic action, and in the stereoisomers of propranolol while the (+) isomer is nearly devoid of β-blocking activity it is a potent antiarrhythmic. **Practolol** is also used. Recently it has been shown that **phenytoin** (*Dilantin*) is effective in ventricular ectopic rhythms and in paroxysmal atrial tachycardia.

In summary, the desirable antiarrhythmics appear to be local anaesthetics with minimal central action.

Antiarrhythmics are used to control paroxysmal tachycardia, the showers of extrasystoles that may arise in cardiac infarction, and to convert atrial fibrillation and flutter to normal rhythm. In this case the heart rate is first controlled by doses of digitalis adequate to depress the bundle of His. Conversion is easiest in atrial arrhythmias of recent origin, but these also revert to the arrhythmia rather readily.

Quinidine is a rather dangerous drug due mainly to its marked tendency to cause hypersensitivity-type toxic reactions.

FURTHER READING

DAWES, G. S. (1952) Experimental cardiac arrhythmias and quinidine-like drugs, *Pharmacol. Rev.*, **4**, 43.

GLYNN, I. M. (1964) The action of cardiac glycosides on ion movements, *Pharmacol. Rev.*, **16**, 381.

PICKERING, G. W. (1961) *The Treatment of Hypertension*, Springfield, Ill.

ROWE, G. G. (1968) Pharmacology of the coronary circulation, *Ann. Rev. Pharmacol.*, **8**, 95.

SEKERES, L., and PAPP, J. G. (1968) Antiarrhythmic compounds, *Prog. drug Res.*, **12**, 292.

SONNENBLICK, E. H., BRAUNWALD, E., and MORROW, A. G. (1965) The contractile properties of human heart muscle, *J. clin. Invest.*, **44**, 966.

STOLL, A. (1949) The cardioactive glycosides, *J. Pharm. Pharmacol.*, **1**, 849.

TRAUTWEIN, W. (1963) Generation and conduction of impulses in the heart, *Pharmacol. Rev.*, **14**, 277.

WILBRANDT, W. (1963) *New Aspects of Cardiac Glycosides*, London.

10

BODY TEMPERATURE AND THE ANTIPYRETIC-ANALGESICS

Although it is generally recognized that body temperature is regulated it is less commonly recognized that the temperature of the body is not uniform; for instance, the skin temperature is variable over different parts of the body surfaces being lowest at the extremities and is in general much cooler than the core temperature measured in the interior of the thorax or abdomen. Furthermore, surface temperature will vary markedly with environmental conditions. It is difficult to know which should be adopted as the reference temperature of the body since, for example, liver temperature is influenced by the rate of metabolism in that organ and rectal temperature by bacterial metabolism in the rectal contents. There is a lot to be said in really accurate studies for measuring temperature at the ear drum by a thermocouple placed in the external auditory meatus. However, in experimental situations, rectal temperature is usually accepted as a reasonable measure of core temperature.

Heat is produced in the body as an inevitable by-product of metabolic processes and the mechanical work of muscular contraction. Heat is exchanged with the environment by the processes of radiation, convection and conduction, and by the evaporation of water from the skin and respiratory passages. In a resting individual whose temperature regulation mechanisms are inactivated the body temperature remains constant if the environmental temperature is about 30° C., but at lower temperatures the body temperature cools at a rate proportional to the difference of temperatures from 30° C. and conversely rises if the ambient temperature is above this level.

In the normal individual, body temperature is conserved over a wide range of temperature by regulatory mechanisms affecting both heat production and heat loss. Heat production is increased in response to a fall in body temperature almost entirely by an increase in muscular activity in the form of involuntary shivering or by voluntary action such as swinging the arms, whereas heat loss is altered by change in surface temperature and blood flow and by sweating. In a cold environment the blood flow through the skin is reduced and blood is shunted into the deep vessels in the core of the limb; this reduced carriage of heat to the skin allows the skin temperature to fall while reducing heat loss from the body core—the converse occurs in hot environments where radiative and conductive losses are made more effective by a rise in skin temperature.

Temperatures are sensed both by central thermoreceptors in the hypothalamus and in the periphery where the sensitivity is mainly to the temperature gradient. Regulation is integrated by two interconnected centres in the hypothalamus, the more anterior of which brings in compensatory mechanisms for hot environments whereas the posterior region is concerned with heat conservation.

Little is understood of the mechanisms which determine that the core temperature is normally regulated at the level of 36°–37·5° C. However, in fever the regulation is set to a higher level. At the onset of a fever shivering occurs, the skin is pale, and the individual feels cold, i.e. heat production has been increased and heat loss diminished and in consequence the temperature rises rapidly. As the temperature rises the usual heat loss mechanisms come into play, and the skin vessels dilate, but heat production remains high in part due to the increased rate of metabolism secondary to the rise in temperature. The subject feels hot at this stage. Fever is usually due to infection with micro-organisms and can be reproduced by the injection of extracts of bacteria containing substances called pyrogens. These are of several kinds but the most active are lipopolysaccharides. They are of importance in pharmacology because solutions prepared for injections should be free of them. Pyrogen-free water is prepared by doubly distilling water and collecting under strictly aseptic conditions.

Body temperature is raised by drugs causing an increase in metabolism. Examples are **2,4 dinitrophenol** and **3,5 dinitro-orthocresol** (DNOC); the latter is a pesticide. These substances uncouple phosphorylation and stimulate tissue respiration. The result is an uneconomical process by which more oxygen and substrates are used and hence more heat produced with little return in the form of high energy phosphate compounds (ATP, ADP, phosphagen, etc). Many phenols have this property including salicylic acid which paradoxically increases body temperature in high doses. Thyroxine also raises temperature by increasing metabolism in part by an uncoupling action, but it has other actions on metabolism as yet ill defined.

Convulsants increase temperature secondary to the excessive muscular activity and hence increase in heat production; lesser rises in temperature result from drugs that cause restlessness, such as **adrenaline, amphetamine, cocaine**, and **β-tetrahydronaphthylamine**. In atropine poisoning hyperthermia may be present due to similar causes. Atropine in ordinary doses does not raise the body temperature except when the ambient temperature is high or during exercise when heat loss by sweating is dominant.

Body temperature is lowered by many drugs having central actions: for instance, in deep general anaesthesia temperature regulation is almost completely lost so that if the operating room temperature is low hypothermia can develop; equally the wraps covering the patient may interfere with heat loss. **Alcohol** also interferes with temperature regulation partly by its central action and also by causing vasodilatation of skin vessels. It is for this reason that alcohol gives the feeling of warmth while simultaneously lowering the temperature. This combination of properties can make it dangerous medication in severe cold weather. **Morphine** and other narcotic analgesics have a similar effect. More striking still is the fall of body temperature induced by **chlorpromazine** and some other phenothiazine drugs. This seems to be mainly due to vasodilatation in the skin but there is an undoubted central component. These actions have been of use in producing hypothermia for cardiac and intracranial surgery. If one attempts to cool an individual by surface cooling, the degree of cooling is restricted by the reactive vasoconstriction and increased metabolism; chlorpromazine largely eliminates these reactive effects and enables cooling to be smoother and more rapid. Naturally all these responses to hypothermic drugs are seen in heightened degree in pyrexial patients, and formerly opium and alcohol were both given to induce sweating and lower the body temperature.

A response of quite a different character is produced by the miscellaneous drugs of the antipyretic–analgesic group such as **acetylsalicylic acid (aspirin), acetanilide, paracetamol, phenacetin, phenazone,** and **phenylbutazone**. These substances do not lower the body temperature in normal individuals, indeed as pointed out earlier if the dose is large enough they may raise the temperature by increasing metabolism. However, in pyrexia, they produce peripheral dilatation, abundant perspiration, and a prompt fall of temperature. Identical effects are produced with fever due to injected pyrogens.

It is commonly said that these drugs can reset the thermostat when it is set too high by infection but this is merely conjuring with words and the mechanism of action is really not

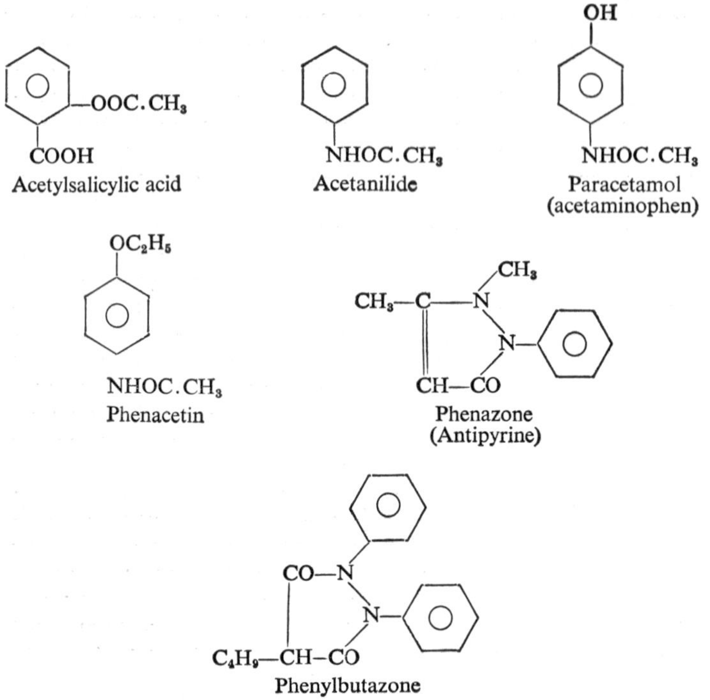

FIG. 10.1. Antipyretic-analgesics.

Acetylsalicylic acid

Acetanilide

Paracetamol (acetaminophen)

Phenacetin

Phenazone (Antipyrine)

Phenylbutazone

understood. Furthermore, while these drugs will make the fevered patient more comfortable it is still not clear whether they favour or retard recovery from the infection itself.

Salicylates

The salicylates are an example of a drug of very simple chemical structure but with complex and perplexing pharmacology.

The antipyretic action of willow bark (*Salix alba*) was known to the ancients, and in the early nineteenth century a glucoside of salicylic acid, salicin, was isolated from it and this was followed shortly by the isolation of salicylic acid which was then shown to be antipyretic. Widespread use followed the recognition of its analgesic activity and the development of a cheap synthesis.

The analgesic action of salicylate is of a different character from that of the opiates, for whereas the latter do not truly eliminate the sensation of pain, but rather alter the psychological reaction to pain, so that the individual becomes indifferent to pain, the salicylates within their limitations cause a genuine analgesia. They are especially effective in aching low-grade pain, e.g. headache, toothache, joint pain and do not have much effect in visceral or wound pain.

There seems to be a ceiling to the intensity of pain that can be suppressed as there is also for opiates. As pointed out in Chapter 3, the experimental assessment of pain and analgesics is very unsatisfactory and this is especially the case with the salicylate type of analgesic. Almost the only test in which their analgesic action has been demonstrated unequivocally is tooth pain produced by electrical stimulation of the dental pulp. There is no question that salicylates are also effective in reducing the malaise accompanying infections and are widely believed to have a tranquillizing effect. However, analgesia by salicylates is not accompanied by any really striking changes of mood, especially not by euphoria, unlike that produced by the opiates. The paucity of overt central effects has led to the suspicion that at least part of the action is a peripheral one on sensory endings. In particular the anti-inflammatory action of salicylate and its effectiveness in countering some of the actions of bradykinin which is generally believed to have a significant role in the phenomena of inflammation have tended to support this proposition. However, it is rendered more dubious by comparison with paracetamol or acetanilide, on the one hand, which are good analgesics but practically devoid of anti-inflammatory action, and phenylbutazone, a poor analgesic, but a powerful anti-inflammatory agent, on the other hand. This does not suggest a close correlation between anti-inflammatory action and analgesia. The anti-inflammatory action is an important feature of salicylate action and leads to a decrease in swelling and heat; in the inflamed joints of rheumatic fever, a similar and more powerful effect is produced by adrenal corticoids. It is interesting that although the action of salicylates in this disease has been a major part of therapy for more than 50 years it is still quite uncertain whether the evolution of rheumatic carditis is favourably influenced by it.

Salicylates have well-marked metabolic effects the most prominent of which is the uncoupling of oxidative phosphorylation, which raises the basal metabolic rate; it also has a hyperglycaemic action possibly mediated by adrenaline released through hypothalamic stimulation, and the formation of glycogen is reduced and the glycogen content of muscle and liver is depleted. This is not an unmixed effect and in some circumstances the blood sugar may be lowered; for this reason salicylates have been used in diabetes but are not very effective.

The commonly used preparations of salicylates are **aspirin** (acetylsalicylic acid) and **sodium salicylate**, although combinations with other drugs such as **phenacetin, paracetamol, codeine**, and **caffeine** are popular. There is little evidence of genuine potentiation in these mixtures, which can be replaced without loss by a larger dose of aspirin or paracetamol.

The pK of salicylic acid is 3·0 so that in the stomach much of the acid is in the non-ionized form. Since this is the form most readily absorbed, it would be expected that absorption from the stomach would be rapid. However, this is limited by the low solubility of the acid (0·3 per cent.) so that absorption will be limited by the rate of dissolution; in the case of tableted preparations the rate of absorption is increased if the particles in the tablets are very small. A considerable part of the salicylate will be absorbed in the small gut despite the tiny proportion (< 0.01 per cent.) that is un-ionized. The major route of metabolism is by conjugation to give salicylglycine (salicyluric acid) and glycuronides. Conversion to gentisic acid (2,5 dihydroxybenzoic acid) is minimal. Of the total excreted in the urine more than half is in the form of unchanged salicylic acid.

Aspirin is absorbed in the same way as salicylic acid but it is rapidly deacetylated in the blood stream, so that after absorption it is equivalent to free salicylate.

The excretion of salicylates is such as to give a half-time of about 4–8 hours for the plasma concentration.

Toxic Effects. Considering the enormous scale on which they are used (in the United States the average annual consumption is about 200 tablets per head) major toxic effects are uncommon, but minor toxic effects largely of gastro-intestinal type are very common.

Epigastric discomfort is common as is minor bleeding due to gastric erosion. If gastroscopy is undertaken after a dose of aspirin, injection and small haemorrhages may be seen in the neighbourhood of the undissolved aspirin particles deposited on the gastric mucosa. Occasionally major gastric bleeding occurs. With large doses there may be ringing in the ears, dizziness, deafness, drowsiness, and confusion.

This syndrome is called salicylism and is similar to the pattern of toxicity produced by quinine. Salicylates may also produce allergic disorders and, for instance, may precipitate asthma in susceptible individuals. They may also produce renal damage as evidenced by increased urinary excretion of epithelial cells and leucocytes.

The major toxic effects of large doses of salicylates are due to disturbances of respiration and acid–base balance. Respiration is stimulated and air hunger may occur which is difficult to distinguish from that in diabetic ketosis, the overbreathing leads to a fall in the arterial pCO_2 and a respiratory alkalosis. Compensation occurs by bicarbonate loss in the urine so that the plasma bicarbonate falls. In addition lactic acid and keto acids accumulate in the blood due to interference with normal carbohydrate and fat metabolism. The patient will also be hyperthermic. The blood concentration of salicylate will usually be greater than 50 mg. per cent. ($\sim$ 4 mEq./l.). The removal of the excessive body burden of salicylate is favoured by administration of sodium bicarbonate which increases the urinary excretion. Salicylates are not uncommonly taken in large amounts in suicidal attempts.

Phenacetin and Paracetamol

These two drugs have the same application as salicylates to the relief of minor pain and malaise, are as effective and are less likely to cause gastric upsets, but they have their own toxic effects. In particular phenacetin is under a cloud at present owing to reports from Sweden, where the drug is very popular, of the development of interstitial nephritis with papillary necrosis. Paracetamol appears to be free from this toxic effect. Both of these drugs may cause cyanosis due to methaemoglobin formation and may shorten red cell life and hence lead to anaemia.

Mefenamic acid and **flufenamic acid** are recent drugs with aspirin-like activity whose usefulness is still to be determined. **Phenazone** (antipyrine) is little used because of its great liability to produce hypersensitivity reactions.

Phenylbutazone

The anti-inflammatory actions of phenylbutazone were discovered by accident when the drug was used to increase the solubility of amidopyrine. It is much more effective in rheumatoid arthritis and gout than salicylates but it is a poorly tolerated drug with a wide range of toxic effects, notably gastro-intestinal disturbances, including peptic ulceration, hypersensitivity reactions, and bone marrow disorders including fatal aplastic anaemia. It is reserved for cases that are unresponsive to other drugs and then used in short courses to reduce the risks.

Indomethacin has similar effects to phenylbutazone and similar indications. It also produces severe gastro-intestinal side-effects and vertigo but does not produce bone marrow depression.

FURTHER READING

EULER, C. VON (1961) Physiology and pharmacology of temperature regulation, *Pharmacol. Rev.*, **13**, 361.

GROSS, M., and GREENBERG, L. A. (1948) *The Salicylates*, New Haven.

HARDY, J. D. (1955) Control of heat loss and heat production in physiologic temperature regulation, *Harvey Lect.* **49**, 242.

NEWBURGH, L. H. (ed.) (1949) *Physiology of Heat Regulation and the Science of Clothing*, Philadelphia.

SMITH, M. J. H. (1959) Salicylates and metabolism, *J. Pharm. Pharmacol.*, **11**, 705.

SMITH, M. J. H. (1963) in *Salicylates*, ed. Dixon, A. St. J. *et al.*, London.

11

ALIMENTARY CANAL

GASTRIC SECRETION

GASTRIC juice has a high concentration of hydrogen and chloride ions. Hydrions are highly concentrated in the parietal cells of the stomach, the basic reaction being:

$$H_2O + CO_2 \rightarrow HCO_3^- + H^+$$

Because hydrions are being removed from the extracellular fluid, a surfeit of HCO_3^- is left behind and if gastric fluid is lost by vomiting, then a metabolic alkalosis will result.

The digestive properties of gastric juice are due mainly to the presence of pepsin and the secretion of gastric acid provides an environment of pH 1·5–4 which is optimal for pepsin activity.

The secretion of gastric acid and of pepsin is controlled by both humoral and nervous factors. Stimulation of the vagus nerve, or the action of muscarinic drugs, increases gastric secretion and, through this nerve, secretion is affected by various reflexes initiated by gustatory, olfactory, and other stimuli. The vagus is also important in controlling and potentiating the action of the hormone **gastrin** on the oxyntic acid-secreting cells and the pepsin-secreting cells of the stomach.

Gastrin is secreted from the antral region of the stomach in response to the stimulus of food in the stomach and it has a powerful stimulating effect on gastric secretion.

Gastrin has been purified and found to consist of two polypeptides, known as gastrin I and gastrin II, both of which are potent stimulants of gastric secretion. The composition of gastrin I is Glu–Gly–Pro–Tyr–Met–Glu–Glu–Glu–Glu–Glu–Ala–Tyr–Gly–Tyr–Met–Asp–Phe(NH$_2$). Gastrin II is identical except for the addition of an —SO$_3$H group on the 12th amino acid (tyrosine).

Although these peptides are normally both stimulants of gastric acid secretion, they may, under some conditions, actually inhibit acid secretion but at the same time increase pepsin secretion, pancreatic secretions, and gastric tone. Whether these effects of gastrin are of physiological importance is not yet known.

Injected histamine is also a powerful stimulant of gastric acid secretion but it is not known whether endogenously released histamine plays a role in the excitation of oxyntic cells or whether gastrin stimulates histamine release near or within oxyntic cells to cause their secretion. The possibility of histamine being the final link in the excitation of oxyntic cells cannot be decided with our present meagre knowledge of the mechanism of action of, and interaction between, gastrin, histamine, and acetylcholine released from the vagus.

Peptic Ulcers

Gastric juice, with its high acidity and high pepsin content, is highly corrosive, but normally the stomach and upper intestinal walls are protected from its action by a mucosal layer. The development of an ulcer does not appear to depend on any one clear factor but seems frequently to be precipitated by stress conditions occurring over long periods. The patient with a duodenal ulcer has a resting secretion of hydrochloric acid at least twice that of the normal person and the gastrin content of the antrum is also raised. In patients with gastric ulcers, however, the resting acid release is often below normal levels.

Despite much discussion, the usual primary treatment of peptic ulcers is with antacids.

Undoubtedly antacids relieve the pain of the ulcer but this does not necessarily mean that the drug allows the ulcer to heal unless the gastric pH is constantly monitored and not allowed to fall lower than 4. The most effective antacids are the nonsystemic inorganic ones, particularly calcium carbonate and magnesium carbonate.

Since pepsin is probably involved in producing ulcers considerable work has been done to find specific anti-pepsin compounds. Some success has been obtained with a sulphated amylopectin and carbenoxolone, an extract of liquorice, appears to aid the healing of ulcers.

In more serious cases of ulceration other types of treatment are usually considered. A low protein content in the diet reduces secretogogue effects, and large meals, which would mechanically distend the stomach, should be avoided.

The use of anticholinergic compounds is controversial because of the side-effects accompanying any reduction in acid secretion, the most important of these is a reduction in gastric motility and emptying time and, while this may be an advantage in the case of a gastric ulcer, it does not speed the healing of a duodenal ulcer.

Surgical intervention in the form of vagotomy to reduce gastric secretion or antrectomy and gastric resection are only used in the most difficult cases.

Probably the most important advances in the treatment of peptic ulcers will result from our knowledge of the structure of gastrin and the synthesis of gastrin antagonists. Already a promising compound, thioacetamide, has been developed.

ANTACIDS

The normal concentration of hydrochloric acid in the gastric secretion is about 0·5 per cent. The volume secreted in 24 hours is about 1·5 litres and so there is no way to replace a deficiency in the acid of gastric juices by mouth. On the other hand, it is comparatively easy to neutralize the gastric acid, and pain which is due to hyperchlorhydria can be relieved in this way. Antacids are used for this purpose when the acid secretion is producing an irritant action or in order to allow the healing of damaged or ulcerated parts of the stomach, oesophagus, or duodenum. A good antacid should sufficiently neutralize free acidity but at the same time it should not cause systemic alkalosis or unpleasant side-effects such as the generation of very large quantities of gas. Food and milk are both useful non-systemic antacids.

Sodium bicarbonate is a systemic antacid used to secure quick relief from the discomfort of heartburn and dyspepsia. The reaction which occurs in the stomach is as follows:

$$NaHCO_3 + HCl \rightarrow NaCl + H_2O + CO_2$$

The neutralizing action does not last long and sodium bicarbonate is not usually the antacid of choice, especially if an antacid is to be administered for long periods. The evolved carbon dioxide distends the stomach and causes belching and protein digestion is impaired because pepsin is inactivated in alkaline and neutral solution. A more serious feature of prolonged sodium bicarbonate treatment is the possibility that large numbers of hydrions may be removed, causing systemic alkalosis.

Magnesium trisilicate acts as a non-systemic antacid and an adsorbent. As an adsorbent it is able to reduce the effects of acidity by forming a colloidal adsorbent gel in the stomach.

The hydrated silicic acid, formed in the stomach, passes into the intestine and its gelatinous nature may protect ulcerated tissue from attack by gastric acid. The antacid action of magnesium trisilicate is slow in onset but is prolonged and the stomach contents are usually stabilized at pH 4–6.

This compound is widely used in the treatment of peptic ulcers and it is non-toxic but may, in large doses, produce diarrhoea due to the action of soluble magnesium salts in the intestinal tract.

Other magnesium compounds used as antacids include **magnesium oxide** and **magnesium hydroxide**.

Aluminium hydroxide is widely used as an antacid or absorbent in the form of a suspension, powder, or tablets.

After administration of this compound the pH of the stomach contents lies between pH 3·5 and 4·0. This is sufficient to inactivate pepsin. It is not absorbed through the intestine and so there is no risk of systemic alkalosis.

Aluminium hydroxide may cause constipation and is therefore often used in combination with magnesium hydroxide.

VOMITING

The act of vomiting is primarily protective and is designed to remove unwelcome substances from the stomach. Some animals, such as rodents, are not endowed with this faculty but in many animals, such as dogs and pigeons, it is well developed. Vomiting involves many parts of the body but is controlled by the vomiting centre in the medulla. The premonitory sensation, which is felt when this centre is being stimulated, but has not yet acted, is known as nausea. It is generally accompanied by salivation, bronchial secretion, sweating, and inhibition of gastric secretion, and many drugs have these effects in small doses and cause vomiting in large doses. In other words they act as sialagogues, expectorants, diaphoretics, and inhibitors of secretion in small doses and as emetics in large doses.

If the medullary vomiting centre is destroyed, vomiting cannot occur whatever stimulus is used. A second centre, known as the chemosensitive trigger zone of the medulla, appears to be the primary site of action of emetic drugs and if this region of the brain is destroyed these drugs no longer cause vomiting. Though the natural stimulus for vomiting is the presence of irritating substances in the stomach, the same effects can be produced by strong enough stimulation of almost any kind; overstimulation of the labyrinth (as occurs in motion-sickness), or of the sensory nerves from the heart or other viscera, and strong emotion, may all cause vomiting.

Many compounds cause vomiting by a central action but they are not used for this action. They include the cardiac glycosides, the veratrum alkaloids, anti-tumour drugs, apomorphine and related compounds. If it is necessary to produce vomiting in a person in order to eject toxic substances from the stomach, the most simple methods are to give the patient a salt solution to drink or to place a finger in his oesophagus.

Reflex vomiting is caused by irritation of the gastro-intestinal tract and is abolished by destruction of the chemoreceptive trigger zone. Drugs which cause reflex vomiting when taken by mouth include copper sulphate, zinc sulphate, and mercuric chloride. When vomiting is due to irritation of the gastric mucosa it may cure itself by the removal of the irritant, but local methods to protect the mucous membrane are also sometimes effective. The neutralization of excess acid with alkalis may stop vomiting, particularly if it is associated with acidosis.

Many drugs with antihistamine actions act also as anti-emetics perhaps by virtue of their atropine-like action and their sedative effects.

Chlorpromazine is a potent anti-emetic and prevents vomiting caused by drugs, pregnancy, and inner ear disease. It has no effect in the prevention of motion-sickness.

DRUGS WHICH RELIEVE MOTION-SICKNESS

The number of remedies for motion-sickness is legion, and none of them cure all cases, since some people are sea-sick by suggestion, some by stimulation of the labyrinth, some by stimulation of sensory nerves in the abdominal viscera, and some by other causes.

The agents which are most effective against motion-sickness often share with atropine the property of antagonizing the actions of muscarine on peripheral tissues and it is possible they act by paralysing cholinergic systems in the CNS.

The most effective drug in the treatment of motion-sickness is **hyoscine**. This is now widely used. It is taken before motion-sickness is likely to be encountered and its effects last 6 or 7 hours. High doses produce extremely unpleasant side-effects. Compounds of this type will also protect against vomiting induced by drugs.

Promethazine is effective against motion-sickness and vomiting induced by drugs. It is an antihistamine with atropine-like properties and may cause side-effects, including a dry mouth and blurred vision.

Other compounds used in the treatment or prevention of motion-sickness include:

Antazoline (*Histostab, Antistin*), **chlorcyclizine** (*Di-paralene, Derazil, Histantin*), **dimenhydrinate** (*Dramamine*), **diphenhydramine** (*Benadryl*).

The last two compounds are particularly effective and useful anti-emetics.

THE BILE

The bile is continuously excreted by the liver and collected in the gall-bladder, where it is concentrated about ten times. Bile contains bile salts which are emulsifying agents and aid the absorption of fats and fat-soluble vitamins in the intestine. It also contains bile pigments which come from haemoglobin, inorganic salts, water, mucin, cholesterol, and lecithin. It may contain many other substances in small quantities, including many drugs which are excreted in this way.

The bile salts are reabsorbed from the intestine, so that they may circulate and be used again. In their absence, fats are not emulsified and are only poorly absorbed. When food is present in the duodenum the gall-bladder contracts and empties its contents down the bile-duct. This contraction is partly under nervous control and is partly due to circulating hormones. Stimulation of the vagus or the administration of drugs with muscarinic actions causes contraction of the gall-bladder and relaxation of the sphincter of Oddi at the lower end of the bile-duct.

A complicated train of events is involved in the hormonal control of bile secretion. The presence of fats in the duodenum causes the liberation of **cholecystokinin,** which causes a contraction of the gall-bladder. This throws the bile salts into the duodenum where they stimulate the liberation of **secretin,** which causes not only pancreatic secretion but also bile secretion in the liver, so that the gall-bladder is refilled. There are thus several ways in which drugs may act as cholagogues (choleretics) to increase the flow of bile.

The most effective choleretics are the bile salts themselves and they may be used to flush out the biliary ducts to remove small gallstones or infections. They may occasionally be used to aid digestion. Preparations which contain the bile salts are: extract of ox bile, **sodium tauroglycocholate,** and **bilein** and all these may be used as choleretics. **Dehydrocholic acid** produces a watery bile and is used to treat flatulence and abdominal discomfort due to gall-bladder disease. It is also used to treat inflammatory conditions of the biliary system but is not used in the presence of obstructive jaundice.

PURGATIVES

The intestine makes movements of various kinds. Rhythmic contractions of the longitudinal muscles are called pendulum movements and they pull the mucous membrane back and forwards over the food. Rhythmic movements of the circular muscles cause segmentation which mixes the food. The progression of food down the intestine is not increased by either of these movements and is entirely due to peristalsis. This is controlled by Auerbach's plexus, which causes the circular muscle to relax below the food and contract above it and so force the intestinal contents along.

Peristalsis is increased by the presence of bulky substance in the intestine which excites sensory receptors in the mucous membrane.

All these movements are increased by stimulation of the vagus or the administration of eserine or drugs with muscarine-like actions, and these effects are antagonized by atropine.

Sympathetic stimulation and the administration of adrenaline have the opposite effect. The response of the ileocolic sphincter to both nerve stimulation and drugs is the opposite of the rest of the intestine.

The purgative group of drugs include a very large number of compounds which act in a number of different ways. They all cause defaecation and are in wide use, often unnecessarily, in all parts of the world. Terms which are used synonymously with purgative include laxative, cathartic, purge, drastic evacuant, and aperient and, although they may suggest different degrees of purgative action, they all mean the same thing in the end.

Depending largely on the dose used, a purgative may have a gentle action and well-formed stools will be produced. In larger doses, badly formed stools will be produced, and in still larger doses the stools will be watery.

The purgatives act either by a bulk effect, by lubrication, or by irritation.

Bulk Purgatives

The presence of bulky substances in the intestine provides the normal stimulus for peristalsis by stretching the wall of the intestine.

Fruit and vegetables contain cellulose which is not normally digested, and this acts as roughage and increases intestinal mobility. **Bran,** which is often taken as a cereal, contains a large proportion of insoluble fibres and prunes, in addition to providing cellulose and fibre, also contain **diphenylisatin** which is a stimulant purgative.

Numerous substances act as bulk purgatives because they are not absorbed through the intestinal wall but swell by the absorption of fluid.

Agar is a dried extract of Japanese seaweed and consists largely of an insoluble carbohydrate, which swells up with water to form a jelly. If flakes of it are taken by the mouth they swell up in the alimentary canal and increase peristalsis. It is not normally used as a purgative alone because large quantities have to be ingested to be effective.

Magnesium sulphate is isotonic in 3·5 per cent. solution and is a commonly used, bitter-tasting purgative. The bitter taste is usually disguised with a variety of additives. Both magnesium and sulphate ions are only very slightly absorbed and other salts containing them make effective purgatives. These include **sodium sulphate, heavy magnesium oxide,** and **heavy magnesium carbonate** and the corresponding light salts.

Tartrates and phosphates are both only partly absorbed from the intestine and may act as mild saline purgatives.

Lubricant Purgatives

Liquid paraffin (mineral oil) is an inert, oily liquid consisting of a mixture of aliphatic hydrocarbons that is used as a mild laxative. It acts as a lubricant and increases the bulk and softness of the faeces. In reasonable doses it is useful in the treatment of chronic constipation and for patients with haemorrhoids and heart disease who should avoid straining at stool.

It is liable to leak past the anal sphincter and large doses may delay the absorption of carotene, calcium, phosphates, and vitamins D and K.

Dioctyl sodium sulphosuccinate is a wetting agent and is used to soften the stools. It appears to have little effect on intestinal mobility. It has not yet been fully tested but may be useful for patients who must avoid straining at stool.

Enemas

The bulk effect of about one pint of warm soapy water causes rectal distention with stimulation of muscle activity in the rectum and colon and so promotes defaecation.

Irritant Purgatives

These compounds have a local irritant or stimulant action on the intestinal wall and so excite Auerbach's plexus and cause peristalsis. They may act at any part of the intestinal tract and are commonly used when a patient is being treated with drugs that cause constipation and after food poisoning or the administration of anthelminthics.

Bisacodyl was developed as a result of studies of compounds structurally related to the purgative, phenolphthalein. The purgative action of bisacodyl resembles that of other irritant purgatives but it is more active on the large bowel than on the small intestine. Unlike other irritant purgatives, it can be given rectally as well as by oral administration.

This compound is sometimes known as a 'contact purgative' because it acts directly on sensory nerve endings in the mucosa to stimulate peristalsis. This effect can be blocked by the topical application of cocaine.

Mercurous chloride (calomel) has a prolonged irritant action on the intestinal mucosa and was once used as a purgative. Although mercurous chloride itself is almost insoluble and is therefore not absorbed, a proportion of the mercurous salt may be converted to the mercuric form. Mercuric ions are absorbed and may cause mercury poisoning.

Castor oil is a triglyceride consisting of glycerides of ricinoleic acid and isoricinoleic acid. It is expressed from the seeds of the castor-oil plant of tropical Africa.

The oil itself is soothing and is used as eye-drops to protect the eyes from irritation, but in the small intestine it is hydrolysed by lipase to produce ricinoleic acid which stimulates the small intestine. If bile is deficient the oil is not properly emulsified, so that the lipase cannot hydrolyse it and there is no purgation. Castor oil is safe and it is useful in acute constipation but its use may be followed by a period of constipation. It is used to rid the bowel of irritants and infections.

Phenolphthalein is colourless in acids and goes red in alkalis. Its purgative action was discovered as the result of the proposal that it should be added to adulterated wines so that they could be identified by adding alkali to them. Phenolphthalein does not act directly on the small intestine, its effect is due to an action on the colon, which is followed by reflex stimulation of peristaltic activity in the small intestine. The drug is absorbed in the small intestine but some is then secreted into the bile and the colon. This, and its indirect stimulant action, makes its effect slow to appear and prolonged in duration.

Since it is active in small doses, an overdose is easily taken and harm may be done when the compound is distributed in laxative chocolate or in chewing gum form among irresponsible people. It produces diarrhoea and some individuals are unusually susceptible to its action.

Anthracene Purgatives

Aloes, cascara, rhubarb, and **senna** are popular drugs for treating chronic constipation. They

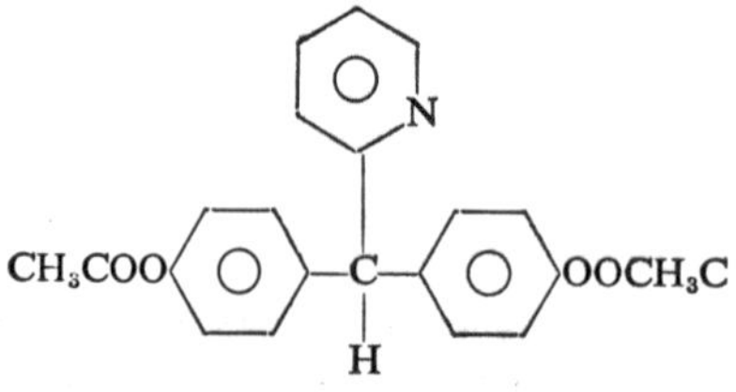

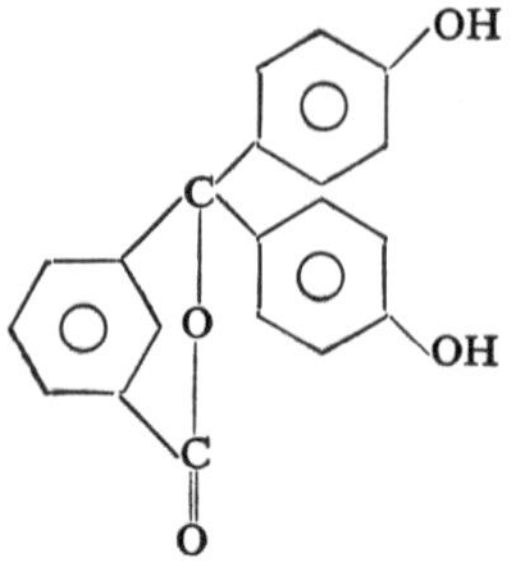

FIG. 11.1. The structures of bisacodyl and phenolphthalein.

are classed together because they contain the anthracene group, usually combined with two atoms of oxygen to form anthraquinone, and with other groups to form emodine. In the crude drug the anthracene group is also combined with sugars to form glycosides. These glycosides are themselves inactive but the active emodine is liberated in the body.

Anthracene purgatives act after a comparatively long latent period (about 10 hours). This is because, like phenolphthalein, they do not act directly on the small intestine. They are absorbed in the small intestine and their active principle is re-secreted in the bile and the colon. **Emodine,** the active principle, then acts directly on the colon and the reflexes arising from this stimulus cause reflex stimulation of the small intestine. The active substances are partly converted in the body to chrysophanic acid, which is very similar to emodine in chemical structure.

PROTECTIVES, DEMULCENTS, AND ASTRINGENTS

Protectives are used in medicine to remove undesirable substances from the intestine and also when gases or poisons have been produced in the intestine itself and are causing flatulence and diarrhoea. Protectives act as adsorbents and are used in a form in which they have a large surface area. Adsorbents are not specific in their action and they may adsorb enzymes and nutrients as well as noxious substances. Activated charcoal is an extremely efficient adsorbent of gases and substances in solution. It is used in the form of a powder or as lozenges in the treatment of food poisoning and diarrhoea.

Kaolin is a natural aluminium silicate with great absorptive power. It is practically insoluble and when taken by the mouth it protects the gut by covering it. Its value in the treatment of diarrhoea may be partly due to this mechanical action, but is mainly due to the absorption of toxins.

Other protectives include **magnesium trisilicate, kieselguhr, fuller's earth, zinc oxide, chalk,** and **starch.**

A demulcent is a colloidal solution of a high molecular weight gum or protein, the molecules of which are adsorbed on surfaces where they form a thin, but fairly consistent, protective film.

They are used in the form of mouth washes and gargles, and as pastilles and lozenges to treat inflamed surfaces of the mouth and throat. They are also used to protect inflamed regions of the gastro-intestinal tract.

Gums consist of complex carbohydrates which yield sugars on hydrolysis with acid: colloidal solutions of gums in water are known as mucilages. **Tragacanth** and **acacia** are gums used for making emulsions and suspensions, and as a basis for pills. Demulcents include **glycerin, propylene glycol,** and the **polyethylene glycols.**

Astringents are compounds which precipitate proteins, and this effect can easily be demonstrated by adding the astringent to a protein solution in a test-tube. They are applied locally to mucous membranes and the skin where their actions are confined to the surface layers. They form a protective layer of precipitated protein and inhibit exudations and the secretion of mucous glands. The membrane looks pale and the word astringent (drawn together) denotes the fact that it has a puckered appearance. In the intestine they tend to check diarrhoea and cause constipation. Many of the heavy metals are astringents. Aluminium, copper, zinc, iron, and lead are all applied as astringents to the skin or used as mouth washes and gargles. Substances of vegetable origin containing tannin possess astringent properties. Tannic acid, which is liberated from these preparations, produces water-insoluble protein precipitates which can be dissolved in acids or alkalis with the reformation of the tannic acid.

Preparations containing **tannic acid** have limited therapeutic uses but, in combination with silver nitrate, they have been used externally for the treatment of burns and skid ulcers. Tannic acid also precipitates alkaloins and heavy metals and has found a limited use in cases of poisoning by these substances. Other forms of treatment for burns and poisoning are usually preferred because they are more effective and precipitated tannates may be absorbed to cause general toxic effects.

FURTHER READING

BRODY, M., and BACHRACH, W. H. (1959) Antacids I. Comparative biochemical and economical considerations, *Amer. J. dig. Dis.*, **4**, 435.

GREGORY, R. A. (1965) Secretory mechanisms of the gastrointestinal tract, *Ann. Rev. Physiol.*, **27**, 395.

JAMES, A. H. (1957) *The Physiology of Gastric Digestion*, London.

WANG, S. C. (1965) Emetic and antiemetic drugs, in *Physiological Pharmacology*, ed. ROOT, W. S., and HOFFMANN, F. G., Vol. 2, p. 256, New York.

12

VITAMINS

THE vitamins are organic compounds which must be supplied in the diet or injected into the body in order to maintain health. Essential amino acids, which are required in larger quantities, are not usually called vitamins, but the daily dose separating vitamins from other dietary essentials has not been defined and the exact boundaries of this chapter depend upon convention. Vitamins are classified as water or fat soluble.

THE WATER-SOLUBLE VITAMINS

[see TABLE 12.1 and FIG. 12.1]

Vitamin C (Ascorbic Acid)

This is a white crystalline solid related to the hexoses. The natural active isomer rotates polarized light to the right, but it is called L-ascorbic acid because it is related to other sugars which are L-isomers.

Vitamin C is a strong reducing agent and is rapidly oxidized by oxygen, especially in alkaline solutions or in the presence of traces of copper. It is easily destroyed by cooking and by an enzyme present in plant tissue.

The first product of oxidation is dehydroascorbic acid and this compound contains all the biological activity of the vitamin and will cure scurvy. Further oxidation is irreversible and abolishes biological activity.

Ascorbic acid is readily absorbed from the intestine and is stored in various tissues, particularly the liver, adrenals, pituitary, and the corpus luteum.

Large doses of vitamin C produce no observable effects in the normal individual but in the vitamin C-deficient person there is immediate alleviation of the deficiency symptoms.

It is likely that ascorbic acid and dehydroascorbic acid play a part in cellular respiration. Ascorbic acid can be oxidized by cytochrome oxidase in the presence of cytochrome C while dehydroascorbic acid can be reduced by glutathione. Ascorbic acid can serve as a hydrogen donor in respiratory systems and may help to maintain —SH activated enzymes in their reduced forms.

Ascorbic acid is concerned in carbohydrate metabolism and deficient animals tend to be hyperglycaemic and to have a diminished glucose tolerance.

A lack of ascorbic acid causes scurvy in man, monkeys, and guinea-pigs, but other animals such as dogs and rats do not get scurvy because their intestinal bacteria can synthesize ascorbic acid. The fundamental lesion caused by a lack of ascorbic acid is that the intercellular cement is weakened because the collagen fibres, normally embedded in it, disappear. Scurvy develops slowly and is associated with weakness and a general appearance of illness. The strength of the capillaries is diminished and haemorrhages occur all over the body and particularly in the skin, gums, periosteum, joints, and intestine. The patient often becomes anaemic due to the presence of numerous small haemorrhages and blood losses into the gastro-intestinal tract and urine. There are characteristic changes in the teeth and the bones become weakened. During infections more ascorbic acid is used by the body and, unless the intake is large, the stores become depleted. Wounds heal slowly or not at all

TABLE 12.1. THE WATER-SOLUBLE VITAMINS

VITAMIN	OTHER NAME	APPROX. DAILY REQUIREMENT (ADULT)	MAIN NATURAL SOURCE	DEFICIENCY DISEASE	THERAPEUTIC USE
C	Ascorbic acid	70–75 mg.	Fruit, vegetables, potatoes, rose hips, etc.	Scurvy	Prevention and treatment of scurvy
P	Rutin, Citrin	..	Fruit, vegetables, potatoes, rose hips, etc.	None in man	Treatment of purpura (?)
B_1	Aneurine, Thiamine	1·6 mg.	Yeast, wheat germ, pork fat, rye bread	Beriberi	Thiamine deficiency and some kinds of neuritis
B_2	Riboflavine, Lactoflavin	1·8 mg.	Yeast, liver, meat extract, human milk, beef	Ariboflavinosis	Riboflavine deficiency
B_6	Pyridoxine, Adermine	1·5 mg.	Yeast, potatoes, liver	Rare in man	Pyridoxine deficiency
Nicotinamide	Niacin, Nicotinic acid	20 mg.	Meat extract, yeast, liver, bread	Pellagra	Treatment of pellagra
Pantothenic acid	..	10 mg.	Yeast, liver	Unknown in man	No established use
Folic acid	..	50 µg.	Yeast, liver, vegetables	Megaloblastic anaemia, sprue	Folic acid deficiency
B_{12}	Cobalamin, Cyanocobalamin	10 µg.	Liver	Pernicious anaemia	Cobalamin deficiency
H	Biotin	..	Yeast, chocolate, intestinal bacterial flora	Rare in man	No established use
Choline	..	250–600 mg.	Eggs, meat, cereal, milk, etc.	Fatty liver (?)	Some forms of liver disease (?)

and the scars lack strength. Minor degrees of vitamin C deficiency are common, though outright scurvy only occurs when the diet is markedly deficient in fresh fruit and vegetables. Milk is not a good source of ascorbic acid, and if it is boiled it loses its activity, so that infants should always be given orange juice or some such other supplement.

Ascorbic acid has been used to treat various diseases in which haemorrhages are particularly likely to occur. The fact that the body tends to become unsaturated during fevers has led to its administration in various infections.

Vitamin P (Citrin, Rutin, Hesperidin)

The existence of vitamin P was suggested when it was found that crude extracts of ascorbic acid were more effective than the pure substance in prolonging the lives of scorbutic animals. Several substances share the biological action of vitamin P in reducing capillary permeability and all are related to flavone. Substances called vitamin P are sometimes also known as flavonoids.

Vitamin P has not been chemically identified but rutin has the same biological properties and its structure is shown in FIGURE 12.1.

Little, if any, vitamin P is absorbed from the gastro-intestinal tract and experiments designed to show an antiscorbutic action for this vitamin require its parenteral injection. For this reason there is some doubt as to whether vitamin P should be considered a natural vitamin.

The substances included under the term 'vitamin P' have a direct constrictor action on

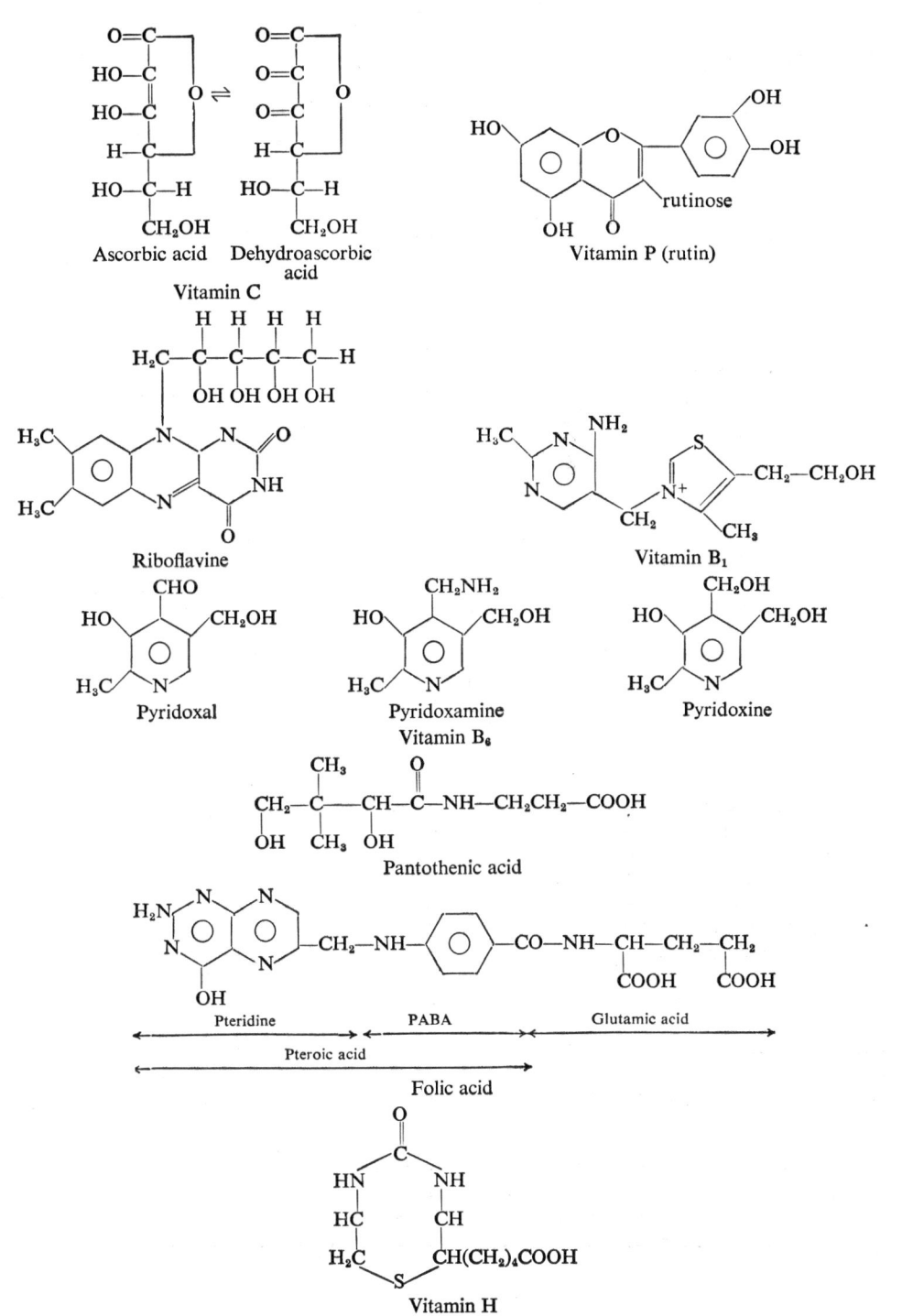

FIG. 12.1. The structures of the water-soluble vitamins.

capillaries and reduce their fragility and permeability.

The status of vitamin P as a natural vitamin is not well established and deficiency symptoms have not been demonstrated but it has been used widely for a variety of therapeutic reasons. It is usually given orally even though it is probably not absorbed by this route. It has been chiefly used to treat diseases where there is capillary bleeding and increased capillary fragility, i.e. allergic states and diabetes mellitus.

THE VITAMIN B COMPLEX

The vitamins in this group comprise a large number of chemically different compounds with a variety of actions. They are commonly grouped under one heading because they are all water soluble and may be extracted from liver and yeast.

The substances forming the vitamin B complex are **aneurine** (thiamine, vitamin B_1), **riboflavine** (vitamin B_2), **pyridoxine** (vitamin B_6), **nicotinic acid, pantothenic acid, cyanocobalamin** (vitamin B_{12}), **folic acid, biotin** (vitamin H), and **choline**.

Vitamin B_1 (Aneurine, Thiamine)

Vitamin B_1 is more stable than ascorbic acid, but less stable than the other vitamins. In neutral solutions a little less than half of it is destroyed in 4 hours at 100° C. Certain bacteria can synthesize vitamin B_1 and they may occur in the intestine and protect an animal from deficiency diseases.

The vitamin contains a pyrimidine ring and a thiazole ring and is active in the body as the coenzyme thiamine pyrophosphate. The formation of this coenzyme requires the presence of adenosine triphosphate. Antimetabolites to thiamine have been synthesized and these include **neopyrithiamine** (pyrithiamine) and **oxythiamine**.

Thiamine pyrophosphate is the coenzyme necessary for the decarboxylation of pyruvic and α-keto-glutaric acids and is therefore important in carbohydrate metabolism. Animals fed on a thiamine-deficient diet suffer from deficiency of this coenzyme so that pyruvic acid accumulates, and this causes an accumulation of lactic acid, since lactic acid is normally converted to pyruvic acid. Both acids accumulate, and abnormally high concentrations are found in the blood.

The accumulation of lactic acid deranges the earlier phases of carbohydrate metabolism, and the animal is unable to tolerate normal quantities of carbohydrate in the diet. The fact that a carbohydrate-rich diet was liable to accentuate beriberi has been known for a long time, but the detailed explanation of this effect has only become evident fairly recently.

Thiamine deficiency eventually leads to the condition known as beriberi. Beriberi was one of the first deficiency diseases to be recognized and, although it can now be easily diagnosed and treated, it is still widespread in some parts of the Far East.

The symptoms of this deficiency disease include polyneuritis, cardiac failure, and reduced growth.

Thiamine is used therapeutically in the treatment of beriberi, and various kinds of neuritis, including alcoholic neuritis and neuritis of pregnancy, both of which may actually be due to a lack of this vitamin.

Vitamin B_2 (Riboflavine)

Riboflavine consists of an orange-yellow pigment, lumiflavin, combined with ribose. It can be made synthetically, and is fairly stable, but is destroyed by alkali or by light, in which it gives off a bright green fluorescence.

Riboflavine acts in the body in the form of riboflavine phosphate or flavine adenine dinucleotide. These coenzymes act as hydrogen carriers between pyridine nucleotides and cytochrome systems and play an important part in metabolism.

Rats fed on a riboflavine-deficient diet do not grow, and eventually develop inflammation of the skin, and cataracts. Deficiency in man causes pallor followed by inflammation of the tongue (glossitis) and skin (seborrhoeic dermatitis). The cornea becomes vascularized, apparently because it is normally dependent on riboflavine for its metabolism. Riboflavine is also necessary for the growth of certain kinds of bacteria.

Riboflavine is used therapeutically only for the correction of deficiency disease.

Vitamine B$_6$ (Pyridoxine)

Like nicotinic acid, pyridoxine is a simple derivative of pyridine. It can be estimated chemically and is present in yeast, wheat germ, liver, muscle, and various vegetables.

Pyridoxine is only one of three forms in which vitamin B$_6$ can exist naturally, the other forms are pyridoxal and pyridoxamine. The active forms of the vitamin are pyridoxal phosphate and pyridoxamine phosphate whose formation is catalysed by pyridoxal kinase. An important role for pyridoxine is as a coenzyme for decarboxylases.

Isonicotinic acid hydrazide (isoniazid) antagonizes the pyridoxal kinase reaction and so has an anti-vitamin-B$_6$ action by blocking the formation of the active form of the vitamin.

Lack of pyridoxine in the diet of rats makes their extremities red, swollen, and oedematous. This condition was once thought to be identical with pellagra, and was known as rat pellagra. It is said that this is worse in cold weather and is analogous to chilblains. Prolonged deficiency may cause anaemia and fits.

Pyridoxine may be given to people receiving isoniazid in order to prevent peripheral neuritis. It is not certain whether man can become pyridoxine-deficient but this vitamin is usually given if there is any deficiency of B complex vitamins.

Nicotinamide (Niacin, Nicotinic Acid)

Nicotinic acid has a more simple molecule than other vitamins, and can easily be synthesized. Its presence in yeast was discovered in 1912, but its function as a vitamin was not known until 1938. Its amide (**nicotinamide**) has the same action.

In the body nicotinic acid is converted to diphosphopyridine nucleotide (NAD) or to triphosphopyridine nucleotide (NADP) and these compounds have an important role as coenzymes for many proteins involved in tissue respiration. Nicotinic acid but not nicotinamide has a direct action on blood vessels causing vasodilatation.

A deficiency of nicotinic acid in the diet produces pellagra, a disease which still occurs among poorly nourished populations in Egypt, the southern states of North America, and other countries in the same latitude. The classical signs of the disease are dermatitis, diarrhoea, and dementia. The most obvious changes are in the skin, which becomes particularly susceptible to sunburn, so that all exposed parts become inflamed and blistered. The nervous symptoms include disturbances of the brain, the spinal cord, and the peripheral nerves.

Most of these symptoms are the result of a deficiency of nicotinic acid and the disease is particularly liable to occur among alcoholics, partly because alcoholics do not usually choose their food carefully, and possibly also because they lose the power of absorbing nicotinic acid.

Nicotinic acid and nicotinamide are used in the treatment of pellagra. High doses may be needed initially and nicotinic acid, in these doses, may cause vasodilatation with flushing and itching of the skin.

Pantothenic Acid

Pantothenic acid is converted to coenzyme A in the body and is active in this form. Pantothenic acid was first recognized as the factor whose absence was responsible for a form of dermatitis in chickens. The effects of deficiency in rats are a loss of weight, grey hair, inflammation of the nose with a red discharge containing porphyrin, and haemorrhages and atrophy in the adrenals. It is essential for the growth of yeast and some bacteria.

Coenzyme A is essential in metabolism as a coenzyme for many enzyme-catalysed reactions involving the transfer of acyl groups.

There is no accepted therapeutic use for pantothenic acid.

Folic Acid (Pteroylmonoglutamic Acid)

Folic acid got its name from the fact that it is commonly present in green leaves. It appeared first as vitamin M and then as vitamin B_c, vitamins which were necessary for the health of monkeys and chickens respectively.

Studies of the nutritional requirements of *Lactobacillus casei* led to the isolation of folic acid in 1945. It contains $2NH_2$-4-OH-pteridine, para-aminobenzoic acid, and glutamic acid [see FIG. 13.2]. Natural folic acid is found conjugated with several molecules of glutamate attached to it in peptide linkages.

Folic acid is converted in the body to dihydrofolate and tetrahydrofolate by folate reductase and these compounds accept a transferable one-carbon group which plays an important part in the synthesis of purine rings and some amino acids. If there is a shortage of purine compounds this means there is a shortage of materials from which nucleic acid is made, and it is therefore not surprising that the production of new cells may depend on the presence of folic acid.

Vitamin B_{12} (Cyanocobalamin)

Liver extracts do not contain enough folic acid to account for all their therapeutic effects in megaloblastic anaemia. Fractions had been prepared which were more active, in smaller doses than folic acid, and which cured lesions of the spinal cord on which folic acid had no effect. These fractions were further purified in Britain but a comparatively quick microbiological assay was developed in America and vitamin B_{12} was isolated there in 1948, just before it was isolated in Britain. The original vitamin B_{12} is known as cyanocobalamin. Other cobalamins, with groups other than cyanide, are known, but can easily be converted to cyanocobalamin which is the one generally available.

Cyanocobalamin is a complex porphyrin-like ring structure called cobamide with a co-ordinate cobalt atom [see FIG. 13.1]. Cyanocobalamin is concerned in the biosynthesis of the methyl groups of thymidine and methionine and, through these, most of the N-methyl, S-methyl, and O-methyl groups of naturally occurring compounds. It is thus associated, at least indirectly, with every known metabolic system.

It is essential for normal growth, haematopoiesis, and for the production of epithelial cells and the maintenance of myelin in the nervous system.

Its action on the blood-forming elements and the results of deficiency are described in Chapter 13.

Vitamin H (Biotin)

Biotin acts as a coenzyme for several enzyme-catalysed carboxylation reactions and therefore plays an important role in CO_2 fixation.

The effects of deficiency include loss of weight and hair, exfoliative dermatitis, hyperkeratosis, and spasticity. This condition is rare in man, but a striking case has been described. An Italian labourer had a passion for raw eggs, and ate about ten a day. Raw egg white contains a protein known as avidin which combines with biotin and prevents its absorption. His blood biotin fell and he had dermatitis. The administration of biotin reversed this condition.

Choline

Choline cannot be classed as a true vitamin because it is present in the body in much larger amounts than are usually associated with vitamins, and because no co-factor concerned in enzymic reactions and containing choline has been found.

Choline has qualitatively similar pharmacological actions to acetylcholine but is very much less potent. It is involved in fat metabolism and is important as a methyl donor in intermediary metabolism. It is also a precursor for acetylcholine.

In order to produce a choline-deficient animal it is necessary to deprive it, not only of choline, but also of methionine. This is because choline can be synthesized from

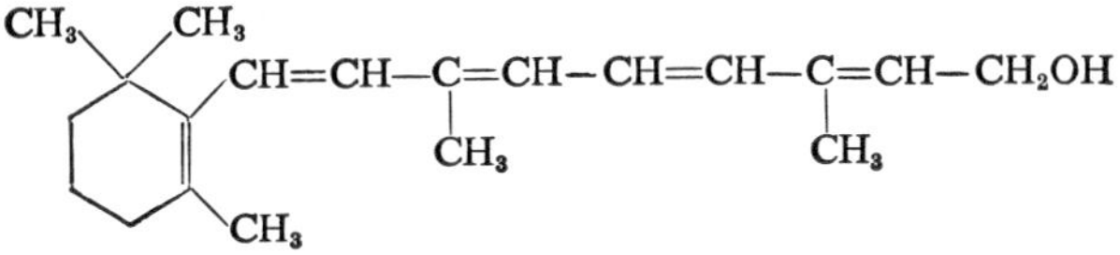

Vitamin A

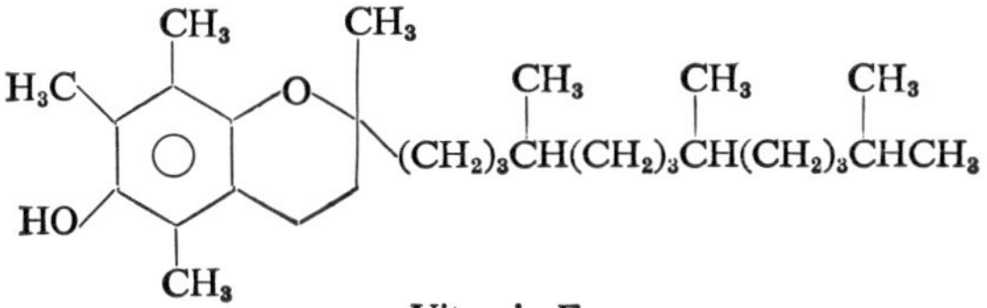

Vitamin E

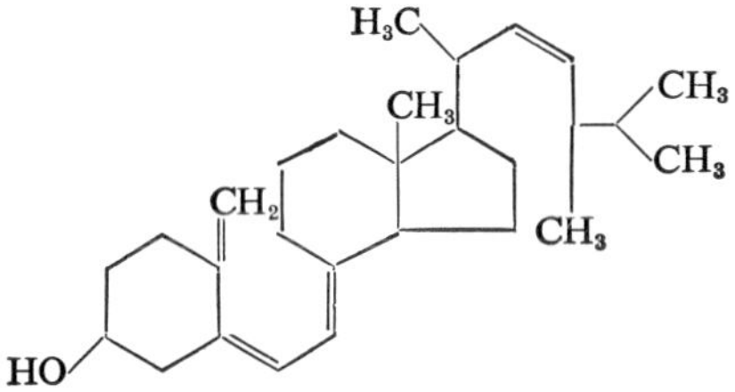

Vitamin D_2

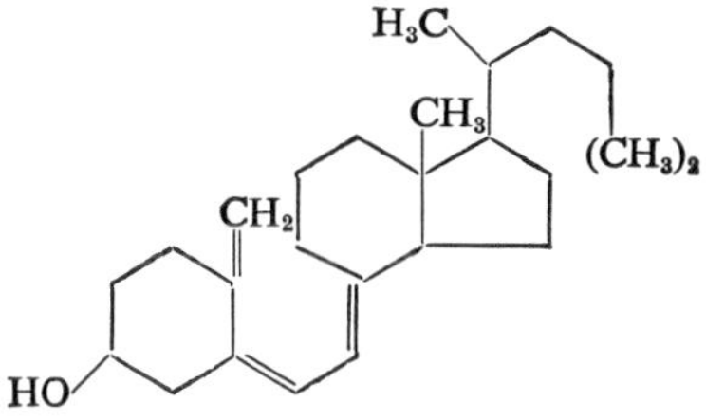

Vitamin D_3

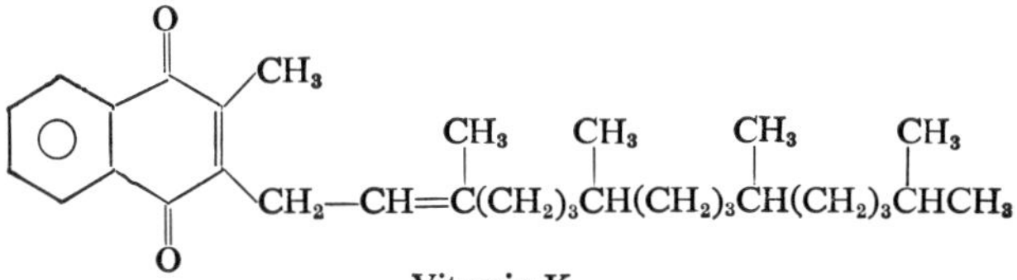

Vitamin K_1

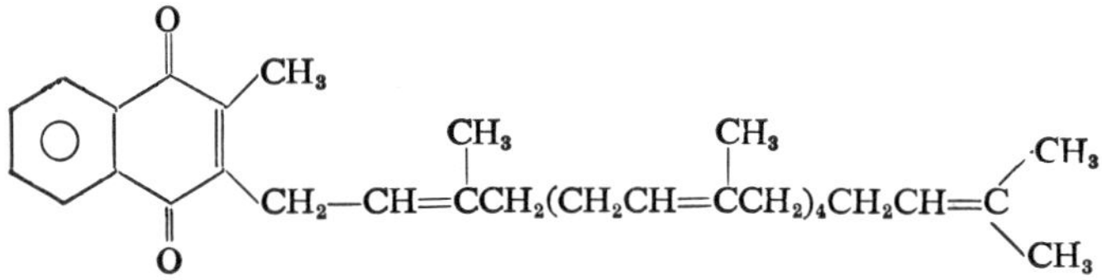

Vitamin K_2

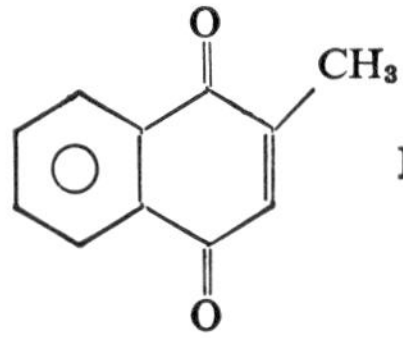

Menaphthone (menadione)

FIG. 12.2. The structures of fat-soluble vitamins.

phosphatidylethanolamine with methionine acting as a methyl donor.

As a result of choline deficiency the fat content of the liver increases and hepatic cirrhosis may result. It seems unlikely that this ever happens in man and no effects of choline deficiency have been observed on cholinergic mechanisms.

Choline and methionine have sometimes been used in the treatment of liver disease.

FAT-SOLUBLE VITAMINS

[see FIG. 12.2]

Vitamin A

Vitamin A is a long-chain alcohol with five double bonds and is obtained from fish-liver oils. If two such molecules are joined together by a double bond with the elimination of two molecules of water at the place where the hydroxyl group is, the result is β-carotene. Carotenes form the red pigment in carrots; they are converted by the body to vitamin A, each molecule of carotene forming one molecule of vitamin A.

Vitamin A is fairly stable at temperatures up to 120° C. in the absence of oxygen, but it is oxidized by aeration even at room temperature, and is destroyed by light. Neither vitamin A nor carotene is destroyed by ordinary cooking.

Vitamin A is well absorbed through the wall of the gastro-intestinal tract, and only if an amount exceeding the daily requirement is ingested does any appear in the faeces. Since the vitamin is fat soluble, its absorption will be related to lipid absorption and in cases of disordered fat absorption it may be necessary to use water-miscible solutions of the vitamin.

Vitamin A plays an essential role in the function of the retina, in the maintenance of epithelial cells, and probably in the synthesis of glucocorticoids. There is also evidence that it may be a growth-promoting factor.

Deficiency of vitamin A reduces vision in dim light because adaptation of the retinal rods to poor illumination is affected. The chemical concerned with dim light vision is rhodopsin which is a combination of a protein, opsin, and a prosthetic group, retinene (11-cis-vitamin A aldehyde). During the synthesis of rhodopsin, cis-vitamin A is converted into cis-retinene and this then combines with opsin to form rhodopsin. The action of light on rhodopsin converts the retinene part of the molecule into the trans-isomer, trans-retinene.

The trans-retinine then dissociates from the opsin and nerve impulses are generated.

The trans-retinene can be reconverted to rhodopsin, via cis-retinene, or may be reduced to trans-vitamin A and then back to vitamin A.

In vitamin A deficiency the retinal rhodopsin concentration falls because it can no longer be synthesized in adequate amounts.

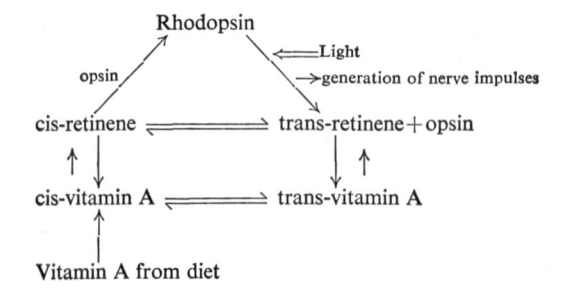

FIG. 12.3. The rhodopsin cycle.

The failure to dark adapt as a result of vitamin A deficiency is quickly overcome by administering the vitamin.

Reserves of the vitamin in the tissues are usually sufficiently large to prevent deficiency except in cases of disordered fat absorption.

Because vitamin A deficiency, when it does occur, leads to epithelial lesions and infections, the vitamin is sometimes given to combat infections but this use is unjustified. The only legitimate use of vitamin A is to treat a deficiency of this vitamin. It may be given as **cod-liver oil** or as **halibut-liver oil**.

Vitamin D

Several substances, all derived from steroids, cure or prevent rickets.

The name 'vitamin D' is applied to two fat-soluble compounds, calciferol (vitamin D_2) and activated 7-dehydrocholesterol (vitamin D_3).

If the bond joining C_9 and C_{10} atoms in steroids is broken by ultra-violet irradiation the resulting compound will often prevent or cure rickets.

When steroids are irradiated, a whole series of products is formed, the amounts of each depending on the prevailing conditions. If ergosterol is irradiated then vitamin D_2 (calciferol) is formed and irradiation of 7-dehydrocholesterol forms vitamin D_3 (activated dehydrocholesterol) the natural vitamin. These two products do not differ greatly in their antirachitic potencies in man.

These substances are soluble in fats and fat solvents. They are reasonably stable and keep in cod-liver oil for several years; they are not destroyed by ordinary cooking. Absorption from the alimentary tract depends on the presence of bile and does not occur if this is absent.

The level of calcium and phosphate in the blood is dependent on the level of vitamin D in the blood. Although vitamin D plays an important part in the regulation of these ions the major role is played by the parathyroid hormone and a smaller part by thyrocalcitonin, ion absorption in the gastro-intestinal tract, skeletal metabolism, and excretion through the kidneys. The part played by vitamin D is further complicated because it is itself required in order to maintain full parathyroid activity [Chapter 14]. The level of calcium ions in the blood is also influenced by the blood pH and by the concentration of plasma proteins.

Calcium salts are important components of the skeletal system and calcium ions are necessary for the functioning of nerves and muscles and for the coagulation of blood, Abnormal levels of calcium in the body may cause malfunction of these systems and so signify a possible deficiency of vitamin D.

In rickets, the calcification of bone is deficient. Dogs or humans get rickets whenever they lack vitamin D. Vitamin D cures rickets by increasing the absorption of phosphate and of calcium from the intestine.

Rickets is a disease of the young. Osteomalacia is a similar disease, due to similar causes, occurring in adults and particularly in pregnant women, who are more susceptible than others because they lose calcium and phosphorus to the foetus.

One result of the action of vitamin D is an increase in the calcium and phosphate in the blood, but the action of vitamin D must be distinguished from that of parathyroid extracts, which also increase the blood calcium, but do so by causing the absorption of calcium from the bones.

The signs of vitamin D deficiency are: (1) The bones are deficient in calcium and phosphorus, soft and liable to bend, so that the person becomes bow-legged or knock-kneed, and the thorax and pelvis are deformed. (2) The teeth are badly formed and liable to become diseased. (3) If the blood calcium falls very low, tetany is produced, and this may occur among children with rickets. (4) The parathyroids become overactive to maintain the blood calcium by liberating calcium from the bones; this tends to make the rickets worse.

Hypervitaminosis D is not uncommon. It occurs in any person who receives excess of the vitamin, often during the treatment of vitamin D deficiency.

Vitamin E

There are several active tocopherols, known collectively as vitamin E. They are fat-soluble alcohols, which have been synthesized, and are associated with reproductive processes. Vitamin E is unstable in rancid fats, being easily oxidized, but stable to ordinary cooking. It is stored in the body, and signs of deficiency take many months to develop. An important chemical property of vitamin E is that it is an anti-oxidant and forms reversible oxidation–reduction systems.

Vitamin E is absorbed through the gastro-intestinal tract in the same way as other fat-soluble vitamins. It is stored in the tissues and the body can be supplied from these stores for a long period. For this reason a vitamin E deficiency can only be obtained by the prolonged ingestion of a vitamin E-deficient diet.

Despite numerous investigations into the action of vitamin E in the body, the subject is still controversial. Even animals whose tissues contain no vitamin E are able to reproduce normally and bear normal offspring.

It may be that vitamin E merely mimics and supplements a naturally occurring coenzyme with similar properties. Where vitamin E acts as an anti-oxidant it is likely that other, unrelated anti-oxidants can take over its role during periods of deficiency.

Vitamin K

Vitamin K is essential for the synthesis in the body of several factors concerned with the clotting of blood. Animals which are deficient in vitamin K tend to bleed easily and this has been shown to be due to a fall in the circulating level of prothrombin.

Vitamin K is fat soluble and consists of at least two naturally occurring substances (vitamins K_1 and K_2), both of which are derivatives of naphthoquinone. More simple substances which contain this group, e.g. **menaphthone** (menadione), have the same effect as the natural vitamins and are slightly more water soluble.

Vitamins K_1 and K_2 are only absorbed from the gastro-intestinal tract if bile salts are present. A deficiency of the vitamins may arise when bile is held back in obstructive jaundice. Other conditions which reduce its absorption include ulcerative colitis, sprue, or large doses of liquid paraffin. Menaphthone is absorbed in the absence of bile salts and enters the blood directly, unlike the natural vitamin K which is absorbed via the lymphatic system.

Vitamin K in the intestines is partially derived from the food and is partly formed by intestinal flora. When rats are raised under sterile conditions, without vitamin K in their diet and without bacteria in their intestines, haemorrhages occur but they disappear in a few days if the normal intestinal flora is allowed to develop.

There appears to be no significant storage of vitamin K in the body.

Vitamin K is concerned in the synthesis of prothrombin and factors VII, IX, and X in the liver and this is described in detail in Chapter 13.

FURTHER READING

HARRIS, J. L. (1955) *Vitamins in Theory and Practice*, Cambridge.

SEBRELL, W. H., and HARRIS, R. S. (1954) *The Vitamins: Chemistry, Physiology, Pathology*, New York.

WEISSBACH, H., and DICKERMAN, H. (1965) Biochemical role of vitamin B_{12}, *Physiol. Rev.*, **45,** 80.

13

BLOOD

RED blood cells are formed in the bone marrow from stem cells which divide and give rise to more mature cells which show two prominent changes as they mature, the acquisition of the iron-containing respiratory pigment haemoglobin and the dissolution and disappearance of the nucleus so that the mature cell when released into the circulation is a biconcave disc of about 7·5 μ diameter and containing 33 per cent. haemoglobin (0·1 per cent. Fe). The cells survive in the circulation for some 120 days before degenerating and being removed from the circulation, the released pigment is metabolized, the iron set free, and returned to the stores. This means that a little less than 1 per cent. of the circulating red cells are being replaced daily. The circulating red cell mass is controlled by homeostatic processes probably mediated by both central nervous and renal mechanisms that control the secretion of a glycoprotein, erythropoietin, which stimulates red cell production. Normal red cell formation depends also on an adequate supply of iron and of the coenzymes, coenzyme B_{12} and tetrahydrofolate which are necessary for nucleotide synthesis.

The total iron pool of the body is composed of that in the red cell mass (2·5 g.), tissue iron (myoglobin, haemenzymes, etc. 0·3 g.), that in iron stores (1 g.), and the small amount circulating in the plasma (4 mg.). The iron stores are mainly in the form of ferritin, a complex of ferric iron with a protein apoferritin found mostly in the liver, spleen, and bone marrow. Iron is transported in the plasma in ferric form in another complex with a special plasma protein transferrin, so that virtually no free iron is normally present, indeed whereas the plasma iron concentration is about 1·2 mg./l. the binding capacity of the transferrin present is about 3·2 mg./l. so that the plasma is capable of accepting a further 2 mg./l. of iron (a total of 10 mg. iron) without its binding capacity being saturated. Since 1/120 of the red cells are being broken down and newly formed each day the amount of iron required each day is about 20 mg. but nearly all of this is recycled from the stores and the normal amount absorbed from the diet is only about 1 mg. a day, this being balanced by excretion in the urine and by the gut.

Because such a small proportion of the iron is obtained from dietary intake extra losses of iron are very important. These are especially so in women who lose iron in menstruation, pregnancy, and lactation and are therefore much more susceptible to iron deficiency than males. The effects of dietary deficiency of iron take a long while to develop—if there were no iron at all in the diet and the loss remained at 1 mg. a day it would take 3 years to drain the iron stores. Iron loss can occur much more rapidly with acute or chronic blood loss, thus the loss of 1 litre of blood is equivalent to the loss of 0·5 g. Fe or half the reserve. In chronic iron deficiency the red cells are reduced in numbers and they are small and deficient in haemoglobin content. On administration of iron in adequate amounts rapid restoration can occur at rates of up to 15 g. haemoglobin (50 mg. Fe) per day.

Iron is not very well absorbed from food, the over-all absorption being about 5–10 per cent. and may be lower owing to natural chelators such as phytate in the diet. Inorganic iron salts administered orally are well absorbed (20–30 per cent.) when given in small amounts but the fraction absorbed decreases as the total amount is increased. In iron

136 Blood

deficiency absorption is considerably improved but it is still not clear why this should be so.

ORAL IRON PREPARATIONS

The most commonly used are **ferrous sulphate, ferrous gluconate, ferrous fumarate,** and **ferric ammonium citrate**. In severe iron deficiency the amounts given must be quite large, i.e. of the order of 100–300 mg. a day with lesser amounts in milder cases. All these preparations are liable to cause such gastro-intestinal disturbances as epigastric pain, colic, and diarrhoea and these side actions may make it impossible to give adequate doses by mouth. Serious toxicity is rare in adults but it is not uncommon and highly dangerous in children, who are attracted by iron tablets which are sugar coated and brightly coloured. Iron toxicity demands energetic treatment including sequestration of the iron by the chelator desferrioxamine given by gavage and intravenously and supportive therapy must be given to deal with the accompanying shock. Desferrioxamine is a hydroxypeptide isolated from *Streptomyces pilosus*, each molecule of which can bind one molecule of trivalent iron.

In patients who are unable to tolerate oral iron preparations, iron may be given by intramuscular injection as the non-ionic complexes **iron sorbitol** and **iron dextran**. Iron dextran and iron dextrin may be given intravenously. The amount of iron given by these routes is commonly 20–50 mg. Since this exceeds the plasma iron binding capacity there is considerable risk of systemic toxicity. There may be anaphylactic-like effects with dizziness, tachycardia, sweating, nausea and vomiting, and circulatory collapse. Moreover, delayed allergic type responses may also occur. Because of the unpleasantness and danger of these responses parenteral iron should be restricted to those who really need it, i.e. those really intolerant of oral iron and those who are refractory to oral preparations.

MACROCYTIC ANAEMIAS

When there is a dietary deficiency of **cobalamins** or **folates** the erythrocytes are decreased in numbers but increased in size and some nucleated cells may escape into the circulation. The defect appears to be one of nucleic acid synthesis which retards cell division. Both of these substances form coenzymes concerned in the transfer of one carbon unit in the biosynthesis of purines and pyrimidines. The effects of deficiency are not confined to the bone marrow, effects also being seen on epithelia in the gut, skin, and hair. Cobalamins are also necessary for the survival of neurones in the CNS and

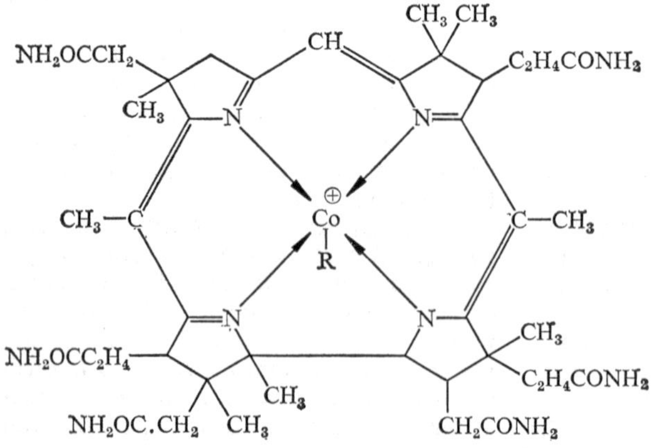

Fig. 13.1. Cobalamin (vitamin B_{12}).

in deficiency a characteristic syndrome, subacute combined degeneration, develops.

The role of cobalamins in erythrocyte development stems from the discovery by Minot and Murphy that liver had a curative effect in pernicious anaemia (the commonest form of macrocytic anaemia in temperate climates) and the finding by Castle that there was no dietary deficiency *per se* but a failure to absorb a dietary factor due to the lack of the absorption promoting factor, 'intrinsic factor', a mucoprotein secreted by the gastro-intestinal epithelium. Purification eventually led to isolation and characterization of cyanocobalamin. This was greatly aided by the finding that the liver factor was a growth factor for some bacteria such as *Lactobacillus lactis*. The vitamin is red in colour, and it was noticed that cultures of *Streptomyces* var. gave pink-coloured culture fluids which were found to be rich in cobalamins. This is now the source of the material used therapeutically.

Cobalamins are not synthesized by animals, which are therefore dependent on dietary sources; deficiency can occur from inadequate intake but is much more frequently due to gastro-intestinal disturbances interfering with absorption [see Chapter 12]. The estimated daily requirement is about 10 μg. In normal individuals cyanocobalamin is rapidly and efficiently absorbed (> 50 per cent.) and is stored in the tissues, notably in the liver, which may contain about 1 mg./kg. wet weight.

Cobalamin has a very complicated chemical structure based on a ring structure closely related to the porphyrins with a cobalt atom held in co-ordinate linkage at its centre. The cobalt also may bind an additional group of which the most important are cyanide in **cyanocobalamin,** hydroxyl in **hydroxocobalamin,** and deoxyadenosine in the biochemically active form **coenzyme B$_{12}$**.

The former two are used therapeutically and differ mainly in their duration of effect. Excess cyanocobalamin is rapidly excreted in the urine because the plasma binding capacity for cyanocobalamin is low so that after giving large doses most is unbound to plasma protein, is filtered in the glomerulus, and cleared rapidly. On the other hand, hydroxocobalamin is bound to a greater extent and is rather more slowly excreted. The therapeutic advantage is debatable.

Since cobalamins are readily available and reasonably cheap, massive doses may be given at infrequent intervals. In treating pernicious anaemia, for instance, it is common to give 1 mg. twice weekly by intramuscular injection until the blood picture is normal and then the same dose once a month. Oral absorption in the enterogenic anaemias is too irregular and uncertain to be relied upon.

Folic Acid

Folic acid is another dietary factor necessary for normal erythrocyte formation but its deficiency does not lead to subacute combined degeneration of the spinal cord. It is available in many foods including green vegetables and deficiency is due either to a poor diet, this is the usual reason in tropical areas (tropical sprue), or to deficient absorption (non-tropical sprue, coeliac disease) frequently associated with intolerance to the protein gluten present in wheat flour [see Chapter 12]. Utilization of folic acid may be defective during chronic administration of anti-epileptic drugs such as phenobarbitone and phenytoin.

Folic acid itself is not the active coenzyme of one carbon transfer but must first be reduced to tetrahydrofolic acid by the enzyme folic reductase. Like the cobalamins, folic acid is efficiently stored so that only small amounts of administered doses are lost by excretion. In the treatment of true dietary deficiency satisfactory responses occur with as little as 25 μg. a day although usually 1–5 mg. is given. In coeliac disease larger doses are necessary to compensate for the poor absorption and usually 10–30 mg. are given. An effective folic acid deficiency is produced by the antifolic drugs which are specific inhibitors of the enzyme folic reductase [see Chapter 18]. In this case reversal of the untoward effects cannot be achieved with folic acid but

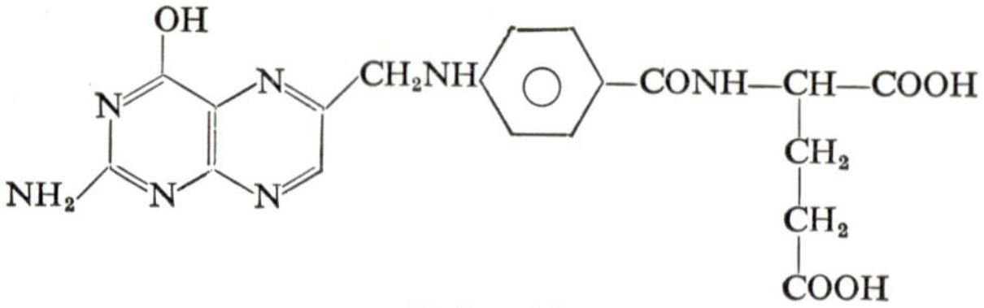

FIG. 13.2. The structures of folic acid and folinic acid.

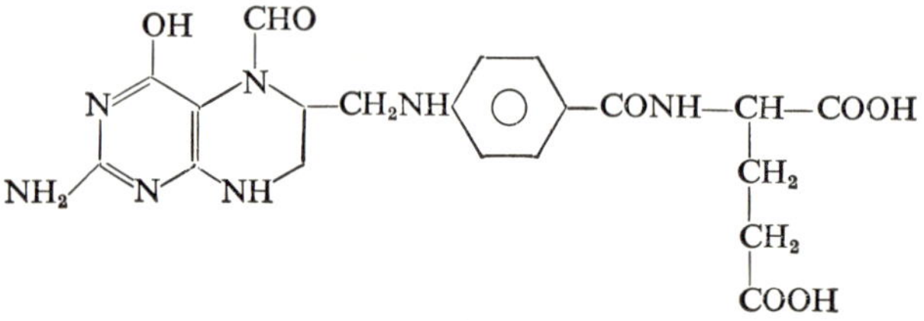

Folic acid

Folinic acid

requires a tetrahydrofolate such as folinic acid (N^5 formyltetrahydrofolinic acid).

POLYCYTHAEMIA VERA

In this condition the number of red cells produced is greater than normal due to a low-grade neoplastic change in the erythropoietic cells. The excess cells can be removed by **acetylphenylhydrazine** which causes haemolysis but this is rather dangerous. Alternatively cell production may be depressed with radioactive phosphorus, but the simplest procedure is to carry out periodic bleeding; while this reduces the cell volume directly it would in itself have only transient effects, but if the bleeding is sufficient to deplete the iron stores and this is combined with moderate restriction of dietary iron intake, the red cell mass becomes dependent on availability of iron and the red cell count remains low for long periods.

BLOOD COAGULATION

Blood coagulation involves a very complicated series of reactions ending in the conversion of the soluble plasma protein fibrinogen into a polymerized meshwork of the insoluble derivative fibrin.

The process can be initiated either in shed blood, or in the body by tissue factors, in both cases leading to the generation of factors called thromboplastins which react with prothrombin in the presence of Ca^{++} to form thrombin [TABLE 13.1].

Thrombin is a peptidase which splits off a peptide fragment fibrinopeptide from fibrinogen, leaving fibrin which then polymerizes to produce the clot.

Blood is kept fluid in the circulation by antagonists which either inhibit the steps referred to above or are able to remove or destroy the small amounts of active materials being produced. When activation of the system occurs a positive feedback ('autocatalytic') reaction develops.

Heparin

Heparin is a natural anticoagulant found in many tissues (first isolated from the liver and hence the name). It is especially concentrated in the mast cells which are basophil cells found in tissues and blood. With certain basic dyes, such as toluidine blue, the granules in these cells alter the colour of the dye from blue to purple. This metachromatic reaction is characteristic of heparinoids. Heparin has been extracted from tissues and purified; it is a polymer containing the repeating unit O,N,sulphato-glycosamino-glucuronate. Heparins extracted from different tissues and by different processes differ in their degree of polymerization and sulphation. Concentrations of heparin must still be specified in Units related to an international standard ($\sim$ 120 Units/mg.).

Heparin prevents the coagulation of blood when added *in vitro* as well as when administered systemically; the mechanism is complex, it certainly inhibits the effects of thrombin on fibrinogen provided that a co-factor is present, but it also has effects on various stages of thromboplastin generation. While clotting time is prolonged by heparin, bleeding time is little affected and the risk of haemorrhage is not great. A further interesting effect of heparin is to cause the clearing of turbid lipaemic serum by activation of the enzyme lipoprotein lipase. The physiological role of heparin is uncertain. Heparin is inactive when given orally in part due to its polyanionic character and in part to instability in the gastric juice. Injected subcutaneously or intramuscularly absorption is irregular probably due to tissue binding and local tenderness and induration may develop. It is, therefore, usually given intravenously, intermittently, or by infusion. The effects of a single intravenous injection are brief, the half-time being of the order of 0·5–2 hours. This is not due to rapid excretion since only traces are found in the urine, but due to rapid metabolism in the liver by desulphation and depolymerization.

Heparin readily forms compounds with bases. It has already been noted that toluidine blue reacts forming a molecular complex, this is inactive as an anticoagulant. A similar complex is formed by the basic polymer hexadimethrine. Proteins also form complexes with heparin that are especially strong if the protein is rich in the basic amino acids arginine and lysine. An example is the low molecular weight nuclear protein protamine. Both protamine (as the sulphate salt) and

TABLE 13.1. BLOOD CLOTTING FACTORS

	BLOOD THROMBOPLASTIN	TISSUE THROMBOPLASTIN
Ca^{++}	+	+
Factor V	+	+
Factor VII	–	+
Factor VIII	+	–
Factor IX	+	–
Platelet factors	+	–
Tissue factors	–	+

$$Prothrombin \xrightarrow[Ca^{++}]{Thromboplastin} Thrombin$$
$$\downarrow$$
$$Fibrinogen \longrightarrow Fibrin$$

hexadimethrine can be used to reverse heparin actions *in vivo* and approximately 1 mg. of either will neutralize the effects of 1 mg. heparin. They both have anticoagulant effects themselves and overdosage must be avoided. In addition, they are both liable to produce hypotension, bradycardia, flushing, etc., perhaps by releasing histamine and other vascularly active autocoids.

Heparin itself is of low toxicity and is an excellent anticoagulant whose use is largely restricted by the inconvenience of the intravenous route, the short duration of action, and high cost. Synthetic sulphated polysaccharides have been shown to be active but up to the present have shown undesirable toxicity.

The most important use of heparin is in cardiovascular surgery, in keeping blood fluid for heart–lung machines, and for brief postoperative periods to prevent mural thrombi developing at sites of surgical injury. It is also necessary in plasma dialysis (artificial kidney machines).

It is widely used in acute thrombotic disease such as cardiac infarction, pulmonary embolism, and venous thrombosis as a stopgap until longer-term anticoagulant therapy can become effective.

The Coumarin Group

The action of this group was discovered during the investigation of a haemorrhagic disease affecting cattle fed on improperly cured sweet clover. It was found that the active agent was 3,3 methylene-bis (4-hydroxycoumarin) which was given the trivial name of **dicoumarol.** Dicoumarol has no action on blood clotting *in vitro* nor does it have any immediate effect when given *in vivo* but following its administration there is a gradual decline in the concentration of both prothrombin and some of the thromboplastin components notably Factors VII, VIII, and IX; the most important of these is Factor VII. The maximum effect is produced in 1–2 days. The slowness of the effect is related to the usual turnover of these proteins. The evidence is strongly in favour of dicoumarol acting by depressing the synthesis of these proteins in the liver, so that their levels in the plasma decline as the circulating proteins are catabolized. The effects of dicoumarol can be antagonized by vitamin K in what appears to be a competitive manner. Indeed, a similar pattern of defective coagulation appears in vitamin K deficiency. Consideration of the chemical structure of vitamin K and the dicoumarol group suggests that these are structural analogues. It is not known what role vitamin K plays in the synthesis of these proteins, although vitamin K appears to be related to the important quinone coenzymes called ubiquinones which are concerned with hydrogen transfer. Dicoumarol itself has drawbacks as a therapeutic agent mainly due to its poor and irregular absorption. Many analogues have been prepared, some of which, **warfarin,**

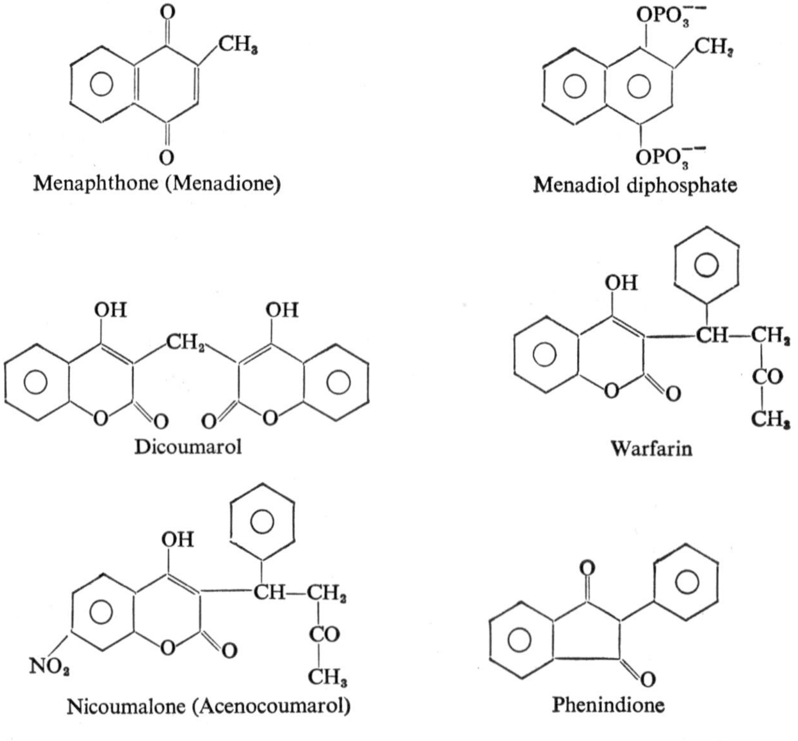

Menaphthone (Menadione)

Menadiol diphosphate

Dicoumarol

Warfarin

Nicoumalone (Acenocoumarol)

Phenindione

FIG. 13.3

phenindione, and **nicoumalone (acenocoumarol)** are most used. Warfarin acquired its name in a curious way. Rats are very susceptible to this group of drugs and die from haemorrhage if the dose is large enough. This led to their introduction as rat poisons and the most widely used was called warfarin. Later it was found that warfarin was a very satisfactory anticoagulant for clinical use.

The toxicity of the dicoumarol group is low and is mainly attributable to overdose leading to haemorrhage particularly from mucous membranes and the genito-urinary tract. Because the effects of the drugs of this group are rather long lasting, when rapid reversal of the effect on blood clotting is required, this can be achieved by intravenous vitamin K as a water-soluble derivative such as **menadiol diphosphate.** Although the clotting factors begin to rise in concentration almost immediately, a significant effect as far as stopping haemorrhage is concerned may take several hours, and if the haemorrhage is serious it may be wise to supply the missing factors by a transfusion of fresh blood or fresh frozen plasma. The usage of phenindione is decreasing because sensitivity reactions involving a rash, leukopenia, and fever are not uncommon.

The long-term use of dicoumarol-type anticoagulants in thrombotic disease is a hotly debated issue at present. It is very difficult to establish that such therapy reduces the long-term risks of further thrombotic incidents. However, there is fairly general agreement that the short-term mortality is reduced, almost certainly due to a reduction in deep vein thrombosis which is a frequent accompaniment of confining elderly people to bed.

FURTHER READING

BOTHWELL, T. H., and FINCH, C. A. (1962) *Iron Metabolism*, Boston.

DOUGLAS, A. S. (1962) *Anticoagulant Therapy*, Oxford.

ELLENBOGEN, L., and HIGHLEY, D. (1963) Intrinsic factor, *Vitam. and Horm.*, **21**, 1.

ENGELBERG, H. (1963) *Heparin*, Springfield, Ill.

FRIEDKIN, M. (1963) Enzymatic aspects of folic acid, *Ann. Rev. Biochem.*, **32**, 185.

GIRDWOOD, R. (1960) Folic acid, its analogs and antagonists, *Advanc. clin. Chem.*, **3**, 235.

GROSS, F. (ed.) (1964) *Iron Metabolism*, Berlin.

INGRAM, G. I. C. (1961) Anticoagulant therapy, *Pharmacol. Rev.*, **13**, 279.

MOLLIN, D. (ed.) (1971) *Haemopoietic Agents*, Oxford.

O'BRIEN, J. S. (1962) The role of folate coenzymes in cellular division, *Cancer Res.*, **22**, 267.

SMITH, E. L. (1960) *Vitamin B_{12}*, London.

14

HORMONES

THE word 'hormone' was introduced by Starling in 1905 to denote 'chemical messengers' and was applied to substances liberated by special glands of internal secretion and which were carried in the blood to produce effects in other parts of the body.

Hormones may be used therapeutically in conditions of hormone deficiency or to affect physiological functions. Drugs may be used to increase or reduce the release of hormones and to antagonize the actions of individual hormones.

The hormones themselves may act at one or more sites, including cell membranes, enzyme systems, subcellular structures, or on nucleic acids, but although most of the hormones were isolated in a pure form between 1920 and 1935, it is still impossible to decide their precise mechanism of action. For many years it was thought that they worked by activating enzymes, a view which was supported by the knowledge that vitamins were a part of coenzymes, but this hypothesis has not yet been fully substantiated.

A more recent suggestion is that hormones may act by regulating the activity of certain genes. The evidence for this type of action has been obtained using the metamorphosis hormone (ecdysone) of insects. This is a steroid hormone which can be shown to influence the giant chromosomes in the salivary glands of midge larvae. The injection of ecdysone into mature larvae causes 'puffing' at one or two gene loci. These puffs contain and synthesize RNA and this RNA is assumed to act as messenger-RNA, the first transcript of the genetic message. The puff is thought to be the region in which genetic information is read and transferred to the cytoplasm to direct the synthesis of proteins.

There is also good evidence that ecdysone is able to cause enzyme induction. When ecdysone is injected into *Calliphora* larvae there follows a darkening of the cuticle due to the incorporation of a tyrosine metabolite, N-acetyl-dopamine. This substance is produced from DOPA by decarboxylation and the decarboxylating enzyme is induced by ecdysone. Inhibitors of RNA and protein synthesis prevent this synthesis.

Mammalian cells lack giant chromosomes so it is not possible to observe directly the action of a hormone on genetic material but several indirect pieces of evidence strongly suggest that this does occur.

Hydrocortisone [p. 154] appears to be a potent inducer of several enzymes, mainly those which are concerned with gluconeogenesis from amino acids and this action could account for the physiological effect of hydrocortisone on carbohydrate metabolism.

Further evidence suggests that other hormones act in this way. Enhanced RNA synthesis has been demonstrated in the testosterone-treated rat, and growth hormone, oestrogens, and thyroxine seem to act in a similar manner. The effects of oestrogens can be blocked by actinomycin and puromycin which are inhibitors of RNA and protein synthesis. If messenger-RNA mediates hormone action then the action of hormones should be reproduced by injecting the appropriate messenger. This has been done by isolating messenger-RNA from the uterus of oestrogen-treated castrated rats and injecting it into the uterus of ovariectomized rats. This procedure produces clear oestrogenic effects.

It is unlikely that all hormones act in this way. Insulin, for instance, acts primarily on cell permeability as does the antidiuretic hormone. It is also unlikely that hormones with a very rapid action can work by what is, from its very nature, a slow process.

THE PITUITARY GLAND

Although the pituitary gland is not essential for life, the hypophysectomized animal is far from normal. The gland is divided into two major hormone-producing parts, the anterior lobe (adenohypophysis) and the posterior lobe (neurohypophysis). The anterior lobe secretes hormones which regulate the growth of body tissues and the activity of the other endocrine glands. The posterior lobe secretes the antidiuretic hormone and oxytocin.

THE ANTERIOR LOBE

Hormones secreted by the anterior lobe include the growth hormone and the trophic hormones, thyrotrophin (TSH), corticotrophin (ACTH), and the gonadotrophins. The latter group consist of the follicle-stimulating hormone (FSH), the luteinizing hormone (LH), and prolactin.

Most of these substances produce their effects on the body through other endocrine glands and removal of the pituitary causes atrophy of the sex glands, the thyroid, and the adrenals: the injection of anterior lobe extracts has the opposite effect. In adults, suppression of anterior lobe secretion may be fatal as in Simmonds' disease but more often the suppression is not complete.

Control of anterior lobe secretions is exerted, to a large extent, by feedback mechanisms involving an action of the circulating hormones on the hypothalamus. Hypothalamic control of the release of at least four anterior lobe hormones is mediated by 'hormone-releasing factors' which are transported down the hypophysial-portal system.

The hormone-releasing factors so far characterized are the corticotrophin-releasing factor and factors releasing thyrotrophin, luteinizing hormone, growth hormone, and follicle-stimulating hormone.

Thyrotrophin (TSH)

TSH is a glycoprotein which acts on the thyroid causing hyperplasia of the cells and the secretion of thyroxine. The mechanism by which TSH stimulates thyroid secretion is unknown despite many studies on the chemical and enzymatic changes that are produced in the gland or in tissue slices.

The control of TSH secretion is largely regulated by the amount of thyroxine circulating in the blood and if thyroxine is injected into the blood stream, then TSH secretion is reduced by this negative feedback mechanism. Any reduction in circulating thyroxine leads to increased TSH secretion and thence to increased thyroid activity. TSH is not used therapeutically but it may be used in the evaluation of thyroid function in conjunction with radioactive iodine.

Long-acting Thyroid Stimulator

This substance appears in the blood of patients suffering from hyperthyroidism and, when injected into animals, it causes prolonged stimulation of thyroid function. It appears to be a gamma globulin and is probably not liberated from the pituitary.

Exophthalmos-producing Substance

Pituitary extracts injected into animals cause protrusion of the eyeballs. The nature of the substance responsible for this effect has not been determined.

Growth Hormone

Over-production of growth hormone is sometimes associated with an eosinophil adenoma of the anterior pituitary. If it occurs before the epiphyses have united it produces a giant. If it occurs later it produces acromegaly.

If an animal is deprived of its pituitary when young it does not grow, but remains a dwarf. The condition can be prevented by the injection of growth hormone, large and continued doses of which produce giants.

Growth hormone acts directly on all cells and causes a rapid growth of bones, associated with a rise of alkaline phosphatase and inorganic phosphate in the plasma. The amount of protein and water in the organs increases, and the amount of fat generally falls. Nitrogen is retained by the body and there is an increased blood glucose level.

This hormone is species specific and because supplies of human growth hormone are severely limited it is only used to treat a small number of cases of dwarfism.

The growth hormone releasing factor, which is produced in the hypothalamus, has recently been isolated and found to be a small acidic peptide with only fifteen amino acid residues. It should be relatively simple to synthesize this compound and it may prove invaluable in the treatment of dwarfism and similar growth disorders.

Corticotrophin (Adrenocorticotrophic Hormone, ACTH)

Corticotrophin is an anterior pituitary hormone whose chemical structure is known. The hormone from pig, ox, and sheep pituitary contains thirty-nine amino-acid residues and if one amino acid from the N-terminal of the molecule is lost then all biological activity disappears. ACTH stimulates the adrenal cortex to secrete cortisol, corticosterone, and a number of weakly androgenic substances. The gland increases in weight, loses ascorbic acid and cholesterol, and undergoes histological changes, mainly in the zona fasciculata.

The most important therapeutic use of ACTH is as a diagnostic agent in studies of disorders of the anterior pituitary and adrenal cortex, i.e. Addison's disease, but it may also be used in the early stages of some inflammatory diseases, and to increase the output of corticoids in children. An injection of ACTH will result in a reduced excretion of sodium, perhaps leading to oedema, and loss by excretion of potassium, nitrogen, uric acid, and 17-ketosteroids. Blood sugar levels will be raised and there may be a fall in circulating red blood cells.

The release of ACTH is under the influence of the nervous system and the negative feedback effect of circulating corticosteroids. ACTH is released under various conditions of stress including haemorrhage, burning, cold, and after a large injection of almost any drug. Emotional stress is an extremely effective stimulus for the release of ACTH.

Gonadotrophins

The anterior pituitary releases three gonadotrophic hormones which affect the ovary: (1) the follicle-stimulating hormone (FSH); (2) the luteinizing hormone (LH); and (3) prolactin.

FSH stimulates the tissues which form the ova and follicles in the female and LH then causes maturation of the follicle, ovulation, and the formation of the corpus luteum. Prolactin maintains the secretory activity of the corpus luteum. These gonadotrophins initiate puberty and regulate the menstrual cycle in females. Prolactin also initiates the production of milk after parturition.

In the male, FSH stimulates the tissues which produce spermatozoa. LH stimulates the interstitial cells of the testes to secrete androgens which causes enlargement of the prostate and seminal vesicles.

The placenta secretes chorionic gonadotrophin which acts like a mixture of the luteinizing hormone and prolactin. It can be extracted from the urine of pregnant women and is used therapeutically.

The gonadotrophins are used mainly for the treatment of infertility and cryptorchism. They are particularly useful for the induction of ovulation in women who are infertile because of ovarian malfunction, even crude extracts of gonadotrophins often producing ovulation. The main complications encountered have been excessive ovarian enlargement and multiple pregnancies. By the careful adjustment of dosage, the number of cases of multiple pregnancies has now been markedly reduced.

Melanophore-stimulating Hormone
This hormone is released from the intermediate tissue of the pituitary gland. The nature of its action in mammals is not clear but in patients with certain endocrine disorders who show pigmentation changes, an alteration in the circulating level of this compound in the blood may be detected.

This hormone has a marked action in causing darkening of the skin of amphibia through the dispersal of the dark pigment granules of the melanophores.

THE POSTERIOR LOBE (Neurohypophysis)
Extracts of the posterior lobe of the pituitary contain two hormones, the antidiuretic hormone (vasopressin, pitressin) and oxytocin.

The former acts primarily on the kidneys and is described on page 169. The latter hormone causes contraction of the uterus and is particularly effective during the later stages of pregnancy and for a few days after parturition [p. 97].

THE THYROID

Thyroxine and triiodothyronine are the active principles of the thyroid gland; they are both iodine-containing amino acids. Thyroxine was isolated and chemically identified some time before the existence of a second thyroid component was suspected but in 1948 the isolation and synthesis of the second, and more active principle, triiodothyronine, occurred.

The synthesis of thyroid hormone has been studied in considerable detail because most disturbances of thyroid function arise from abnormalities in the synthesis.

Synthesis in the gland takes place in several stages: (1) iodine uptake by the gland; (2) oxidation of iodine and the iodination of tyrosyl groups; (3) formation of thyroxine and triiodothyronine from iodotyrosines; and (4) release of thyroxine and triiodothyronine.

Iodine is taken up from the blood by the thyroid gland and concentrated 20–100 times. This uptake mechanism is an active membrane process and may be inhibited by thiocyanate, perchlorate, or by cardiac glycosides. Once in the gland, the iodine is oxidized and incorporated into the tyrosyl groups of thyroglobulin.

It is this stage in the synthesis which is blocked by antithyroid drugs. These agents produce an enlarged, goitrous thyroid and numerous compounds are now known which have this action and are known to act by inhibition of the synthesis of thyroid hormone.

The antithyroid drugs fall into four groups: (1) the thioamides, i.e. thiourea; (2) aniline derivatives, i.e. sulphonamides; (3) polyhydric phenols, i.e. resorcinol; and (4) miscellaneous compounds.

The structures of some of the compounds which have been used as antithyroid drugs are shown in FIGURE 14.2.

These antithyroid drugs have an almost immediate effect, when there is no reserve of thyroxine, because they act at the first stage of iodine incorporation by the gland. The

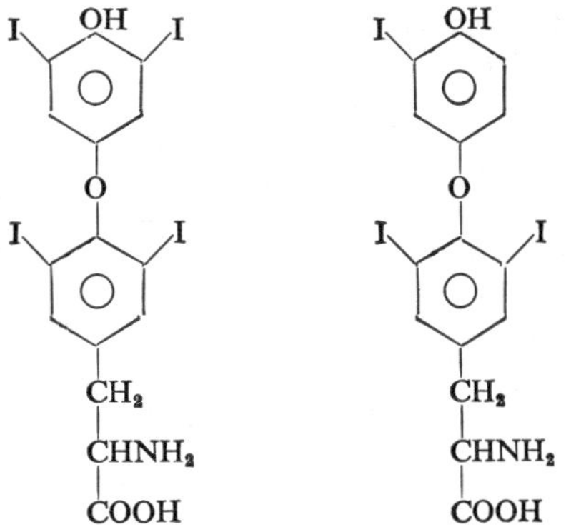

Thyroxine

Triiodothyronine

FIG. 14.1. The thyroid hormones.

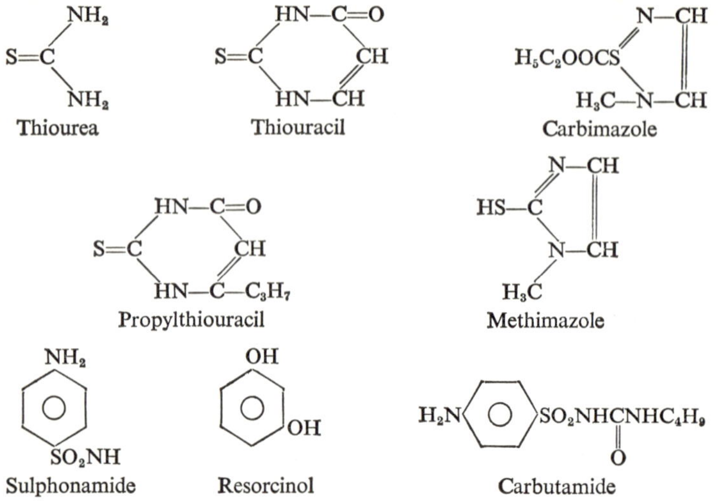

FIG. 14.2. The structures of some antithyroid drugs.

Thiourea
Thiouracil
Carbimazole
Propylthiouracil
Methimazole
Sulphonamide
Resorcinol
Carbutamide

iodine is still concentrated in the gland but these drugs prevent its incorporation into the organic form perhaps by antagonizing the oxidation of iodine which is brought about by peroxidase. It is also possible that they inhibit the synthesis of the thyroid hormone by blocking the coupling of iodotyrosines to form iodothyronines but firm evidence on this is difficult to obtain.

In the normal person, whose thyroid contains much thyroxine, thiouracil has no effect on the metabolism for several months, but in hyperthyroidism there is usually little thyroxine in the gland, and the drug is quickly effective.

While the initial high doses of thiouracil or related compounds are being given, toxic effects may occur, including rashes, fever, oedema, swelling of the lymph glands, and conjunctivitis. The most serious effects are the disappearance of white cells and platelets from the blood; treatment must therefore be controlled with blood counts and stopped if necessary.

The most commonly used antithyroid preparations of this type are **carbimazole** (*Neo-Mercazole*), **propylthiouracil, methylthiouracil,** (*Methiacil, Thimecil*), **methimazole** (*Tapazole*). The drug of choice is probably carbimazole.

The synthesis of thyroid hormone continues with oxidation of the iodine by a peroxidase, and the inactive compounds moniodotyrosine and diiodotyrosine are formed. The next stage of the synthesis, in which two molecules of diiodotyrosine are coupled, produces the active hormone thyroxine. Triiodothyronine, which is also active, is formed at the same time. These active compounds are synthesized and stored as parts of the molecule of thyroglobulin and are released from the gland as free amino acids. Proteases must be concerned in this release process and, as would be expected, moniodotyrosine and diiodotyrosine are liberated as well but they are not secreted into the blood. Instead, they are broken down enzymatically and the iodine, liberated in the form of iodide, is reincorporated into protein.

Thyroxine in the blood is bound to proteins called 'thyroid binding proteins' and this binding can be competitively antagonized by substances which are chemically similar to thyroxine or by a variety of other substances including aspirin and diphenylhydantoin. When this antagonism occurs the thyroxine levels in the blood fall but secretion by the gland is unchanged.

Increased thyroxine binding occurs in pregnancy and this is brought about by circulating oestrogens.

The thyroid hormones act directly on cells and stimulate metabolic activity. The actual changes in the oxygen consumption of cells in different parts of the body vary widely after thyroxine. The testes, for instance, are hardly affected but the oxygen consumption of the heart may double. The thyroid also controls growth and hypothyroid humans do not grow up but become cretins. Because of these various effects it is unlikely that thyroxine acts on a single cellular mechanism. One possible mechanism of action was suggested by the observation that minute amounts of thyroxine caused a swelling of fragmented mitochondria. If the hormone was altering the permeability of the mitochondrial membrane then it could also be regulating the energy output of the cell.

Alternatively, thyroxine may act by increasing protein synthesis and certainly, in rats given thyroxine, there is an increase in the incorporation of amino acids into tissues when their oxygen consumption rises. Tissues like the testes, where the oxygen consumption does not rise, do not incorporate amino acids in the presence of thyroxine.

The finding that the presence of puromycin, which reduces amino acid incorporation, reduces the effect of thyroxine on oxygen consumption, suggests that this results from an action of thyroxine on protein synthesis.

Thyroxine is slowly eliminated from the body and so has a prolonged action and removal of the liver slows elimination even more. The liver conjugates thyroxine with glucuronic and sulphuric acids and excretes these compounds in the bile. These conjugates are hydrolysed in the intestine and the free compounds are reabsorbed so that they return to the liver and the process is repeated.

THYROID DEFICIENCY

Thyroid deficiency causes myxoedema (Gull's disease), in which the skin is dry, the hair loose, the body cold, the pulse is slow, and mental functions are impaired. The metabolic rate falls and a mucoid substance accumulates in the subcutis giving the patient a puffy appearance (myxoedema). Cholesterol accumulates in the blood. Failure of the thyroid early in life produces a cretin, who, in addition to the above symptoms, fails to grow either mentally or physically.

The cure of myxoedema by the administration of thyroid was the first, and one of the most dramatic, triumphs of hormone therapy.

Various reports of the effects of grafting thyroids in thyroidectomized animals were published in 1890, and the next year G. R. Murray successfully treated myxoedema with crude extracts of sheep thyroids. Providing the right dose of thyroid hormone is taken, a patient with myxoedema can look forward to a perfectly normal and full life. Thyroxine and triiodothyronine are also used for this treatment.

Normal secretion by the thyroid requires an adequate intake of iodine and when this is lacking in the diet the thyroxine levels in the blood fall, thyrotrophin is secreted in excess, and the thyroid enlarges. The enlarged gland is about ten times more efficient in concentrating iodine than the normal gland so hypothyroidism does not usually result from an iodine-deficient diet. This condition is known as simple or non-toxic goitre and is treated by adding iodine to the diet, often in combination with salt.

THYROID HYPERACTIVITY

An excessive increase in thyroid secretion often leads to striking changes. The most typical symptoms are staring eyes, often with protrusion of the eyeballs, and a rise in metabolic rate. There is an increase in nitrogen excretion in the urine, the reserves of carbohydrate disappear from the liver, fats from the fat deposits, and cholesterol from the blood. The excretion of water and of calcium in the urine is increased. All these factors lead to a general loss of weight, but the increase in the work of the heart, lungs, liver, kidneys, and adrenals leads to an increase in the weights of these organs. The excitability of the sympathetic receptors is increased, and this is associated with an increase in the pulse rate and a disturbance of the cardiac rhythm.

Thyroxine produces all these effects in the normal, whole animal. In exophthalmic goitre (Graves' disease, Basedow's disease) or in cases of secreting adenomas, the thyroid becomes overactive and the patient shows all the symptoms of an overdose of thyroid hormone.

DRUGS WHICH INHIBIT THYROID FUNCTION

Inhibitors of thyroid function, apart from the antithyroid drugs which interfere with synthesis, may be classified as follows: (1) ionic inhibitors that block the uptake of iodine by the gland; (2) iodide which suppresses the secretion of thyroxine in hyperthyroidism; and (3) radioactive iodine which impairs thyroid function by radiation damage.

Ionic Inhibitors

These substances affect the power of the thyroid to accumulate iodine. The active agents are anions and in some way resemble iodide ions.

Thiocyanate and Perchlorate. Thiocyanate is not concentrated in the gland but inhibits the uptake of iodide and has a weak inhibitory action on iodide binding. Perchlorate is concentrated in the gland and is excreted unchanged in the urine.

Iodide

This is the oldest treatment for hyperthyroidism. If iodide is given to patients with exophthalmic goitre, it causes a temporary cure with disappearance of the symptoms of hyperthyroidism. This is probably because thyroxine is retained in the gland instead of being released into the blood. The beneficial effects usually reach a maximum in 10–14 days and the symptoms then recur in spite of the continuance of the treatment, and though the cure is not permanent, it still serves a useful function in preparing hyperthyroid patients for the operation of thyroidectomy, because it reduces the size and vascularity of the gland.

Often it is used for this purpose after previous treatment with antithyroid drugs.

Radioactive Iodine

This is prepared as sodium iodide (I^{131}) and is used for the study of thyroid function and in the management of hyperthyroidism.

I^{131} emits gamma and beta rays and is rapidly taken up by the thyroid, where the radiation will destroy the tissue of the gland. It is not easy to judge the correct dose to destroy just sufficient thyroid tissue, but nevertheless this treatment is often regarded as the one of choice for the management of hyperthyroidism.

Tracer studies with I^{131} have been widely applied to disorders of the thyroid gland. The uptake of iodine can help the diagnosis of hyperthyroidism and myxoedema and the response of the thyroid to TSH and antithyroid drugs can be judged. Since the thyroid accumulates iodine the position of the gland and its size can be estimated with radiation-detecting equipment after the administration of I^{131}.

THE PARATHYROIDS

The normal function of the parathyroids is to keep the blood calcium level constant. Removal of the parathyroids causes death with tetany due to a fall in the concentration of calcium ions.

The chemistry of the hormone is not yet fully understood. Bovine parathyroid hormone consists of 76 to 83 separate amino acid residues, at least 33 of these residues being necessary for the hormone to have biological activity.

The hormone acts to regulate the blood calcium by several means: (1) it promotes absorption of calcium from the gastro-intestinal tract; (2) it mobilizes the calcium in bone; and (3) it increases renal capacity for calcium reabsorption and regulates the excretion of the ion in the faeces, sweat, and milk. The most important of these effects is that of bone calcium regulation.

Parathyroid injection is used therapeutically only for the early control of the tetany associated with hypoparathyroidism. The hormone acts slowly so calcium is normally given intravenously to obtain immediate relief. The hormone must be used with extreme care in order that hypercalciuria or hypercalcaemia are not produced. Once the tetany is brought under control its recurrence may be prevented by instituting a careful diet and by treating with vitamin D [p. 133].

Thyrocalcitonin

There is now evidence for the existence of a hypocalcaemic hormone in the thyroid which has the opposite effects to those of the parathyroid hormone. Thyrocalcitonin is secreted in response to hypercalcaemia and reduces the circulating calcium level.

THE PANCREAS

INSULIN

Insulin is secreted by the β cells of the islets of Langerhans in the pancreas and is used in the treatment of diabetes mellitus. It plays an important part in the regulation of blood sugar levels and its relation to other regulative factors is shown in FIGURE 14.3.

In 1926, four years after active extracts of insulin were obtained from the pancreas, crystalline insulin was isolated and an investigation into its structure became possible. It has a molecular weight of about 5700 and is made up of two parallel amino acid chains of thirty and twenty-one amino acids crosslinked by disulphide bonds of cystine residues. There are species differences in the structure of insulin which are usually confined to three amino acids in one of the chains. The sequence of amino acids in the chains was worked out by Sanger in 1960 and insulin was synthesized for the first time in 1964 by Katsoyannis.

The diabetic state is characterized by marked changes in all phases of carbohydrate, protein, and fat metabolism. The rise in blood sugar level is a result of the decreased utilization of glucose and also the increased production of glucose. Storage of glucose as glycogen is reduced and glucose production from non-carbohydrate sources, especially fat, is increased. Until 1949 it was believed that insulin acted on the sugar metabolizing systems within the cell but it is now known that its primary action is on the cell membrane itself, and glucose is not utilized because it cannot penetrate the cell at the normal rate. If insulin is provided, the glucose can again cross the membrane and be metabolized. This theory of the action of insulin explains why glucose is not deposited as glycogen and why the rate of glucose oxidation is reduced. There is also strong evidence that insulin has a part in regulating glycogen synthesis by an independent action on the enzyme system involved. It is still not certain whether the impairments in fat and protein synthesis in diabetes are secondary effects of changes in carbohydrate metabolism or whether they directly require the presence of insulin. Insulin has been shown to stimulate the incorporation of amino acids into rat diaphragm bathed in a glucose-free medium so, at least as far as protein synthesis is concerned, insulin must be exerting a direct effect.

When circulating insulin is deficient or not fully effective, symptoms of diabetes mellitus will occur. These include hyperglycaemia, glycosuria, thirst, and alterations in weight. The causes of insulin lack or insufficiency may be: (1) lack of insulin secretion due to absence, degeneration, or poisoning of the islet cells; (2) tissue insensitivity to insulin; (3) excess of

150 *Hormones*

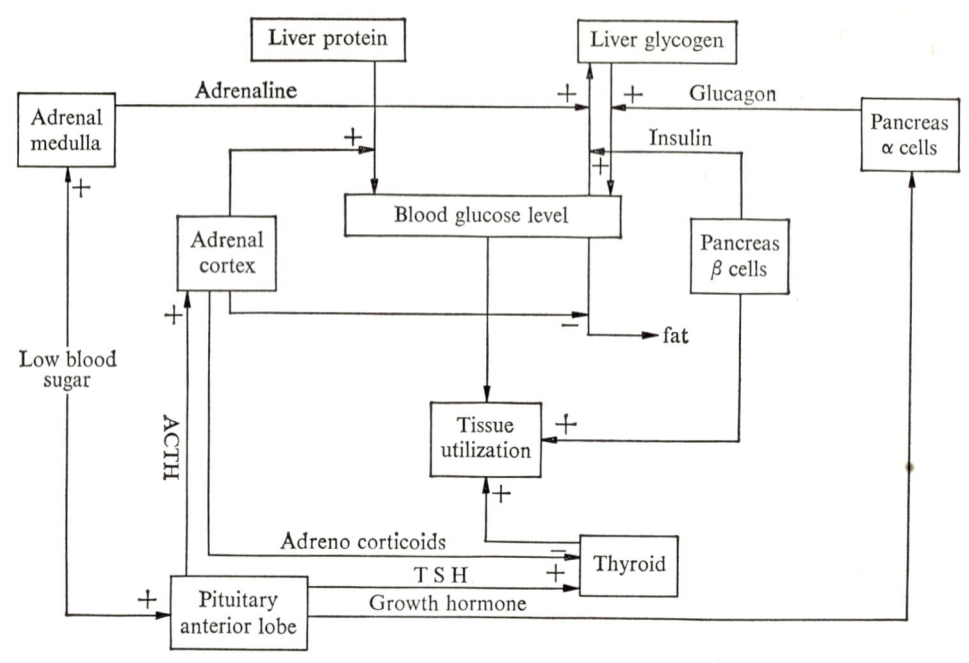

FIG. 14.3. The factors controlling blood sugar levels.
+ potentiation of effect or secretion.
− inhibition of effect or secretion.

insulin antagonists, i.e. adrenocortical hormones, pituitary hormones, glucagon, and insulin auto-immunity; and (4) depressed insulin release or transport.

The diabetic, without treatment, utilizes less glucose than the normal person, and there is an increased formation of new sugar. The storage of sugar is depressed and all these factors tend to increase the blood sugar level so that glycosuria may be present when the renal threshold is exceeded. The metabolism of fat increases to compensate for the decreased sugar metabolism, and this leads to the loss of body fat and to the formation of ketone bodies, which poison the patient, increase his respiration, and may make him unconscious and eventually kill him. Diabetic coma is not always easily distinguishable from hypoglycaemia caused by an overdose of insulin: it may be treated by giving sugar and insulin together, because both these substances tend to increase sugar metabolism and so relieve the fat metabolism and decrease the formation of ketone bodies. The disease is treated by reducing hyperglycaemia and ketonuria and the maintenance of body weight. Obesity, which is often present, may be reduced by a low-calorie diet and the pancreas may be stimulated to produce more insulin by drug therapy. Alternatively, the insulin deficiency may be remedied by giving insulin in a suitable form or the tissue uptake of sugar may be increased by a synthetic drug.

Hypoglycaemia may occur in a diabetic patient treated with insulin or a synthetic hypoglycaemic agent, due to unpredictable changes in the insulin requirement or the failure to eat properly or because of an insulin

TABLE 14.1. THE CHARACTERISTICS OF SOME INSULIN PREPARATIONS

INSULIN TYPE	TIME OF ONSET (HRS.)	DURATION OF ACTION (HRS.)
Soluble (frequent injections required)	1	6–8
Globin zinc (rarely used)	1–2	12–18
Isophane	1–2	18–20
Zinc suspension, lente	1–2	20–24
Zinc suspension (amorphous), semilente	1–2	12–16
Zinc suspension (crystalline), ultralente	4–6	24–30
Protamine	4–6	24–30

overdose. Hypoglycaemia will also result from over-secretion of the islet cells as happens in some types of pancreatic tumours. The symptoms of hypoglycaemia are often heralded by a feeling of hunger or nausea, sometimes accompanied by bradycardia and mild hypotension. There is usually a feeling of apprehension and sweating, faintness, and yawning may occur. The slow heart rate is replaced by a fast rate as adrenaline is released into the circulation and if the hypoglycaemia becomes severe, coma and death may result.

Most of these symptoms may be attributed to the effect of low blood sugar on the CNS, which relies exclusively on glucose as a substrate for its oxidative metabolism and a prolonged period of hypoglycaemia will cause irreversible damage to the brain. The symptoms are promptly and dramatically relieved by glucose. An injection of adrenaline has a similar effect by releasing sugar from the liver.

Absorption

Insulin is generally injected subcutaneously. Intravenous injections are less effective but quicker in their action. Administration by the mouth is ineffective because insulin is destroyed by the gastric juice. A number of attempts have been made to prolong the action of subcutaneous doses, so as to avoid frequent injection [TABLE 14.1]. One successful method is that of Hagedorn, who found that in neutral solutions insulin combines with simple proteins known as protamines to form a precipitate. If a suspension of this precipitate is injected it breaks up slowly in the tissue where it is injected, and produces prolonged effects. If a small quantity of zinc is also added the effect is even more prolonged, and protamine zinc insulin is widely used in the treatment of diabetes. Insulin zinc suspensions (Lente insulins) which contain no protein other than insulin have the advantage that hypersensitivity reactions are rare and a single daily injection gives a smooth control of blood sugar for 24 hours.

ORAL HYPOGLYCAEMIC AGENTS

The management of diabetes mellitus was made very much easier with the introduction of orally effective hypoglycaemic drugs. There are two major types of oral hypoglycaemic agents, the sulphonylureas and the biguanides [FIG. 14.4].

Sulphonylureas

Tolbutamide (*Orinase*) and **Chlorpropamide.** These compounds are arylsulphonylureas with substitutions on the benzene and urea groups. Their hypoglycaemic action is probably mediated by stimulation of insulin release from the islet cells of the pancreas.

Both substances are readily absorbed through the intestinal wall; tolbutamide appears in the blood 30 minutes after ingestion and is bound to plasma proteins and has a plasma half-life of about 5 hours. Chlorpropamide is also bound to plasma proteins and, unlike tolbutamide, it is excreted unchanged.

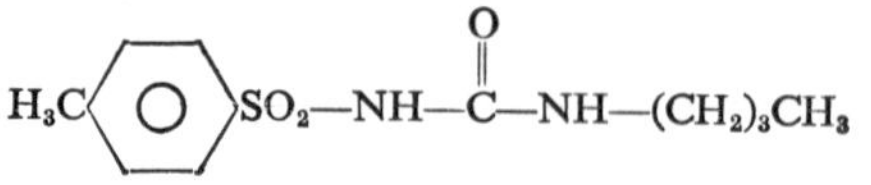

H₃C—⟨O⟩—SO₂—NH—C(=O)—NH—(CH₂)₃CH₃
Tolbutamide

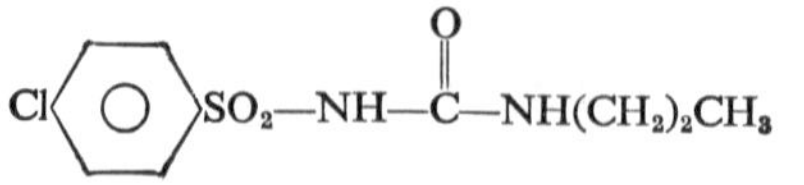

Cl—⟨O⟩—SO₂—NH—C(=O)—NH(CH₂)₂CH₃
Chlorpropamide

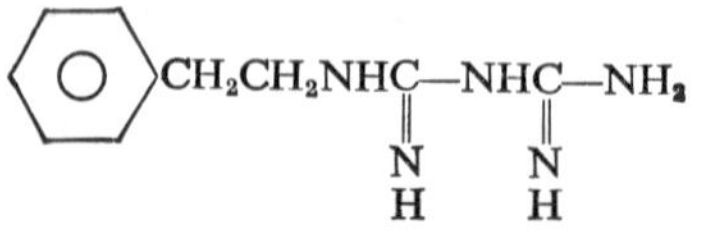

⟨O⟩—CH₂CH₂NHC(=NH)—NHC(=NH)—NH₂
Phenformin

FIG. 14.4. The structures of some oral hypoglycaemic agents.

The drugs should be used with great care in patients with a history of liver disease. Toxic reactions include allergic rashes, gastro-intestinal and haematological disturbances.

Biguanides

Phenformin (*D.B.I.*, *Dibotin*). Phenformin does not stimulate the secretion of insulin by the pancreas and hypoglycaemia is not induced in normal subjects by this drug. The mechanism of action is unknown but it may prevent the degradation of insulin or reduce the effectiveness of an insulin antagonist. The latter possibility would explain why phenformin has a hypoglycaemic action only in diabetic patients. The drug is well absorbed from the gastro-intestinal tract and its effects last from 6 to 15 hours. It is used in the treatment of diabetes which presents for the first time in the mature patient and may be used in combination with the sulphonylureas or with insulin. The usefulness of the latter combination of drugs is still a matter of debate and is still undergoing clinical trial.

GLUCAGON

When commercial preparations of insulin are administered there is a brief period of hyperglycaemia before the prolonged hypoglycaemic effect begins. This, and subsequent experimental observations, suggested the existence of a discrete hyperglycaemic factor in the preparations and this was named glucagon. Glucagon has now been isolated and chemically purified and is a peptide containing twenty-nine amino acids.

Glucagon is present in the pancreas and is probably secreted by the α cells. The administration of glucagon depletes liver glycogen and the glycogenolytic action of glucagon is not, unlike that of adrenaline, blocked by antiadrenergic drugs.

It seems unlikely that glucagon plays an important physiological role but it is used to counteract insulin-induced hypoglycaemia.

THE ADRENAL STEROIDS

Under the influence of adrenocorticotrophic hormone, the cortex of the adrenal gland is stimulated to synthesize a number of separate steroid hormones from cholesterol. The adrenal cortex is essential to life and if it is removed death occurs within a few days.

Under-activity of the adrenal cortex leads to Addison's disease and over-activity produces Cushing's disease or the adrenogenital syndrome. The secretion of the cortex is controlled by the adrenocorticotrophic hormone [p. 144] so the symptoms of adrenocortical abnormality may be secondary to disease of the pituitary.

About forty-three crystalline steroids have been isolated from the adrenal cortex but only seven of these are active in the body. They are usually classified into two groups, the mineralocorticoids and the glucocorticoids. The mineralocorticoids control salt and water balance by acting on the renal tubules to cause the retention of sodium, chloride, and water. The glucocorticoids accelerate the formation of glucose from protein (gluconeogenesis) [see p. 149] and have only slight effects on salt and water balance. The glucocorticoids also inhibit antibody formation and tissue responses to inflammation.

Two features, common to all these steroids, appear essential for biological activity, an $\alpha\beta$ unsaturated carbonyl group in ring A at C_3 and a two-carbon side chain on ring D with a ketone group at C_{20} [see FIG. 14.5]. Differences in activity between these compounds are related to the presence or absence of an α-hydroxyl group at C_{17} and of a ketonic or β-hydroxyl group at C_{11}. The absence of an oxygen atom at C_{11} makes the compound effective in causing sodium retention. When an oxygen atom is present at C_{11} the compound is moderately potent with respect to both electrolyte and carbohydrate activity. When both an oxygen atom at C_{11} and a hydroxyl group at C_{17} are present, the compound has strong carbohydrate regulating activity and has anti-inflammatory actions but little electrolyte regulating activity. For these reasons the term 11-oxycorticoids refers to glucocorticoids and 11-deoxycorticoids refers to the mineralocorticoids. Aldosterone does not fit into this classification.

The adrenal cortex also synthesizes oestrogens, androgens, and progesterone but their importance under normal conditions is not certain. The action of these hormones is described on page 158.

BIOSYNTHESIS OF ADRENAL STEROIDS

By perfusing the adrenal gland with carbon-labelled cholesterol and acetate it was found that some radioactive corticosteroid hormones were produced and it was concluded that cholesterol and acetate can act as precursors.

Cholesterol appears to be the main precursor and the first stage of synthesis involves a cleavage of six carbon atoms in the cholesterol side chain to yield a C_{21} product, pregnenolone. Progesterone is then formed by an $\alpha\beta$ unsaturated 3-ketone oxidation and then

Hormones 153

TABLE 14.2. THE ADRENOCORTICOIDS

MINERALOCORTICOIDS (11-deoxy)	
11-deoxycorticosterone (DOCA) (deoxycortone acetate, desoxycorticosterone acetate)	High sodium retention, slight carbohydrate activity
17-hydroxy-11-deoxycorticosterone	Only slight activity
18-aldocorticosterone (aldosterone)	High sodium retention

GLUCOCORTICOIDS (11-oxy)	
11-dehydrocorticosterone	Moderate sodium and carbohydrate activity
Corticosterone	Moderate sodium and carbohydrate activity
11-dehydro-17-hydroxy-corticosterone (cortisone acetate)	Weak sodium retention, strong carbohydrate and anti-inflammatory activity
17-hydroxycorticosterone (cortisol, hydrocortisone)	Weak sodium retention, strong carbohydrate and anti-inflammatory activity

a number of hydroxylating enzymes catalyse hydroxylations stepwise at C_{11}, C_{17}, and C_{21}.

Of the seven active steriods which are secreted into the blood, only three are secreted in physiologically significant amounts; they are corticosterone, hydrocortisone (cortisol), and aldosterone.

Synthesis of the steroid hormones may be inhibited by drugs which affect the hydroxylation reactions. The most important of these drugs are metyrapone and amphenone B [FIG. 14.7].

Metyrapone and Amphenone B

These compounds suppress the synthesis of aldosterone, corticosterone, and hydrocortisone by inhibiting β-hydroxylase which catalyses the β-hydroxylation of DOCA and deoxyhydrocortisone.

When circulating hydrocortisone levels are reduced in this way there is an increased output of DOCA and deoxyhydrocortisone and so, after giving these drugs, there is a fall in the

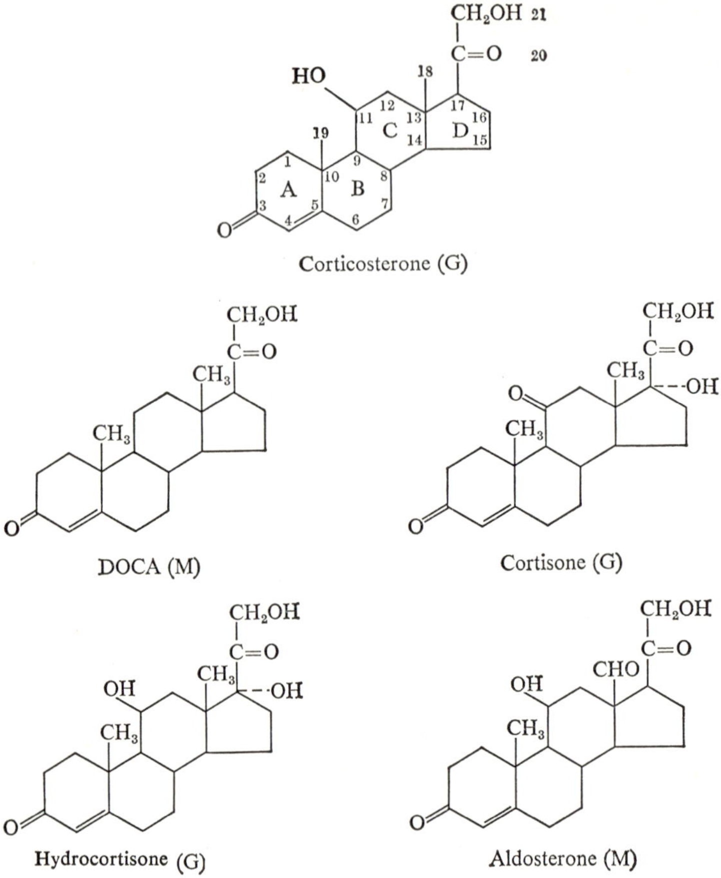

154   Hormones

Corticosterone (G)

FIG. 14.5. Structural formulae of the five most physiologically active steroids.
M, mineralocorticoids; G, glucocorticoids.

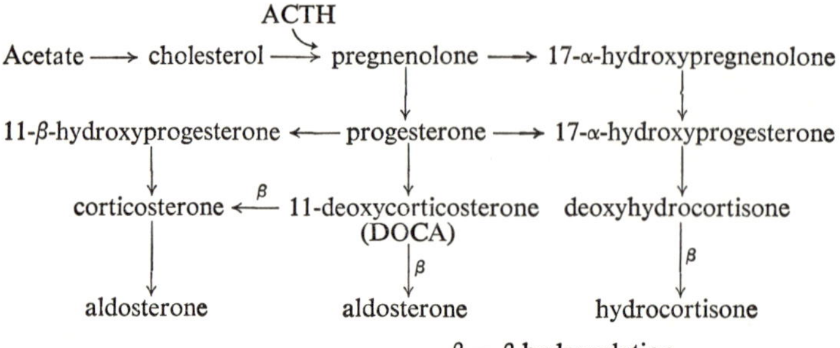

DOCA (M)

Cortisone (G)

Hydrocortisone (G)

Aldosterone (M)

Acetate ⟶ cholesterol $\xrightarrow{\text{ACTH}}$ pregnenolone ⟶ 17-α-hydroxypregnenolone

11-β-hydroxyprogesterone ⟵ progesterone ⟶ 17-α-hydroxyprogesterone

corticosterone $\xleftarrow{\beta}$ 11-deoxycorticosterone   deoxyhydrocortisone
                              (DOCA)

aldosterone   aldosterone   hydrocortisone

β = β-hydroxylation.

FIG. 14.6. The biosynthesis of adrenal steroid hormones and the point of action of ACTH and β-hydroxylation.

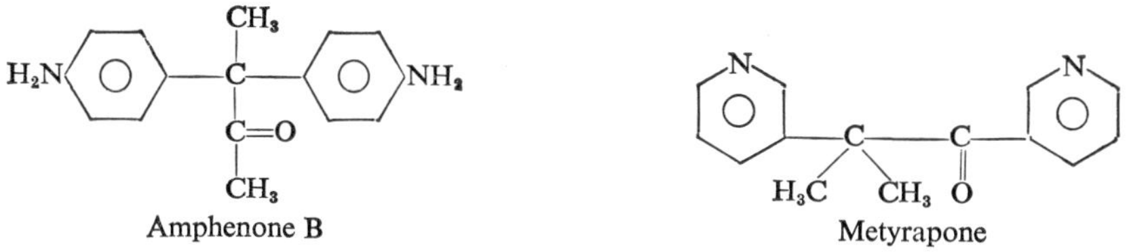

Amphenone B   Metyrapone

FIG. 14.7. The structures of drugs which inhibit the biosynthesis of steroid hormones.

blood levels of hydrocortisone and a rise in 17-hydroxycorticosteroids. The urinary 17-hydroxycorticosteroids and 17-ketosteroids rise and aldosterone falls. Metyrapone is used as a test for hypothalamic-pituitary function. After the drug is administered the urinary 17-hydroxycorticosteroids and 17-ketosteroids are measured. If ACTH release is low then the urinary levels of these compounds will not rise.

Spironolactone

The actions of the mineralocorticoids can be specifically inhibited by certain compounds. Various steroid lactones, e.g. spironolactone, act by competitive displacement of steroids such as aldosterone from receptor sites in the distal renal tubule. This effect is described in Chapter 15.

CONTROL OF CORTICOSTEROID SECRETION

With the exception of aldosterone, the secretion of these hormones is largely under the control of ACTH. The factors affecting ACTH release have been described on page 144.

The control of aldosterone secretion is an extremely complex subject and is still a matter for debate. A wide variety of conditions have been associated with an increased aldosterone secretion including: (1) low sodium diet; (2) high potassium diet; (3) decreased extracellular volume; (4) haemorrhage; and (5) emotional stimuli.

It does seem certain that aldosterone secretion is relatively independent of control by the anterior pituitary and it seems more likely that a trophic hormone, known as angiotensin II, is mainly responsible for increased production of aldosterone by the adrenal cortex.

Angiotensin II is an octapeptide which is formed from the decapeptide angiotensin I in the plasma. Angiotensin I is derived from plasma globulin when the enzyme renin is present. Renin is produced by the kidney and the stimuli for its production include a reduced arterial pressure and probably changes in circulating electrolyte levels [see Chapter 15]. It is possible that angiotensin II also exerts some regulatory influence over the secretion of hydrocortisone.

ACTIONS

The corticosteroids have a great variety of actions in the body; they affect the metabolism of fats, carbohydrates, proteins, and purines; they influence the functions of the cardiovascular system, the kidneys, muscle, and the nervous system; they also help the body overcome conditions of stress.

The corticosteroids increase gluconeogenesis, oppose the action of insulin, and cause hyperglycaemia. Glucose is formed from amino acids released in tissue breakdown and fat is mobilized, often producing ketosis. The adrenalectomized animal is hypersensitive to insulin as is a patient with Addison's disease. Administration of large doses of cortisol over a long period, or cortical hypersecretion as occurs in Cushing's disease, produces metabolic changes which are, in general, the opposite of those occurring in adrenocortical insufficiency.

The regulation of electrolyte and water balance is probably the most important role of the adrenocortical hormones. When secretion

TABLE 14.3. THE CHARACTERISTICS OF SOME CLINICALLY USEFUL NATURAL AND SYNTHETIC CORTICOSTEROIDS

COMPOUND	ALTERNATIVE NAME	ORIGIN	RELATIVE SODIUM RETAINING POTENCY	RELATIVE CARBOHYDRATE REGULATING POTENCY	RELATIVE ANTI-INFLAMMATORY POTENCY	MAIN THERAPEUTIC USE	USUAL ROUTE OF ADMINISTRATION
GLUCOCORTICOIDS							
Hydrocortisone	Cortisol	Adrenal cortex	1	1	1	Acute allergic states / Skin disease	Topical, oral, I.V.
Cortisone acetate	Cortisone	Adrenal cortex	1	0·6	0·6	Adrenal insufficiency	Oral
Prednisolone	Deltahydro-cortisone	Synthetic	<1	3	4	Rheumatoid arthritis	Oral, topical injection
Prednisone	Deltahydro-cortisone	Synthetic	<1	3	3·5	General use	Oral
Methylprednisolone	Medrol	Synthetic	0	5	5	Skin disease	Oral
Triamcinolone	Kenacort	Synthetic	<1	4	3	General use except in adrenal insufficiency	Topical, I.M.
Paramethasone acetate	Haldrone	Synthetic	0	8	10	Anti-inflammatory	Oral
Betamethasone	Celestone	Synthetic	0	?	25	Anti-inflammatory	Oral
MINERALOCORTICOIDS							
Deoxycortone acetate	⎱ DOCA	Adrenal cortex	100	0	0	Adrenal insufficiency	Implant, injection
Desoxycorti-costerone acetate	⎰		125	10	10	Adrenal insufficiency and skin disease	Topical, oral
Fludrocortisone acetate	Alflorone	Synthetic					
Aldosterone	Aldocorten	Adrenal cortex	3,000	0·3	?	None	—

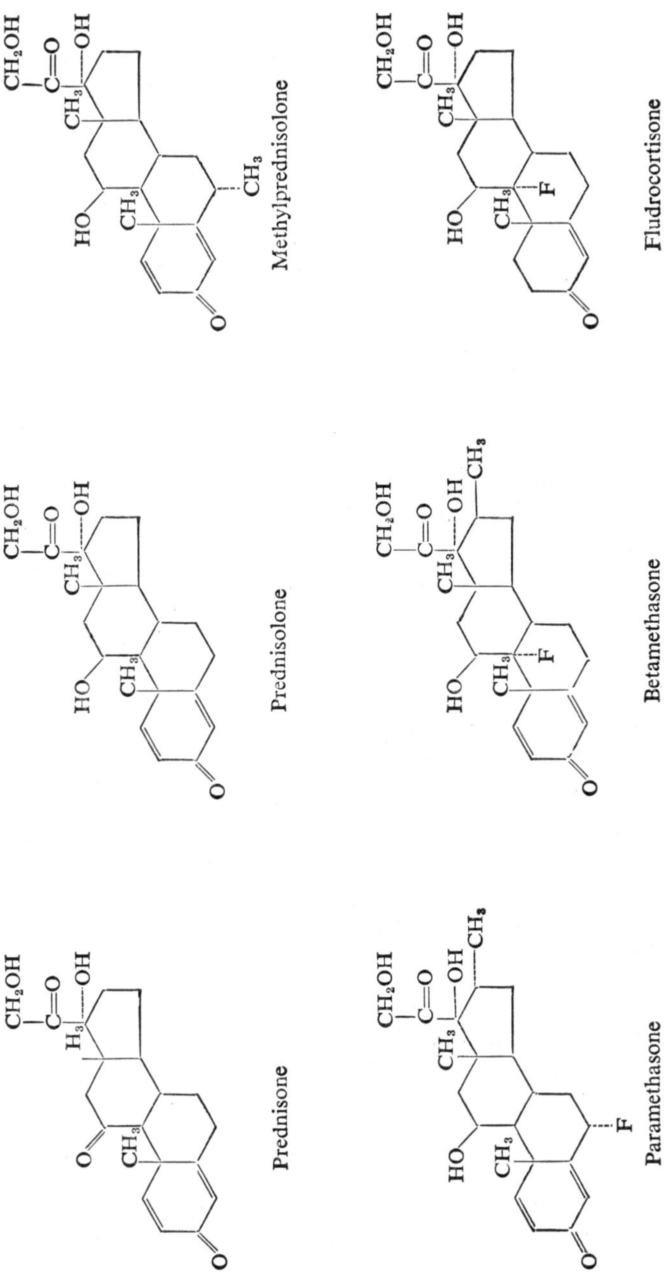

Fig. 14.8. The structures of some synthetic steroids.

is deficient there is sodium loss, hypercalcaemia, reduction of extracellular fluid volume, and the cells take in water. When there is hypersecretion there is sodium gain, hypocalcaemia, and an increase in extracellular fluid volume.

Alterations in electrolyte and water balance caused by adrenal insufficiency will lead to disturbances in the cardiovascular system. The most important changes will be a fall in blood volume and consequent increase in blood viscosity. A lack of adrenocortical hormones also reduces the efficiency of the myocardium and patients with Addison's disease often have small hearts. Hypertension is a common symptom of adrenocorticoid hypersecretion; this is mainly due to the mineralocorticoids and is a common symptom in Cushing's disease.

Hydrocortisone and various synthetic analogues are able to inhibit the development of local inflammation. The mechanism of this effect is not known but may be due to an action of the steroids on the metabolism of the cells involved in the inflammatory process. Steroids are often used locally for a variety of skin complaints and for arthritis.

Corticosteroids act beneficially in some diseases in which hypersensitivity is important. The corticosteroids do not inhibit antibody production in man, nor is the interaction of antigen and antibody, or the release of histamine from sensitive cells affected. It seems reasonable to conclude that the adrenocorticosteroids do not influence the immune reactions that lead to cell injury, but rather reduce the inflammatory reactions of the cell to injury.

TABLE 14.3 summarizes the characteristics of some of the corticosteroids which are used clinically. The structural formulae of some of the more important synthetic compounds are shown in FIG. 14.8.

SIDE-EFFECTS

Prolonged use of adrenal steroids may lead to a Cushing-type syndrome due to:

1. The retention of electrolytes and water. The symptoms include 'moon face', weight gain, oedema, raised blood pressure, and heart failure.
2. Metabolic disturbances. The symptoms include those associated with diabetes.
3. Sexual changes including abnormal hairiness and menstrual disturbances. These changes occur with very low doses but are usually reversible.

Treatment with corticosteroids may suppress the secretion of corticotrophin and so lead to atrophy of the adrenal cortex. Sudden withdrawal of the steroid treatment may then produce acute adrenal insufficiency.

Other side-effects that may occur with prolonged usage include a susceptibility to infection, peptic ulceration, muscle weakness, osteoporosis, increased coagulability of the blood, and psychoses. This last complication is not uncommon and may be dangerous and take the form of manic depression or schizophrenia. These side-effects can usually be eliminated by a careful reduction in steroid dose.

THE SEX HORMONES

The sex hormones are all steroids and are formed mainly in the interstitial cells of testes in the male and in the corpus luteum and placenta of the female.

The natural sex hormones are the oestrogens, progesterones, and the male hormones, the androgens.

THE OESTROGENS

The oestrogens are female sex hormones responsible for the development and maintenance of accessory sex organs and secondary sexual characteristics in the female.

They increase the motor activity of the

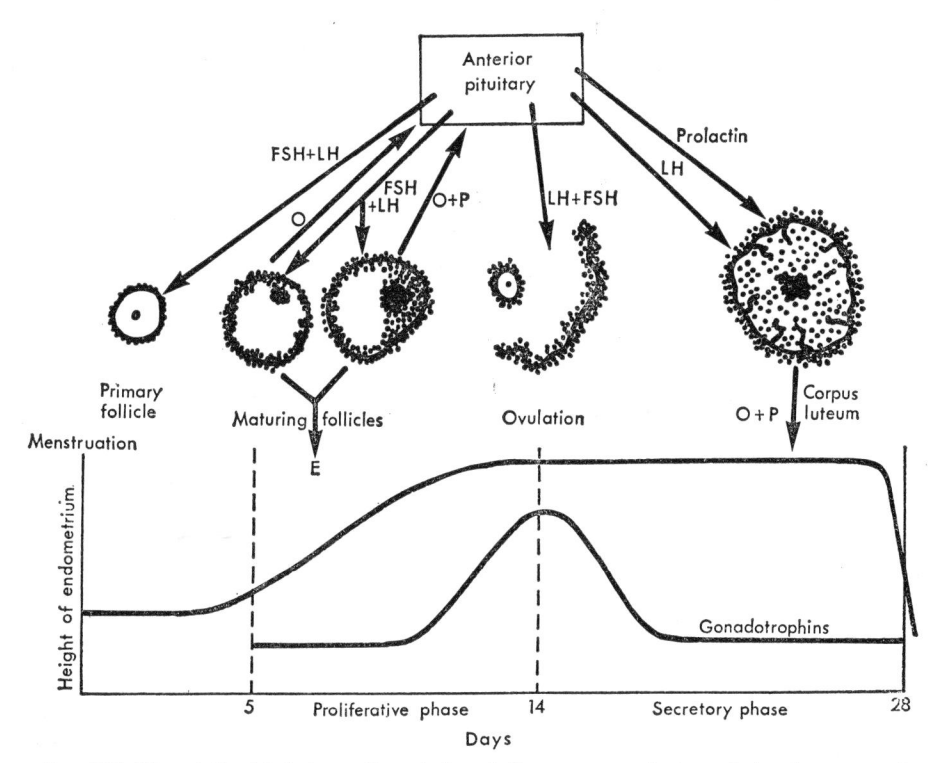

Fig. 14.9. The relationship between the anterior pituitary, ovary, and uterus during the menstrual cycle. O, oestrogen; P, progesterone; LH, luteinizing hormone; FSH, follicle-stimulating hormone.

uterus and increase the size of the mammary glands and induce oestrus. They cause proliferation of the endometrium [FIG. 14.9] and menstruation occurs when they are withdrawn.

The ovary secretes three oestrogenic compounds, oestradiol, oestriol, and oestrone. These compounds are also secreted in small amounts from the adrenal cortex, the testes, and the placenta. Oestradiol is the most potent oestrogen secreted by the ovary and it is readily oxidized in the body to oestrone which can then be hydrated to oestriol. These changes occur mainly in the liver and all three compounds are excreted in the urine as glucuronides and sulphates. In pregnancy the oestrogens originate from the placenta and the urine of pregnant women is rich in natural oestrogens.

Oestrogens are used to correct deficiency states. Probably the most common disorder of this type is the syndrome occurring at menopause when oestrogens are no longer secreted. The syndrome is characterized by hot flushes, weakness, and psychological disturbances and the administration of oestrogens usually secures some relief.

If menstruation ceases for more than 3 months in the absence of pregnancy or disease, a condition of amenorrhoea is said to exist. The normal cycle may be induced to begin again by the careful use of oestrogens and progesterones.

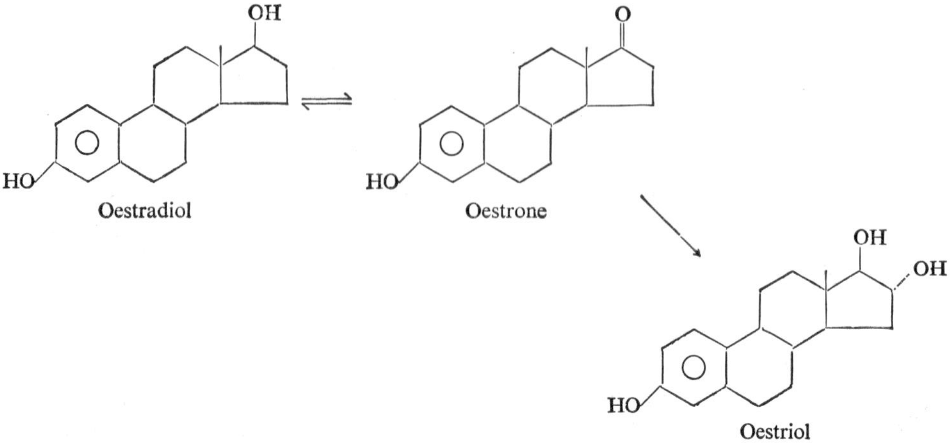

Hormones

FIG. 14.10. The interconversion of the oestrogen hormones.

The progress of carcinoma of the breast and prostate may be inhibited by the use of oestrogens because both these tissues are dependent upon a balance of sex hormones for their growth and function. Oestrogens suppress the growth of the prostate by antagonizing testosterone and inhibiting gonadotrophin which would stimulate the production of testosterone. The mammary gland is not affected by the administration of male sex hormones but testosterone, in combination with cytotoxic or antimetabolite drugs and the removal of other endocrine glands, may influence the course of the disease.

The most common side-effect of oestrogen therapy is nausea, rather similar to the 'morning sickness' of pregnancy. There may also be anorexia, vomiting, and diarrhoea. These symptoms usually disappear as treatment continues.

THE INDIVIDUAL NATURAL AND SYNTHETIC OESTROGENS

Many preparations of naturally occurring and synthetic sex hormones are used therapeutically but the responses produced by all of them are very similar so the choice of drug is often determined by the convenience to the patient. Oral administration is nearly always preferred.

These compounds may all be used for the following complaints: disorders of the menstrual cycle, menopausal symptoms, senile vaginitis, pruritus vulvae, and cervicitis. A few of the oestrogen-type hormones which have found a place in therapeutics are listed in TABLE 14.4 and their structures shown in FIGURES 14.10 and 14.11.

ANTI-OESTROGENS

Progesterones and androgens may be considered as anti-oestrogens and their properties are discussed in relation to oral contraception on page 164.

Two important anti-oestrogens have recently been discovered. They are related to chlorotrianisene and are called **ethamoxytriphetol** (MER–25) and **clomiphene** (MRL–41).

Chlorotrianisene, which is weakly oestrogenic, was found to give no enlargement of the pituitary in rats even when given in high doses. Oestradiol normally causes pronounced enlargement of the pituitary and this effect may also be reduced with chlorotrianisene.

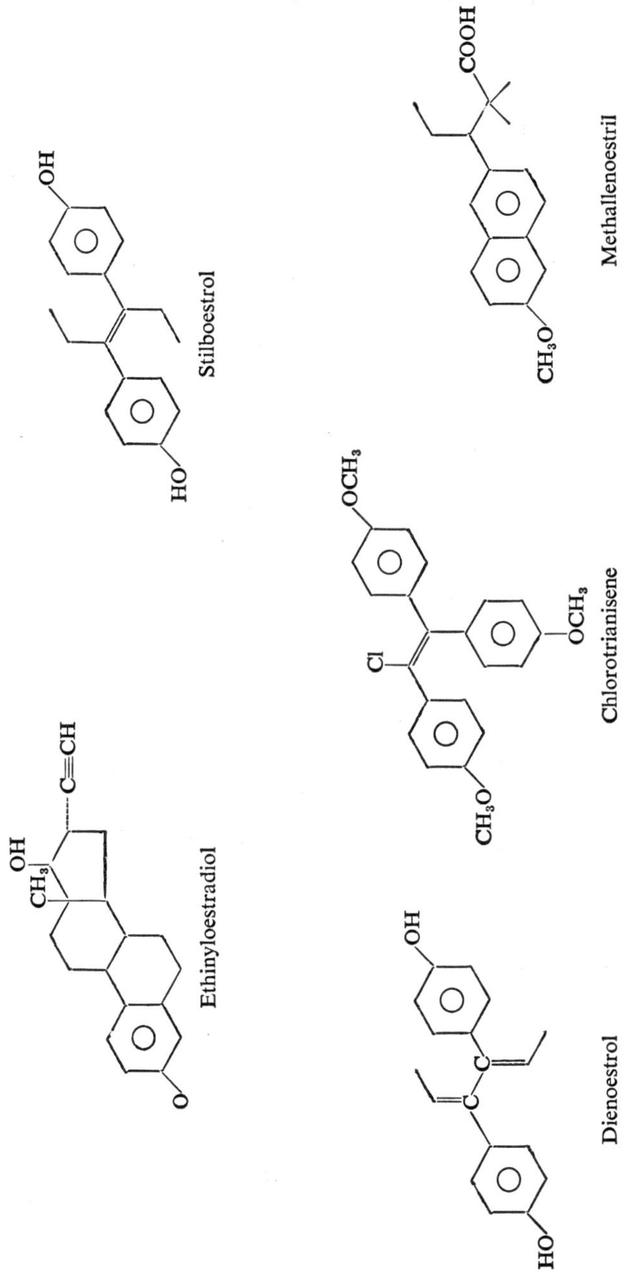

FIG. 14.11. The structures of some clinically useful oestrogens.

TABLE 14.4 SOME CLINICALLY USEFUL COMPOUNDS WITH OESTROGEN-LIKE ACTIVITY

COMPOUND	ORIGIN	USUAL ROUTE OF ADMINISTRATION	COMMENTS
Oestriol	Natural	I.M.	
Oestradiol	Natural	I.M.	
Ethinyloestradiol (Ethinyl Estradiol)	Synthetic	Oral	Very potent
Mestranol	Synthetic	Oral	Very potent
Stilboestrol (Diethylstilboestrol)	Synthetic	Oral	
Dienoestrol	Synthetic	Oral	
Chlorotrianisene	Synthetic	Oral	Stored in adipose tissue, prolonged weak action.
Methallenoestril	Synthetic	Oral	Potent, little withdrawal bleeding.

The chemically related compound ethamoxytriphetol has no oestrogenic activity but is strongly anti-oestrogenic and it inhibits naturally released oestrogens as well as stilboestrol and chlorotrianisene. The action of this compound in man has not been fully investigated.

Clomiphene interferes with the release of gonadotrophins from the pituitary, has no oestrogenic activity and moderate anti-oestrogen potency. Small doses stop the oestrous cycle of normal rats and cause a reduction in the size of the ovaries. Given to humans, this compound causes an enlargement of the ovaries and it has been used in the treatment of infertility.

PROGESTERONES

Progesterone is the naturally occurring progestational hormone and it is secreted by the corpus luteum which is formed in the uterus after ovulation, half-way through the menstrual cycle. Progesterone causes proliferation of the endometrium and the inhibition of its secretion initiates menstruation.

The hormone also reduces the excitability of the uterine muscles and causes the embedding of a fertilized ovum and the development of the placenta and alveolar proliferation in the mammary gland. Progesterone secretion also inhibits ovulation.

Progesterone is only active when given by

TABLE 14.5. COMPOUNDS WITH MAINLY PROGESTERONE-LIKE ACTIVITY

COMPOUND	METHOD OF ADMINISTRATION	PROGESTERONE ACTIVITY	ANDROGEN ACTIVITY	THERAPEUTIC USE
Progesterone	Injection only	High		Habitual abortion, amenorrhoea, uterine bleeding, dysmenorrhoea
Ethisterone	Oral	Delayed, prolonged	+	
Megestrol	Oral	High		Oral contraception
Medroxyprogesterone acetate	Oral	High		
Dydrogesterone	Oral			
Chlormadinone	Oral	Very high		Anti-oestrogen, contraception
Norethisterone	Oral	High, prolonged	+	Contraception
Norethynodrel	Oral	Oestrogen and progesterone activity		Contraception

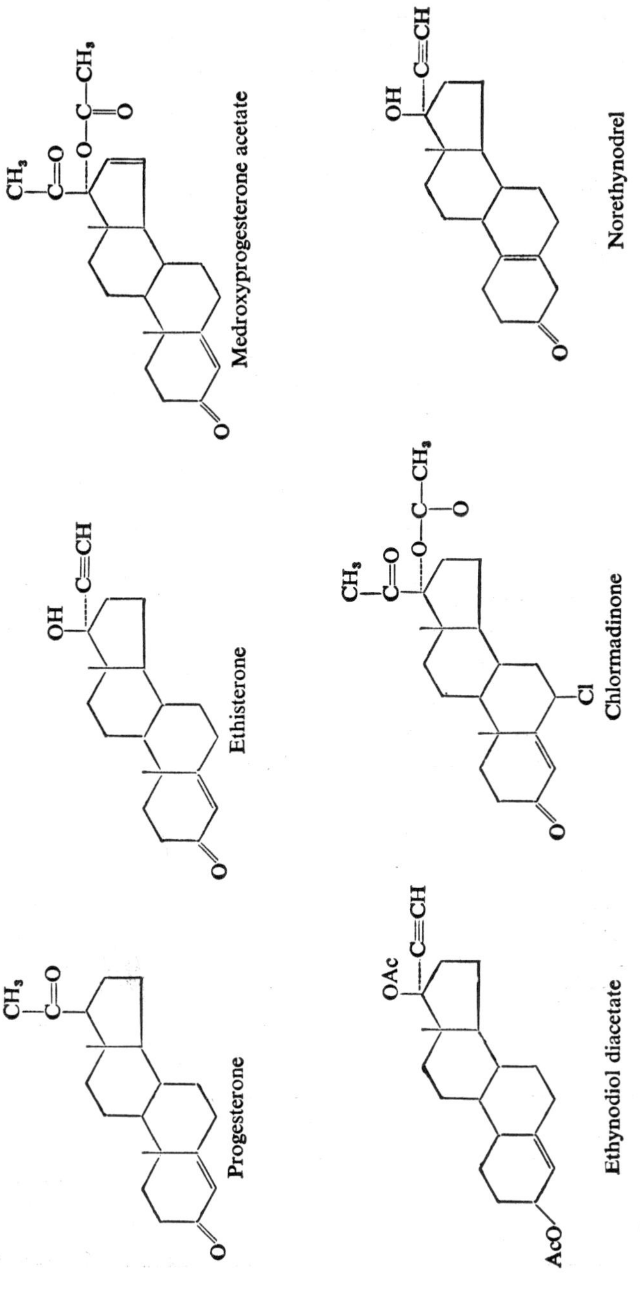

Hormones 163

FIG. 14.12. The structures of some compounds with progesterone activity.

injection but a number of synthetic compounds have now been discovered which can be given orally.

The compounds that are used therapeutically can be divided into two classes, the progesterone derivatives and the compounds related to 19-norsteroids [TABLE 14.5]. Orally active progesterones are used for a number of gynaecological disorders. A common disorder which may be treated is functional uterine bleeding. In this condition there are prolonged and irregular periods of bleeding, probably due to the irregular production of oestrogens with interruption by the secretion of progesterone. Progesterones are specific in alleviating this condition and they are usually most effective when administered with oestrogens.

ORAL CONTRACEPTIVES

Mechanism of Action

Under the influence of progesterone secreted by the corpus luteum, the oestrogen-dominated uterus is able to receive a fertilized ovum and pregnancy will be maintained. During this time the circulating levels of oestrogens and progesterones are high and they act on the anterior pituitary to inhibit the release of gonadotrophins and so stop further ovulation occurring.

The administration of an oestrogen or a progesterone or both will inhibit ovulation and therefore pregnancy.

The mechanism of this effect is probably that oestrogens stop the secretion of FSH from the pituitary and the presence of progesterone prevents the release of LH.

Ovulation can therefore be prevented either by stopping the stimulus to ovulation or by preventing follicle growth and either of the steroids will effectively do this. In theory, therefore, either an oestrogen or a progesterone should alone be sufficient to prevent ovulation. In practice the two steroids are usually combined, the oestrogen inhibiting ovulation and the progesterone being mainly responsible for ensuring that withdrawal bleeding will be of short duration and prompt.

Oral contraceptive preparations containing only progesterones have been used because of the possible unwanted side-effects of long-term administration of oestrogens. Continuous administration of high doses of progesterone abolishes the menstrual cycle and leads to atrophy of the ovarian and endometrial tissue, and lower doses, without having these complications, do not give reliable contraception so this type of contraceptive requires the development of new progesterone compounds.

Because the contraceptive compounds can be taken orally, and because fertility is not impaired and conception can occur normally when the drug is discontinued, it is likely that oral contraceptive techniques will become increasingly popular. There are still obvious improvements to be made to this type of contraception such as the elimination and assessment of side-effects and the production of compounds with long-lasting actions. This latter property now seems a real possibility and there are reports of contraceptive compounds which can be implanted subcutaneously and remain effective for many years.

There is also the possibility that post-coital contraceptives may be developed. One class of compounds that might prove useful here are the prostaglandins, which have been applied

PROGESTIN	OESTROGEN	NAME	
Norethynodrel	Mestranol	*Enavid (Enovid)*	
Norethindrone	Mestranol	*Ortho-Novum, Norinyl*	TABLE 14.6
Norethindrone acetate	Ethinyloestradiol	*Norlestrin, Anovlar*	THE COMPOSITION
Medroxyprogesterone acetate	Ethinyloestradiol	*Provest*	OF SOME ORAL
Ethynodiol diacetate	Mestranol	*Metrulen*	CONTRACEPTIVES

as vaginal pessaries and will inhibit implantation in the uterus.

There are a number of minor side-effects associated with the majority of oral contraceptives. These side-effects include occasional nausea, vomiting, dizziness, and weight gain. These effects do not usually persist and they can be attributed almost entirely to the oestrogen administered. They are similar to symptoms experienced in early pregnancy, a condition in which the normal blood oestrogen levels are also raised.

After contraceptive pills had been in use for a number of years reports began to appear of cases of thrombophlebitis and there is no doubt that there has been an increase in deaths from thrombosis in women of child-bearing age. However, the risk of fatal complications is only 3 per 100,000 women per year, about the same risk of death that a woman runs in her home and less than her risk during pregnancy and labour.

There has been alarm expressed over other side-effects of oral contraceptives and these effects include visual disorders, diabetes, jaundice, and carcinoma of the breast and uterus. Despite vigorous investigation, there is no evidence to justify these fears but the potential hazard of these compounds means they should be used with discretion in women with a history of thrombophlebitis, impaired hepatic function, and any oestrogen-dependent neoplasm.

ANDROGENS

The androgens are the male sex hormones. The naturally occurring one is testosterone and this is secreted by the interstitial cells of the testes under the influence of the luteinizing hormone.

It is continuously secreted during adult life and is responsible for the development, function, and maintenance of the secondary male sexual characteristics, the male accessory sex organs, and for spermatogenesis. Castration causes atrophy of the accessory sex organs but this may be prevented by the administration of androgens. The androgens are also secreted from the adrenal cortex and the ovaries and they cause retention of water, nitrogen, potassium, sodium, calcium, chloride, sulphate, and

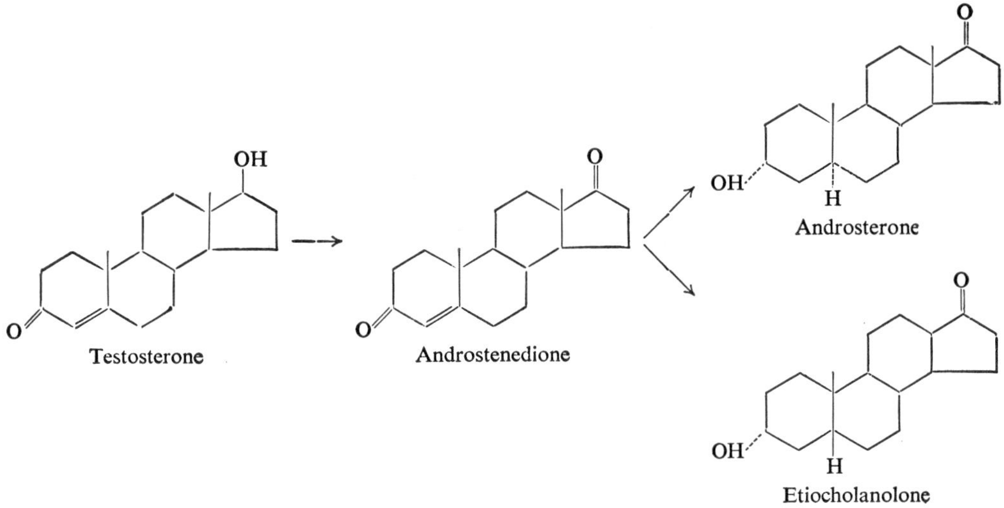

Fig. 14.13. The degradation of testosterone.

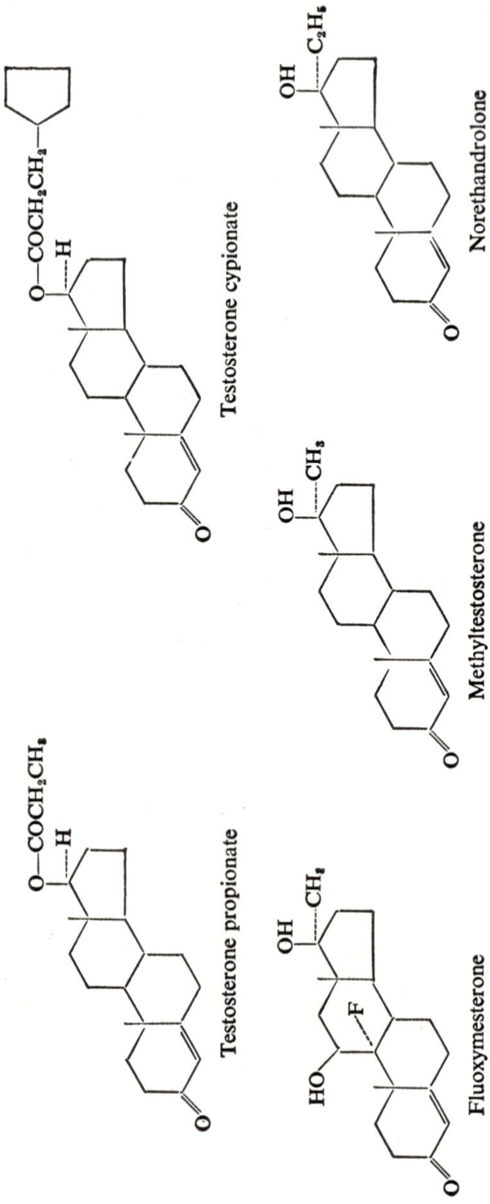

Fig. 14.14. The structures of some compounds with androgen-like properties.

TABLE 14.7 INDIVIDUAL ANDROGEN COMPOUNDS

COMPOUND	ROUTE OF INJECTION	MAIN USE
Testosterone propionate injection (*Androteston*)	I.M.	Androgen
Testosterone cypionate injection	I.M.	Androgen
Testosterone enanthate (*Delatestryl*)	I.M.	Androgen
Fluoxymesterone (*Halotestin*)	Oral	Androgen
Methyltestosterone	Oral	Weak androgen
Testosterone implants	Implantation	Androgen
Nandrolone phenylpropionate (*Durabolin*)	I.M.	Anabolic
Norethandrolone (*Nilevar*)	I.M., oral	Anabolic

phosphorus. They also increase protein anabolism.

Testosterone has both androgenic and anabolic activity but many synthetic compounds have been developed in which the anabolic properties predominate and these have proved useful therapeutically to promote growth and the formation of new tissue.

The hormone is degraded in the liver to androsterone, which is only weakly androgenic, and its inactive isomer, etiocholanolone [FIG. 14.13]. These substances are excreted in the urine as sulphates and glucuronides.

The most important use of androgens is in replacement therapy when normal testosterone secretion is reduced or absent. They are used to treat hypogonadism, hypopituitarism, and osteoporosis.

The use of androgens as anabolic agents is likely to have important applications but at present there are complications, including the difficulty of producing an androgen with high anabolic activity but very low androgenic activity. The use of androgens in women always carries the risk of producing masculinization. This may start by the growth of facial hair and deepening of the voice but these effects are reversible if the drug is quickly withdrawn. More prolonged administration may lead to baldness, acne, excessive body hair, and hypertrophy of the clitoris.

FURTHER READING

BUSH, I. E. (1962) Chemical and biological factors in the activity of adrenocortical steroids, *Pharmacol. Rev.*, **14**, 317.

COPP, D. H. (1964) Parathyroids, calcitonin and control of plasma calcium, *Recent Progr. Hormone Res.*, **20**, 59.

DIXON, H. B. F. (1964) Chemistry of pituitary hormones, in *The Hormones*, Vol. 5, New York.

GUILLEMIN, R. (1964) Hypothalamic factors releasing pituitary hormones, *Recent Progr. Hormone Res.*, **20**, 89.

KARLSON, P., and SEKERIS, C. E. (1966) Biochemical mechanisms of hormone action, *Acta endocr. (Kbh.)*, **53**, 505.

LARAGH, J. H., and KELLY, W. G. (1964) Aldosterone: its biochemistry and physiology, in *Advances in Metabolic Disorders*, New York.

MATSUZAKI, F., and RABEN, M. S. (1965) Growth hormones, *Ann. Rev. Pharmacol.*, **5**, 137.

METZ, R., and BEST, C. H. (1960) Insulin and glucagon, *Practitioner*, **185**, 593.

RALL, J. E., ROBBINS, J., and LEWALLEN, C. G. (1964) The thyroid, in *The Hormones*, Vol.5 New York.

SCHWYZER, R. (1964) Chemistry and metabolic action of non-steroid hormones, *Ann. Rev. Biochem.*, **3**, 259.

YOUNG, F. G. (1960) Insulin, *Brit. med. Bull.*, **16**, 175.

15

RENAL PHARMACOLOGY

The major function of the kidney is to excrete water and electrolytes in such a fashion as to regulate the plasma and extracellular volume and composition. In the glomerulus a protein-free ultrafiltrate of plasma is formed at a rate of about 125 ml./min. corresponding to a filtration of 180 litres per day. Glomerular filtration is independent of arterial blood pressure over a wide range and the action of drugs on urine formation is rarely effected through alteration of filtration rate, an exception being when drugs lower the arterial pressure below about 70 mm. Hg in which case autoregulation begins to fail. In some circumstances vasoconstrictor drugs may reduce filtration rate by constricting the glomerular arterioles. Compared with the filtration rate the usual urine secretion of 1–3 litres per day is small and indicates that a large part of the filtered water is reabsorbed during passage down the renal tubules. It is on the processes causing reabsorption of water and change in electrolyte concentration that renal drugs exert their main action.

In the proximal tubule active sodium reabsorption occurs and the tubule is freely permeable to the main anions, chloride and bicarbonate, which follow passively along the electric potential gradient set up by the sodium movement. The tubule is also freely permeable to water so that water absorption follows electrolyte absorption and the tubule fluid remains isotonic with the plasma. At the end of the proximal tubule some 80–90 per cent. of the filtered water and the electrolyte has become absorbed. It is believed that some regulation of this process must occur but little is known of the mechanism. The loop of Henle is the next part of the tubule and this dips deep into the medulla of the kidney, makes a hairpin bend, and then returns to the cortex and passes into the distal tubule. In the loop of Henle some further reabsorption of electrolyte occurs in such a way as to develop a radial osmotic gradient ranging from 300 milliosmols at the corticomedullary junction to 1,000–1,500 milliosmols at the tip of the renal papilla. This osmotic gradient which is developed by the counter-current multiplier mechanism discovered by Wirz, Hargitay, and Kuhn is communicated to the extracellular fluid of the medulla. In the distal tubule and collecting ducts further electrolyte changes occur which are of a different nature from those in the proximal tubule. The major process is reabsorption of sodium with simultaneous excretion of an equivalent amount of hydrions plus potassium—a process referred to as cation exchange. Secondarily this leads to bicarbonate reabsorption as the hydrions react with bicarbonate in the tubule lumen, converting it into carbonic acid and dissolved carbon dioxide. These are both able to diffuse across the renal tubule with ease and hence are reabsorbed. The hydrions required for exchange with sodium are generated in the renal tubule cells by the hydration of carbon dioxide to carbonic acid followed by ionization into hydrions and bicarbonate. This process is catalysed by the enzyme carbonic anhydrase. The relative amount of hydrions and potassium exchanged for sodium depend on their availability and usually hydrion exchange predominates. However, when the supply of hydrions is reduced by inhibitors of carbonic anhydrase hydrion exchange is depressed and potassium exchange is enhanced. However, the total amount of sodium reabsorbed is also reduced. The exchange process is also influenced by the arterial pCO_2. A portion of the distal sodium reabsorption is regulated by adrenal cortical hormones, notably aldosterone. Water reabsorption in the distal tubule and collecting ducts is regulated independently by antidiuretic hormone (ADH) which controls the water permeability of this part of the nephron. Thus in the absence of ADH the nephron is virtually impermeable to water and the urine is voluminous and very dilute. In the presence of ADH the tubule is freely permeable to water and comes into osmotic equilibrium with the extracellular fluid through outward movement of water. In the distal tubule the osmotic pressure of tubule fluid thus approaches that of the cortical extracellular fluid (300 milliosmols), but in the collecting ducts which pass through the medulla to the papilla the extracellular osmolarity is that set up by the loop of Henle and its counter current process so that the urine becomes concentrated to a maximum of about 1,000 milliosmols and its rate of secretion is slow. The action of drugs affecting the kidney will now be considered against this background of normal function.

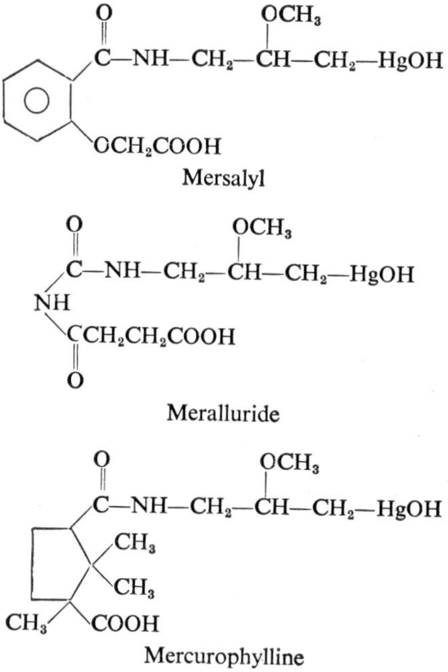

Organic Mercurials

Inorganic mercury compounds have been known to have diuretic properties for several centuries, the discovery of this action being coincidental to their use as antisyphilitics. Their use is very limited owing to excessive toxicity. The first organic mercurial diuretic was discovered in a similar way during the clinical trial of the compound for its antisyphilitic action. It was, however, much more potent than inorganic mercury compounds and of low toxicity. Several organic mercurials have come into general use as diuretics and their structures are shown in FIGURE 15.1.

The major action of the organic mercurials is on the proximal tubule where they reduce the reabsorption of sodium and hence of anions and water and lead to much more fluid being delivered to the distal tubule. The greater amount of sodium delivered to the distal tubule increases the reabsorption there and consequently increases the excretion of hydrions. However, the net effect is to cause

FIG. 15.1. The structures of organic mercurials.

Mersalyl

Meralluride

Mercurophylline

a diuresis and natriuresis. A moderate increase in potassium loss also occurs. The extra excretion of hydrions leads to a systemic metabolic alkalosis. Characteristically the response to mercurials develops rather slowly and this has led to the hypothesis that the organic mercurial is not directly diuretic but slowly liberates divalent mercuric ions in the tubules which are the actual diuretic agent. Support for this idea has come from the finding that much of the mercury is excreted in forms other than the original diuretic, that the diuretic action is enhanced by acidosis as is the liberation of ionic mercury from the diuretics, and further that the effectiveness of organic mercurials as diuretics is related to the ease with which they liberate ionic mercury in acid solution. The pH dependence of their action is of practical importance as with repeated doses the mercurials become less effective. This is due to the alkalosis referred to above and the diuretic action may be restored by correction of the alkalosis with acidifying salts such as ammonium chloride.

The main use of the mercurials is in oedema due to cardiac failure in which they are highly effective. They are also used in ascites due to cirrhosis of the liver and portal obstruction and occasionally in renal oedema. When the glomerular filtration rate is low and tubule function is impaired the action of the mercurials is generally poor.

The normal route of administration is by intramuscular injection. Oral administration is unsatisfactory owing to irritation of the gastro-intestinal tract and it is the desirability of the oral route that has led to a diminishing use of mercurials and replacement by newer orally active compounds. There is no indication for intravenous use of mercurials since they may have cardiac toxicity by this route. Toxic effects are otherwise uncommon and are usually of an allergic type. If the doses of mercurials are excessive in amount and frequency mercury poisoning may ensue.

Carbonic Anhydrase Inhibitors

As pointed out above, when carbonic anhydrase is inhibited the supply of hydrions to the distal cation exchange process is reduced, a smaller amount of hydrions are secreted, and despite a compensatory increase in potassium secretion the total amount of cation leaving the tubule cell is reduced and in consequence the amount of sodium that can be reabsorbed is reduced. Although this is mainly an action on the distal tubule there is some evidence that a similar action is produced elsewhere in the nephron. A secondary effect of the decreased hydrion secretion is a reduced conversion of bicarbonate to carbonic acid and hence reduced bicarbonate reabsorption. A large number of aromatic and heterocyclic sulphonamides are potent carbonic anhydrase inhibitors. Of these **acetazolamide** and **dichlorphenamide** are those in current use. Their administration leads to a brisk diuresis in which the urine is alkaline and rich in bicarbonate and potassium. A systemic acidosis and hypokalaemia result. The response to successive doses of these drugs becomes reduced as the acidosis develops, probably because in acidosis the formation of hydrions uncatalysed by carbonic anhydrase occurs at a rate sufficient to operate the cation exchange process at an adequate level. Both acetazolamide and dichlorphenamide are effective given orally but are little used as diuretics alone; they may, however, be used in conjunction with mercurials and are of especial value in pulmonary heart disease owing to their effects on the alkalosis present in this condition.

Acetazolamide reduces intra-ocular tension by interfering with the secretion of aqueous

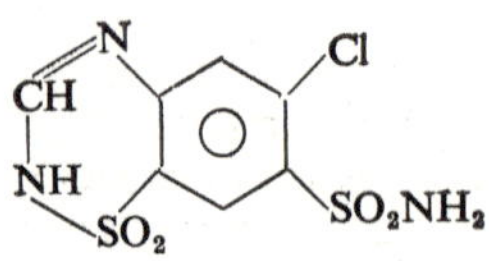

Chlorothiazide

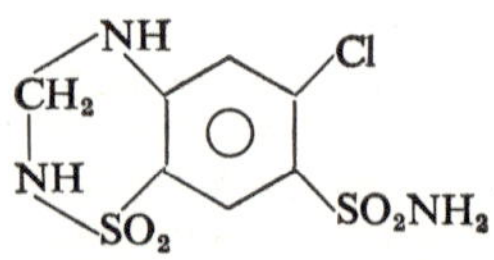

Hydrochlorothiazide

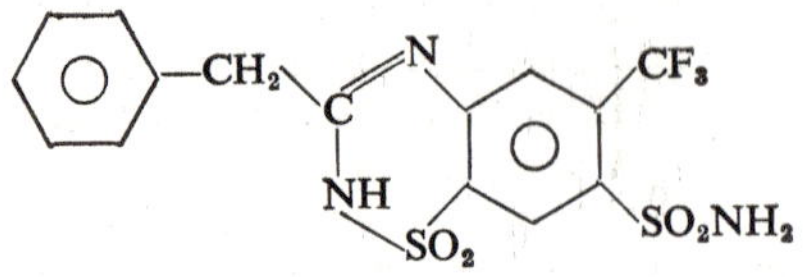

Bendrofluazide

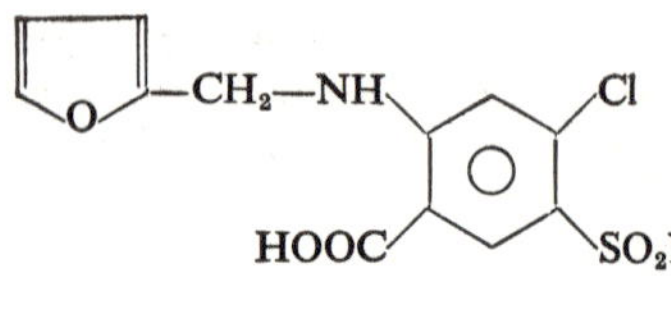

Frusemide

Fig. 15.2

humour and may be used in the treatment of glaucoma. It may also reduce the frequency of attacks in petit mal and grand mal epilepsy. Toxic effects are infrequent.

Thiazides

The carbonic anhydrase inhibitors are all sulphonamides with the amide group unsubstituted. In the search for better drugs of this group the benzthiadiazines were synthesized and found to be diuretics with a different type of action. The derivative first introduced and still the most widely used is **chlorothiazide**, although **hydrochlorothiazide** and **bendroflu-azide** (*Bendroflumethiazide*) [FIG. 15.2] are also used and are more potent. Because of the possession of the sulphonamide group the thiazides are carbonic anhydrase inhibitors and so have in a mild degree the action of this group but having in addition a powerful depressant action on distal tubular reabsorption, and may be said to combine the actions of mercurials and carbonic anhydrase inhibitors. They are powerful orally acting diuretics producing an alkaline urine and potassium loss with hypokalaemia. For this reason they are combined with potassium salts since hypokalaemia is to be guarded against in treating cardiac conditions because of its potentiation of the cardiac actions of the cardiac glycosides.

The thiazides are in wide use as effective diuretics in cardiac disease. They also exert useful mild antihypertensive action. A curious action of thiazides is to *reduce* the diuresis in diabetes insipidus. There is no satisfactory explanation of this action.

Clinical toxicity of the thiazides is infrequent but they tend to cause hyperglycaemia and may precipitate diabetes mellitus. They cause hyperuricaemia by interfering with uric acid excretion and may cause acute attacks of gout in those predisposed to the condition.

Frusemide [FIG. 15.2]

Frusemide is related to the thiazides and produces a similar pattern of electrolyte loss. It is, however, more rapid in action and

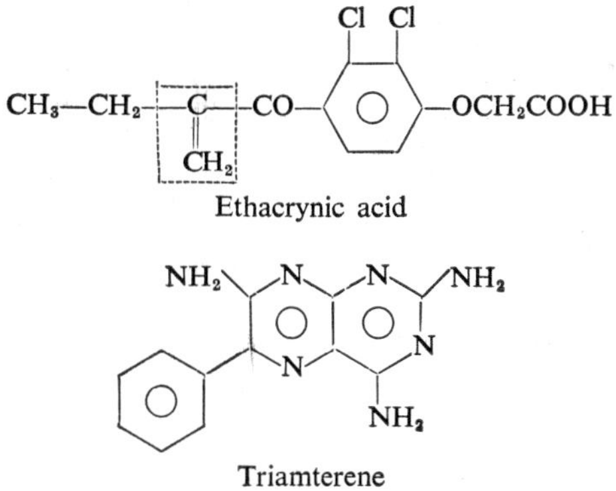

Ethacrynic acid

Triamterene

FIG. 15.3

more potent in the sense that it can produce a greater peak effect than thiazides. It is useful when very rapid effects are needed as in acute heart failure and pulmonary oedema. It should be pointed out here, however, that although power and speed in a diuretic are pharmacologically dramatic, the production of a torrent of urine can be embarrassing to the patient and may lead to an undesirable contraction of the plasma and extracellular fluid space, accompanied by hypotension.

Ethacrynic Acid [FIG. 15.3]

Ethacrynic acid is a diuretic of novel structure with a highly reactive ethylene (boxed in the formula). This group reacts with sulphydryl groups like many other olefins (e.g. maleic anhydride) to form adducts. It is probable that it exerts its action by reacting with sulphydryl groups in the kidney tubules associated with the active transport mechanism for sodium. Since this is basically the mode of action postulated for mercurials it is not surprising that these two diuretics tend not to be additive, nor that their general pattern of action is similar. Ethacrynic acid, however, has a more pronounced action on absorption in the loop of Henle than mercurials and is generally more potent as well as being orally active.

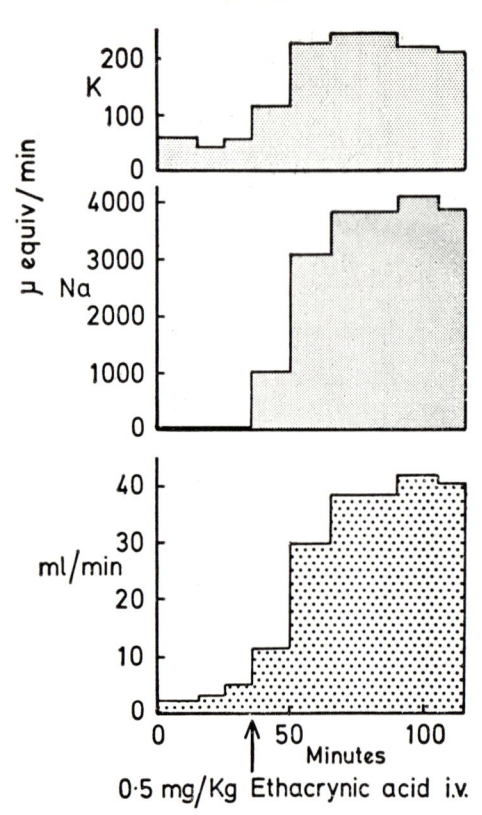

FIG. 15.4. The effects of an intravenous injection of ethacrynic acid on urine production, and sodium and potassium excretion in a patient with oedema due to cardiac failure.

The clinical experience with ethacrynic acid is still slender but it appears highly effective and of low toxicity. Like the thiazides it may precipitate gout.

One of the interesting things about ethacrynic acid is its marked species selectivity. It is highly active in man and the dog, but it is without effect in rats and only weakly active in the guinea-pig.

Triamterene [FIG. 15.3]

Triamterene, in normal animals and subjects, produces a diuresis, increased excretion of sodium and bicarbonate, but a decreased excretion of potassium. At first it was thought that this was due to antagonism of the effects of aldosterone but the effects persist in adrenalectomized animals and in the presence of aldosterone antagonists.

Amiloride has very similar actions. Both drugs are rarely used alone, but in combination with diuretics causing potassium loss, they potentiate the diuresis while reducing the potassium loss.

Aldosterone and Spironolactone

Aldosterone plays a physiological role in regulating sodium and water balance by its action on the renal tubule. Present evidence suggests this is mainly exerted in the distal tubule and stimulates sodium reabsorption and potassium secretion. The mechanism of action of aldosterone has been explored further in the toad bladder where it also increases sodium transfer. It appears that the main limiting factor to sodium transfer in this organ is the rate of passive entry of sodium into the cells and aldosterone increases this after a characteristic delay. This delay is due probably to a process involving the synthesis of a greater amount of a protein constituent of the cell which takes an hour or two to be effected. The amount of aldosterone secreted physiologically is controlled by a complicated process involving renin release by the juxtaglomerular cells of the kidney and the formation of angiotensin which stimulates the cells in the adrenal cortex which form aldosterone. Administration of aldosterone leads to a decrease in sodium excretion and an increase in potassium excretion but this effect rapidly decreases with repeated administration presumably due to a compensatory change in the proximal tubule. However, in adrenal insufficiency in Addison's disease aldosterone corrects the defect in renal handling of electrolytes. Aldosterone is not used clinically because it is inactive by the oral route and **fludrocortisone** (9α-fluorohydrocortisone) which is orally active is used instead. Most other corticoids with the exception of cortexolone have little mineralocorticoid action.

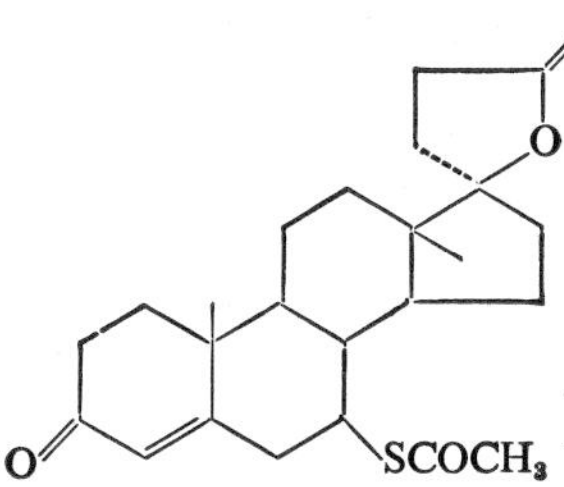

Fig. 15.5. The structure of spironolactone.

Spironolactone

Spironolactone [Fig. 15.5] is one of a series of steroid derivatives having a lactone ring in the spiro arrangement at position 17. It appears to be devoid of direct effects as illustrated by its lack of effect on renal electrolyte excretion in adrenalectomized animals. However, it will antagonize endogenous and exogenous mineralocorticoids apparently by a simple competitive mechanism. Spironolactone is rather disappointing as a diuretic perhaps due to the compensatory processes referred to above. When proximal tubule activity is reduced by other diuretics the effect of spironolactone is enhanced. Its use is restricted to refractory oedema which has not responded to other diuretics.

Osmotic Diuresis

Diuresis can be produced by administration of large amounts of a substance readily filtered in the glomerulus but which is reabsorbed with difficulty in the proximal tubule. A simple example is the hexitol, **mannitol**. Normally, as sodium is reabsorbed in the tubule its concentration remains constant because sodium and its accompanying anions are the major osmolytes of the glomerular filtrate, and hence the passive reabsorption of water by osmotic equilibration maintains the sodium concentrations. When mannitol is present, as sodium is reabsorbed an increasing fraction of the remaining osmolyte in the tubule is mannitol and the sodium concentration falls. As the rate of sodium reabsorption is directly dependent on its concentration and ceases when the concentration falls to ~ 60 mEq./l. a reduced reabsorption of both sodium and water occurs and hence a diuresis rather similar to that produced by mercurials results. A similar diuresis can be caused by excess filtered glucose in uncontrolled diabetes mellitus. Sodium sulphate produces a similar effect in a slightly different way. The sulphate ion is virtually non-absorbed and as it is passively concentrated in the tubules generates a concentration potential retarding sodium reabsorption.

Osmotic diuretics have a limited clinical use in poisoning (salicylates, barbiturates) where they may reduce passive reabsorption by reducing the concentration gradient and may also be used in acute renal insufficiency.

Drugs Affecting Uric Acid Excretion and Metabolism

Uric acid is the main end product of purine metabolism in man and the normal plasma level is precariously near the solubility limit at which crystals precipitate in the tissues. It appears that in the course of evolution man has lost the gene determining the enzyme uricase present in other mammals which metabolizes uric acid further to allantoin but he has retained a mechanism in the kidney for conserving uric acid. This is a complicated process in which both tubular secretion and reabsorption occur but the latter predominates so that urate clearance is normally less than 10 per cent. of the filtration rate.

Gout results when the plasma urate rises and deposition occurs (mainly as monosodium urate) at selected sites in joints, subcutaneous areas (tophi), and the kidney. The increased plasma urate level in gout may be due to excessive urate production from an inborn error of metabolism, may be stimulated by drugs, such as acetazolamide, may be a consequence of increased nucleic acid breakdown in neoplasms, or it may be due to defective excretion by the kidney.

Uric acid excretion can be influenced by a large number of drugs which with one exception are acidic in character and are apparently excreted by the same transport process in the proximal tubule as hippurate, penicillin, the acid dyes of the phenol red type, and the radiographic contrast agents, diodrast, iopanoic acid, and diatrizoate.

Since the tubules both reabsorb and secrete uric acid and both these processes are sensitive to drugs, urate excretion may either decrease or increase. Most uricosuric drugs decrease clearance in small doses and increase it at greater dosage. In looking for improved uricosuric drugs the main objectives have been to favour the latter action and to produce prolonged effects. **Salicylates** decrease urate clearance except at high concentrations and are, therefore, unsatisfactory. The related carboxylic acid **probenecid** is very effective in increasing urate clearance which may increase by 3–10-fold and its effects are sufficiently long lasting that dosage twice a day suffices. **Sulphinpyrazone**, a relative of phenylbutazone, is even more active and selective but is more toxic than probenecid. Uricosuric drugs cause a rapid excretion of urate but the immediate fall in blood level may be disappointing because of the large tissue reservoir of deposited urates in gout. The normal urate pool is only 1–2 g., equivalent to about 48 hours' production, but in gout excess excretion of over 100 g. urate has been found after prolonged use of probenecid.

Recently it has become possible to influence plasma urate level by depressing uric acid synthesis by **allopurinol,** an analogue of hypoxanthine which inhibits xanthine oxidase, the enzyme responsible for the last stages of conversion of purines into uric acid. The levels of hypoxanthine and xanthine in the blood and urine are increased but since these latter are more soluble deposition in the tissues does not occur. Allopurinol is now established as an important drug in the control of gout [FIG. 15.6].

Alteration of Urine pH

It is frequently useful to be able to alter the pH of the urine. This may be required to potentiate the action of a drug such as mersalyl, to provide the best milieu for chemotherapeutic action, or to control drug excretion. The latter action is of growing importance. Drugs that are weak bases exist in equilibrium between the charged, protonated form and the uncharged forms. The charged form is hindered by its hydrophilic character from easy transfer across cell membranes whereas the uncharged form is more hydrophobic and can often diffuse across cell membranes relatively rapidly. When a basic drug is filtered in the glomerular

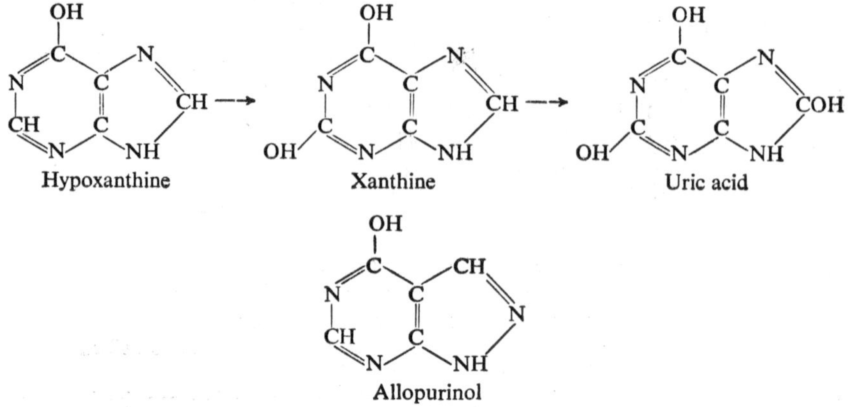

Hypoxanthine → Xanthine → Uric acid

Allopurinol

FIG. 15.6

FIG. 15.7. The structures of some uricosuric drugs.

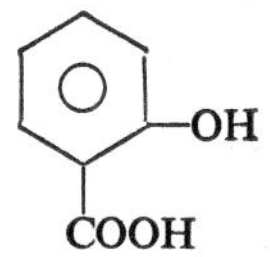

Salicylic acid

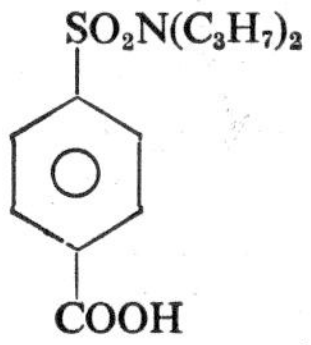

Probenecid

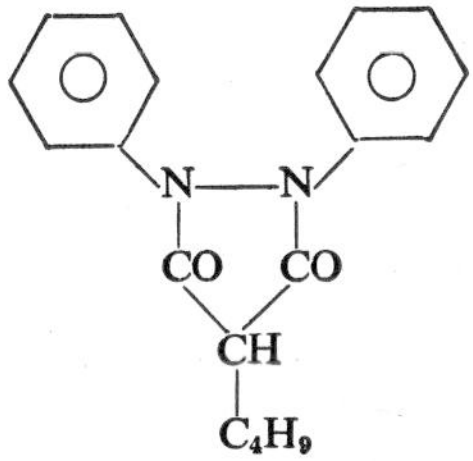

Phenylbutazone

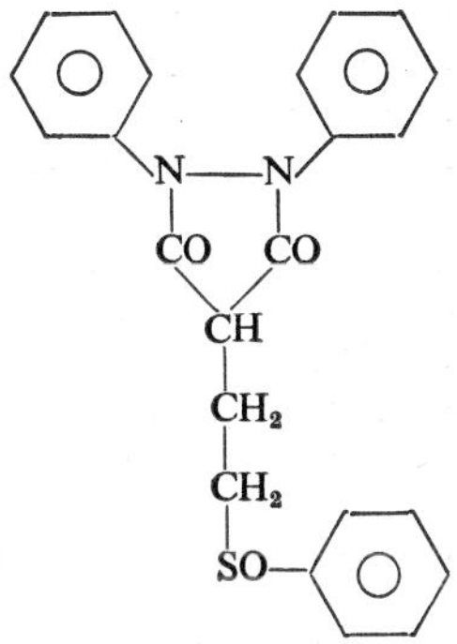

Sulphinpyrazone

filtrate and concentrated in the renal tubules by reabsorption of part of the water in which it is dissolved, the drug will tend to diffuse back into the blood. The rate at which it can do so depends on the fraction which is uncharged and hence on the urine pH. Therefore the blood level of a basic drug that is mainly excreted unchanged will be significantly reduced by lowering urine pH (examples, amphetamine, mecamylamine). In the case of acidic drugs (such as salicylates or barbitone) excretion is increased by raising the urine pH.

The urine pH is most simply raised by giving **sodium bicarbonate, or sodium citrate,** the citrate ion being metabolized so that the final effect is equivalent to giving sodium bicarbonate but without the release of carbon dioxide in the stomach which may be undesirable. Acidification is usually achieved with **ammonium chloride.** In this case the ammonium ion enters into the ornithine cycle in the liver and is converted into urea and yields a hydrion; this reaction occurs rapidly and efficiently so that the administration of ammonium chloride has an effect equivalent to that of giving hydrochloric acid.

FURTHER READING

BABA, W. I., TUDHOPE, G. R., and WILSON, G. M. (1962) Triamterene, a new diuretic drug, *Brit. med. J.*, ii, 756.

BANK, N. (1968) Physiological basis of diuretic action, *Ann. Rev. Med.*, **19**, 103.

BERLINER, R. W., and ORLOFF, J. (1956) Carbonic anhydrase inhibitors, *Pharmacol. Rev.*, **8**, 137.

BEYER, K. H., and BAER, J. E. (1961) Physiological basis for the action of newer diuretic agents, *Pharmacol. Rev.*, **13**, 517.

BEYER, K. H., BAER, J. E., MICHAELSON, J. K., and RUSSO, H. (1965) Renotropic characteristics of ethacrynic acid: a phenoxyacetic saluretic-diuretic agent, *J. Pharmacol. exp. Ther.*, **147**, 1.

DE STEVENS, G. (1963) *Diuretics*, New York.

GUTMAN, A. B. (1966) Uricosuric drugs with special reference to probenecid and sulfinpyrazone, *Advanc. Pharmacol.*, **4,** 91.

KAGAWA, C. M., STURTEVANT, F. M., and VAN ARMAN, C. G. (1959) Pharmacology of a new steroid that blocks salt activity of aldosterone and deoxycorticosterone, *J. Pharmacol. exp. Ther.*, **126,** 123.

ORLOFF, J., and BERLINER, R. W. (1961) Renal pharmacology, *Ann. Rev. Pharmacol.*, **1,** 287.

PITTS, R. F. (1959) *The Physiological Basis of Diuretic Therapy*, Springfield, Ill.

PITTS, R. F. (1958) *The Physiology of the Kidney and Body Fluids*, 2nd ed., Springfield, Ill.

SHARP, G. W. G., and LEAF, A. (1966) Mechanism of action of aldosterone, *Physiol. Rev.*, **46,** 593.

16

CHEMOTHERAPY I: BACTERIA, FUNGI, VIRUSES

HISTORICAL

ALTHOUGH there are many remedies in the literature of folk medicine which purport to cure fevers and infected wounds, few have been found to contain active ingredients. An exception is the infusion of Peruvian bark which contains cinchona alkaloids highly effective in the treatment of malaria.

When this preparation was introduced into Europe, it became used indiscriminately in the treatment of all fevers (as opium was). The rationalization of its use came only after the discovery of the causative agents of infective disease and the subsequent classification of febrile illnesses according to their origin. The focus shifted accordingly from the alleviation of symptoms to the eradication of the cause. It was soon possible to grow bacteria in culture and it was then found that the organisms could be killed by carbolic, iodine, and heavy metal salts like silver nitrate and mercuric chloride. These agents provided the basis for the new antiseptic surgery introduced by Lister. They were used to sterilize instruments and suture material, to cleanse the skin, were sprayed in the air while operations were in progress, and were applied locally to wounds. It soon became apparent that severe limitations to their use were imposed by their toxicity for healthy animal and human cells which was comparable to their toxicity for the infecting organism. What was needed were agents which were selectively toxic against micro-organisms but with minimal toxicity for the host.

It was Ehrlich who first perceived one of the ways in which this might be achieved. In the course of experiments in which he was staining cells with the new synthetic dye-stuffs, he noticed that some of these dyes were taken up selectively by particular cells or by organelles within the cells. He realized that if it were possible to find dyes that were selectively taken up by micro-organisms and were also toxic, then the selectivity of uptake might allow a toxic action on the micro-organism without significant toxicity to the host. While the initial idea applied to uptake of the antibacterial, the underlying general principle was one upon which all chemotherapy is based, viz. the discovery of biochemical difference between the infective agent and the host, and the search for toxic agents that can exploit this difference and are therefore selectively toxic.

Ehrlich's first success with his new approach was with the benzidine-azo dyes, Trypan Red and Trypan Blue. These were able to cure experimental infections with trypanosomes, but the margin between the therapeutic dose and the toxic dose was small. About this time (1905) Thomas found that an organic arsenic compound atoxyl (arsanilic acid) was highly effective in experimental trypanosomiasis and not very toxic. This finding was rapidly exploited by Ehrlich who made and tested many hundreds of organic arsenicals. Out of this programme came tryparsamide, soon shown to be effective in treating African trypanosomiasis in man, the arsphenamines and arsenoxides which revolutionized the treatment of syphilis and were the mainstay of the therapy of this disease until the advent of penicillin. The strategy of finding a lead in therapy, and then synthesizing large numbers of congeneric molecules for test in both culture and experimental infection, is now the general way in which new drugs are developed and it has been extremely successful in the development of chemotherapeutic agents for protozoal and parasitic diseases. It was curiously unsuccessful in bacterial chemotherapy until the discovery in 1932 by Domagk that the azo dye prontosil could cure streptococcal infections in mice, and in a sense this was a throwback to Ehrlich's starting-point, the azo dyes. Clinical trials soon showed its effectiveness in human streptococcal infections, but curiously enough its use was not widely exploited. This was because the medical thinking of the time favoured treatment with specific antisera. One anomalous feature of prontosil was that it was almost wholly ineffective in culture, but was effective in the whole animal. This anomaly was explained by Trefouel and his colleagues who showed that prontosil was metabolized *in vivo* to the simpler substance sulphanilamide which *was* active *in vitro* as well as *in vivo*. This made it clear that the activity of prontosil was nothing to do with its being a dye but depended on the sulphonamide group; the synthesis of congeners proceeded apace and out of the more than 4,000 sulphonamides synthesized came agents of greater effectiveness, lower toxicity, and improved pharmacological properties. The first evidence of how the sulphonamides act came from the discovery by Woods and Fildes that the effectiveness of sulphonamides was much lower in some culture media compared to others. They were able to show that an antagonistic substance was present in these media which turned out to be 4-aminobenzoic acid (PABA), a bacterial growth factor. The structural analogies between PABA and the sulphonamides were evident and suggested that the basis of the chemotherapeutic was the inhibition of a reaction in the bacteria which utilized PABA.

The next great advance came from exploitation of the fact first noted by Pasteur that some bacteria could interfere with the growth of other bacteria. In 1939 the group led by Florey at Oxford started a systematic study of such 'antibiotics'. The second substance they studied had been originally discovered by Fleming in 1929. Fleming found that a green mould of the penicillin species which had contaminated a culture plate seeded with staphylococci caused lysis of the colonies in its neighbourhood. A filtrate of a culture of the mould was highly active in killing a considerable range of bacteria and could cure some infections in mice. The active material was, however, unstable and attempts to purify it failed. Florey's group soon confirmed these findings as well as the very low toxicity of the material to animals. They were able to partly purify the material and obtain enough to try in a patient. The result was spectacular and it soon became clear that penicillin, as the agent had been named by Fleming, was a chemotherapeutic agent of quite extraordinary effectiveness.

Within a short time the problems of large-scale production had been solved, and indeed use of penicillin confirmed that a new age in the treatment of infection had arrived. Widespread search for other antibacterial products produced by micro-organisms has revealed hundreds of new agents often with quite novel chemical structures. The phenomenon is a curious one that may be an evolutionary device that gives the organism that produces the antibiotic a competitive advantage. It is usually found that when organisms are growing in favourable conditions with abundant supplies of nutrients, only a trivial amount of antibiotic is produced, but when conditions are unfavourable to rapid growth the synthesis of antibiotic is increased, i.e. under the very conditions in which an improved survival might result if competitors were eliminated. We have seen that some antibacterial agents are natural products, others result from chemical synthesis, and some again from synthetic variants on natural products. The natural agents are often called antibiotics to distinguish them from the synthetic ones; this seems an absurd relic of a vitalistic past and we will not make this distinction but refer to all as chemotherapeutic agents.

PRINCIPLES OF CHEMOTHERAPEUTIC ACTION

As pointed out earlier the strategy of selective chemotherapy is to take advantage of biochemical differences between micro-organisms

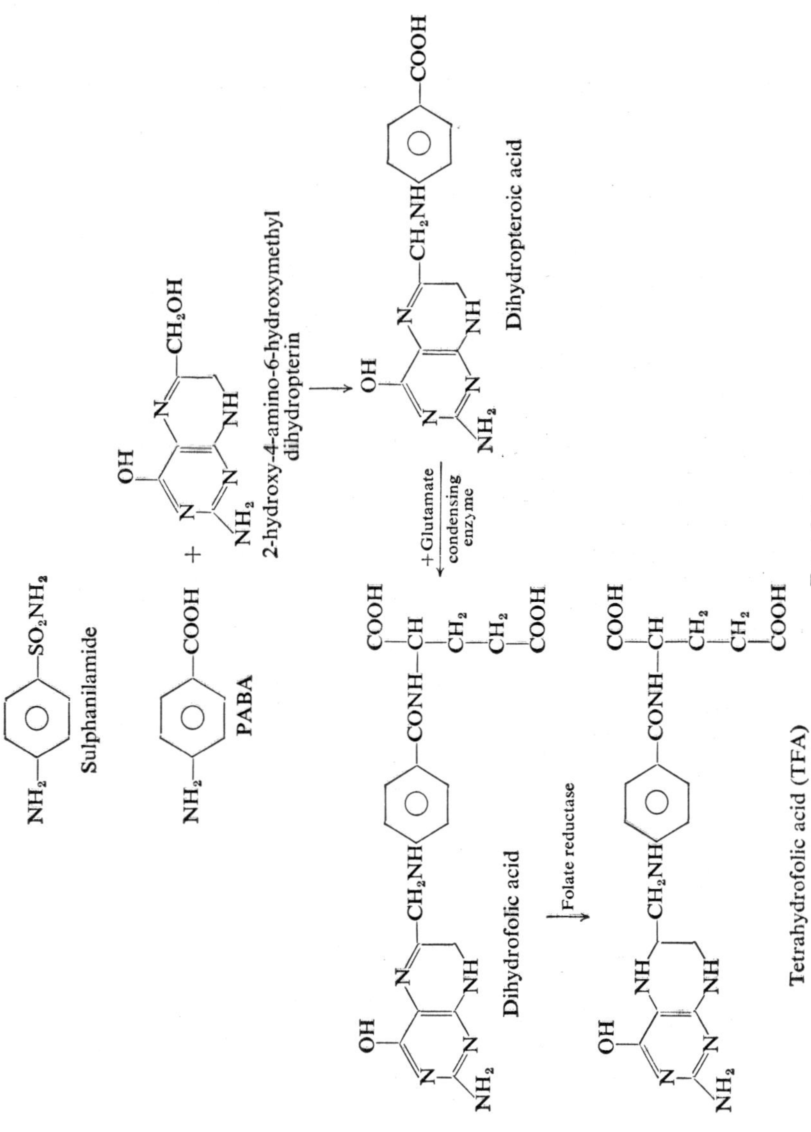

Chemotherapy I: Bacteria, Fungi, Viruses 179

Fig. 16.1

and the host to seek points of attack in the organism that are entirely absent in the higher organisms. Pathogenic micro-organisms represent an enormous range of species and it is, therefore, not surprising to find that antibiotics may attack a very wide or very narrow range of species. We shall discuss later the relative merits of broad- and narrow-spectrum chemotherapeutics. We shall now consider in detail what these biochemical differences amount to.

We saw earlier that sulphanilamide interferes with the utilization of the growth substance PABA by micro-organisms. Further investigation showed that the bacteria condense PABA with a pteridine to form dihydropteroic acid and then add a terminal glutamic acid residue to form dihydrofolic acid. This is then reduced by folate reductase to tetrahydrofolic acid (TFA) which is an important coenzyme essential for the synthesis of nucleotides. In its absence the organism cannot make nucleic acid and is therefore unable to reproduce. Sulphonamides competitively inhibit the first of these steps, and thus reduce or completely block the synthesis of TFA.

The organisms are able to reproduce for a while on the pre-formed stores of TFA but these do not last long due to metabolic losses and dilution and then reproduction ceases, but the bacteria are *not* killed—the action is thus referred to as *bacteriostatic*. Now folic acid is a vitamin essential for the survival of man. Why does the sulphonamide not produce similar effects on the host? The reason is that mammals are unable to synthesize folic acid and are wholly dependent on pre-formed folic acid in the diet. On the other hand, the organisms that are sensitive to sulphonamides are unable to utilize the pre-formed folic acid in the tissue fluids because it is unable to penetrate the bacterial cell wall. Some organisms are able to utilize pre-formed folic acid and are consequently resistant to sulphonamides. The structural resemblance between sulphanilamide and PABA is obvious and it was one of the first inhibitory metabolic analogues to be discovered. For antibacterial action it is vital that an unsubstituted amino group is present in the 4 position but the amide group can be substituted by a variety of aliphatic, aromatic, and heterocyclic groups, thus allowing a considerable variation in potency, solubility, etc. [p. 188].

The metabolic pathway leading to TFA can also be interfered with by inhibition of folate reductase so arresting synthesis at the dihydrofolic stage; neither dihydrofolic acid nor folic acid can be utilized in nucleotide synthesis. The highly potent inhibitor of folate reductase, methotrexate, is a powerful antibacterial when tested *in vitro* and inhibits the growth of *Staph. aureus* at a concentration of 10^{-9} M. It is another very elegant example of a metabolic analogue. However, mammals, while relying on preformed folic acid from the diet, still need to reduce folic acid to TFA and so possess a folate reductase. Alas, methotrexate is equally good at inhibiting human folate reductase and because of this lack of selectivity is useless as an antibacterial. However, after a prolonged search agents have been found that are preferential inhibitors of the bacterial enzyme. For instance, trimethoprim inhibits the *Staph. aureus* enzyme at a concentration 100,000 times lower than acts on the human enzyme [TABLE 16.2]. It is therefore perfectly possible to use

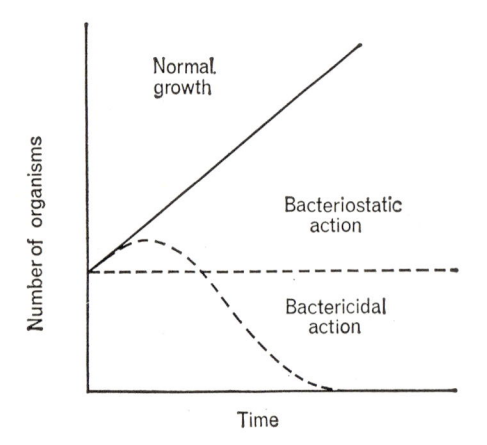

FIG. 16.2. Effects of bacteriostatic and bactericidal agents on bacterial multiplication in culture.

TABLE 16.1. SPECTRUM OF ACTIVITY OF COMMONLY USED ANTIBACTERIAL SUBSTANCES

	BACTERICIDAL				BACTERIOSTATIC	
	BENZYL-PENICILLIN	CLOXACILLIN	AMPICILLIN CARBENICILLIN	STREPTOMYCIN	SULPHONAMIDES	TETRACYCLINES
Gram −ve cocci	+	+	+	−	−	+
Gram +ve cocci	+	+	+	+	+	+
Benzylpenicillin resistant staph.	−	+	+	+	−	+
Gram −ve bacilli	−	−	+	+	+	+
H. influenzae	−	−	+	−	+	−
Pseudomonas	−	−	+	−	−	−
Proteus vulg.	−	−	+	+	+	+
Gram +ve bacteria	+	+	+	−	+	+
Myco. tuberc.	−	−	−	+	−	+
Spirochaetes	+	+	+	−	−	+
Rickettsia	−	−	−	−	−	+
Yeasts and fungi	−	−	−	−	−	−

TABLE 16.2. INHIBITION OF FOLATE REDUCTASE

	Half inhibition of folate reductase (M)		
	Human	E. coli	Staph. aureus
Methotrexate	9×10^{-8}	6×10^{-9}	1×10^{-9}
Trimethoprim	3×10^{-4}	5×10^{-9}	5×10^{-9}

doses that almost totally inhibit the bacterial enzyme, without affecting the human enzyme; trimethoprim is in consequence a useful antibacterial. In this case the selectivity of the action depends on differences in the structure of the human and bacterial enzymes that determine the strength of binding of the inhibitors. The availability of inhibitors acting on two distinct stages in a metabolic pathway raises the important question of how effective the two are in combination. This problem has been extensively studied. The combination is synergistic, i.e. the effects are greater than expected from the sum of the individual effects, so that in combination much smaller amounts of the two drugs are needed than either alone [FIG. 16.3].

Bacteria differ from mammalian cells in having a cell wall in addition to a lipoprotein cell membrane; the latter is probably basically similar to that of mammalian cells. The cell wall provides a strong mechanical support for the cell which not only protects the organism from mechanical damage but also enables it

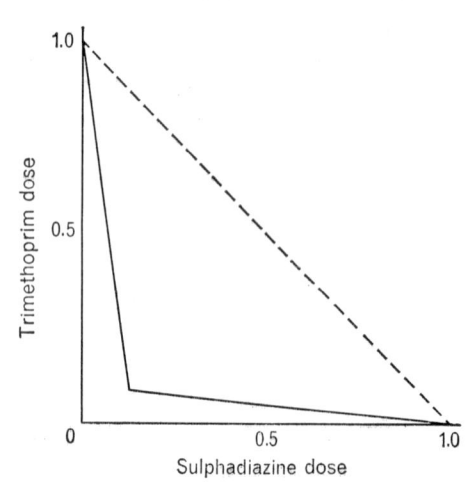

FIG. 16.3. Curative effect of combination of trimethoprim and sulphadiazine on mice infected with *Proteus vulgaris*. The solid line shows the concentration of both drugs needed to cure compared with the doses of either alone. The most effective combination is 8 per cent. of the dose of trimethoprim with 12 per cent. of the dose of sulphadiazine. The dashed line is the result expected if the drugs are just additive. (Hitchings and Burchall (1965) *Advanc. Enzymol.*, **27**, 417.)

to survive in media of low osmotic strength without bursting. When bacteria are grown in sublethal concentrations of penicillin, they are abnormal in shape, being bloated and distorted. This led to the suggestion that the antibacterial effects of penicillin might be due to interference with the synthesis of cell wall structures. It was then found by Park and his colleagues that in these abnormal cells there was an accumulation of large amounts of a peculiar compound containing amino acids (called a 'Park peptide'). The reasonable suggestion was made that this peptide represented a building block for cell wall synthesis which accumulated because the inhibition of a later stage in cell wall production prevented its use.

Gradually the complex story of how the cell wall is made has become unravelled and the way in which penicillin works has become clearer. The Park peptide consists of UDP coupled to N-acetylmuramic acid (NAM) and then to a pentapeptide which in *Staph. aureus* consists of L-Ala–D-Glu–L-Lys–D-Ala–D-Ala. The terminus of the chain consists of the unusual D-isomer of alanine which is not found in animals. The first stage in construction of the cell wall polymer is the coupling of the NAM groups of the peptides by alternating N-acetylglucosamine (NAG) groups, and the second is by coupling of the peptide chains by a transpeptidation reaction in which the terminal D-Ala is lost [FIG. 16.4]. The evidence suggests that it is mainly this latter stage that is inhibited by penicillin although the details still remain uncertain. Other antibacterials also interfere with the cell wall reactions. For instance, D-cycloserine (*Oxamycin*) also causes formation of abnormal cell forms and the accumulation of a different peptide, the product of reaction 3. D-cycloserine is an inhibitor of reactions 4 (*a*) and 4 (*b*) so that D-Ala and D-Ala–D-Ala are not found. Cycloserine [FIG. 16.5] can be regarded as a structural analogue of D-alanine.

Vancomycin and ristocetin have yet another way of interfering with cell wall synthesis; they have specific binding properties for peptides with a D-Ala–D-Ala terminus. The complex of peptide and antibacterial inhibits the cross linking process. Bacitracin also inhibits cell wall formation but the details of the process are obscure.

The inhibition of cell wall synthesis leads to the formation of unstable forms during reproduction which lyse and hence the antibacterials acting in this way are bactericidals. Since cell wall synthesis has no counterpart in mammalian cells the cytotoxic effect is specific. Although all bacterial cell walls appear to contain mucopeptide, those of Gram-negative organisms contain much less and depend mainly on an alternative structure (teichoic acid) which is therefore not susceptible to penicillin-type action. It is also possible that the resistance of Gram-negative organisms is partly due to the failure of the antibiotic to penetrate.

Some chemotherapeutic agents act upon the cell membrane. For instance, the macrolide polymers such as nystatin, amphotericin, and filipin have a specific lytic action on cells whose

1. UDP—NAM+L-Ala → UDP—NAM—L-Ala
2. UDP—NAM—L-Ala+D-Glu → UDP—NAM—L-Ala—D-Glu
3. UDP—NAM—L-Ala—D-Glu+L-Lys → UDP—NAM—L-Ala—D-Glu—L-Lys
4(a) L-Ala → D-Ala
4(b) D-Ala+D-Ala → D-Ala—D-Ala
5. UDP—NAM—Ala—Glu—Lys+D-Ala—D-Ala
  → UDP—NAM—Ala—Glu—Lys—D-Ala—D-Ala (PP)
6. PP+UDP—N-Acetylglucosamine →

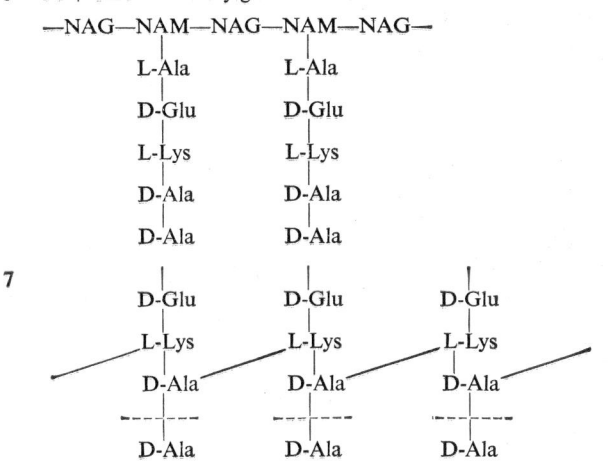

—NAG—NAM—NAG—NAM—NAG—
　　　　　|　　　　　|
　　　　L-Ala　　　L-Ala
　　　　　|　　　　　|
　　　　D-Glu　　　D-Glu
　　　　　|　　　　　|
　　　　L-Lys　　　L-Lys
　　　　　|　　　　　|
　　　　D-Ala　　　D-Ala
　　　　　|　　　　　|
　　　　D-Ala　　　D-Ala

7.
　　　　　|　　　　　|　　　　　|
　　　　D-Glu　　　D-Glu　　　D-Glu
　　　　　|　　　　　|　　　　　|
　　　　L-Lys　　　L-Lys　　　L-Lys
　　　　　|　　　　　|　　　　　|
　　　　D-Ala　　　D-Ala　　　D-Ala
　　　　---|---　---|---　---|---
　　　　D-Ala　　　D-Ala　　　D-Ala

FIG. 16.4. Synthesis of bacterial cell wall.

membranes contain cholesterol. Bacterial cell membranes do not contain appreciable amounts of cholesterol and are not affected but the cell membranes of fungi are rich in cholesterol, so that these substances are fungicides. Unfortunately, mammalian cell membranes also contain cholesterol, so that toxicity confines the use of these agents mainly to topical application. Gramicidin and tyrothricin have a more general action on cell membranes and are also only used topically.

The second major group of chemotherapeutic actions is on protein synthesis. So far actions on amino acid activation have not been seen and the site of action has been localized to the ribosome. A particularly clear action is that of puromycin which is a structural analogue of the terminal adenylic acid of a t-RNA.

It appears that puromycin binds to the ribosome in place of the aminoacyl end of t-RNA, and then peptidyl transferase attaches it to the growing end of the peptide by its amino group. Since its structure is inappropriate for further growth of the peptide it acts as a terminator and the short peptide chain then detaches from the ribosome. The cell accumulates peptide fragments each terminated by puromycin. Since puromycin acts equally well on protein synthesis in mammalian cells, it is not a practical antibacterial.

FIG. 16.5. Cycloserine.

A related mechanism is that of chloramphenicol and tetracycline which bind directly to the ribosome preventing the peptide bond-forming reaction. These agents are selective for bacterial ribosomes and do not bind to the larger ribosomes of animal cells.

Both chloramphenicol and tetracycline are bacteriostatic and their effects are quite rapidly reversible. Streptomycin and the related neomycin, kanamycin, and gentamicin also inhibit protein synthesis as a result of binding to the ribosome and in this case the binding has been shown to depend on a single structural protein (P10) on the 30S subunit. The binding of streptomycin distorts the ribosome so that t-RNA binding is defective, and not only is the rate of amino acid incorporation slowed but a mis-reading of the genetic code occurs. This means that errors are made and the wrong amino acids incorporated; the proteins produced are useless and it is probable that these abnormal proteins account in some way for the fact that streptomycin is bactericidal unlike the other inhibitors of protein synthesis.

COMBINATIONS OF ANTIBACTERIALS

We have already referred to one case, sulphonamides and trimethoprim, where combined use is synergistic. This is a common feature when antibacterials act on the same process, e.g. penicillin and ristocetin, or chloramphenicol and tetracycline, but when the drugs act on entirely different systems the results are often more difficult to predict. For instance, sulphonamide and penicillin are often less effective in combination than either alone and chloramphenicol also reduces the effectiveness of penicillin. In general it is not wise to combine bacteriostatic and bactericidal drugs.

RESISTANCE

The development of resistance to chemotherapy is a major problem not only as a source of failure in a particular case but because it will lead to the state where the majority of organisms that are isolated in disease are resistant to one or more antibacterials, as is now the case with staphylococci isolated in hospitals. Resistance develops as a result of the presence of natural mutants which are selected out as a result of the killing of the susceptible population. Resistance is *not* caused by the drug. Resistant strains are readily obtained by culturing in the presence of the antibacterial drug. Commonly, if a high concentration of drug is used no resistant colonies are found and it is necessary to culture in the presence of successively rising concentrations, so that resistance is then the result of a number of mutations. In the case of streptomycin, completely resistant strains can be isolated from mixed populations.

Resistance can be due to several causes. It may be that in the resistant strain the target enzyme is produced in greatly increased amounts so that, even though strongly inhibited, enough residual total activity remains. This is the major cause of resistance to folate reductase inhibitors; the enzyme concentration may be several thousand times as great in resistant as in sensitive strains. A more radical change is where as a result of a change in its structure the target molecule is no longer able to bind the antibacterial. This is clearly the case with streptomycin, where ribosomes from resistant organisms no longer bind streptomycin and this is due to a mutation affecting the P10 binding protein. Reconstitution of ribosomes from resistant organisms with P10 from sensitive organisms restores sensitivity. Binding of chloramphenicol to ribosomes of resistant strains is similarly lost. In the case of sulphonamide resistance the pteroic synthetase seems to become less sensitive to inhibition, although this may not be the only cause of resistance. In some instances it appears that resistant organisms are less permeable to the antibacterial. This has been reported with tetracyclines, sulphonamides, methotrexate, and some antitrypanosome drugs. In other cases the organism develops the ability to detoxify the antibacterial, a classic example being in the case of penicillin where resistant strains of staphylococci contain the enzyme penicillinase which opens the β-lactam ring of penicillin to form the inactive product penicilloic acid. The enzyme can be so active that resistance is very great. Inactivation of chloramphenicol can occur as a result of O-acetylation, and streptomycin can be converted to an adenylate.

A recent discovery has been the development of transferable resistance. This was first noted in Japan where dysentery organisms became resistant simultaneously to three or four antibacterials (sulphonamides, streptomycin, tetracycline, chloramphenicol). This was shown to be due to exchange of genetic material between bacteria in a manner similar to the transfer in bacterial sexual conjugation. The transfer of DNA probably occurs through conjugation tubes (pili) and can rapidly infect a sensitive population. These R-factors can also cross species so that for instance R-factors in coliforms may infect other enterobacteria such as *Shigella* or *Salmonella*. The resistance from R-factors is due either to increased metabolism, i.e. the R-factors carry the genes for the metabolic enzymes, or to reduced permeability. There are few organisms that will not develop resistance under appropriate conditions and it is very important that therapy should be designed to minimize the evolution of resistance. The most important factor is adequate dosage over a relatively short period (normally less than 7–14 days). Frequently two or more chemotherapeutics together may reduce the risk of resistance. If resistance depends on mutants, the chances of a mutant resistant to two or more antibacterials appearing is extremely small (this is not true with infective R-factor resistance). A case where multiple therapy has especial significance is in the chemotherapy of tuberculosis. These sluggish organisms multiply very slowly and prolonged therapy for periods up to 2 years is needed. This provides very favourable conditions for development of resistance when either streptomycin or isoniazid is used alone but is rare when they are used in combination and especially so when the weak antimycobacterial p-aminosalicylic acid is added to the combination.

CHEMOTHERAPEUTIC SPECTRA

Some chemotherapeutic agents act only on a single species or a limited group of organisms. These are referred to as narrow-spectrum. Examples are isoniazid active only against mycobacteria, nystatin active only against yeasts, or griseofulvin active against fungi. At the other extreme are drugs which affect a very wide range of species and are referred to as broad-spectrum. Examples are tetracycline and ampicillin. Other agents may have an intermediate range, such as penicillin, which kills cocci and Gram-positive bacilli, but is ineffective against most Gram-negative bacilli. The purported advantage of the wide-spectrum agents is that they reduce the need for identifying the causal organism and testing it for sensitivity. On the other hand, they violently alter the normal saprophytic bacterial flora as well as attacking the pathogens and are liable to lead to serious problems from superinfection by organisms such as *Candida* which are normally kept in check by the competitive pressure of surface saprophytes.

The present view is that except where treatment is very urgent it is better to isolate the organism to test its sensitivity to a range of antibacterials and select the most appropriate one even if of narrow spectrum.

PENICILLINS

Penicillins are acyl derivatives of 6-amino penicillanic acid. The original penicillin introduced by the Oxford workers was a mixture in which the most effective component was the phenacetyl derivative of 6-APA referred to as **benzylpenicillin** (or penicillin G). It was then found that by adding phenylacetic acid to the culture medium a greatly increased yield of virtually pure benzylpenicillin was obtained. This is a very active antibacterial which kills a wide range of Gram-negative and positive cocci; streptococci remain highly sensitive, but the majority of staphylococci isolated nowadays are resistant penicillinase-producing strains. Most strains of gonococci and pneumococci are sensitive. *Clostridia, B. anthracis,*

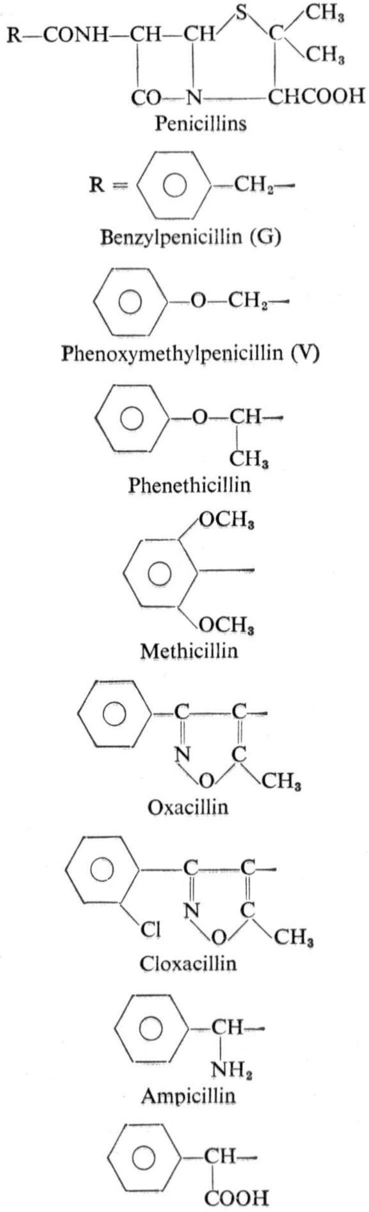

186 *Chemotherapy I: Bacteria, Fungi, Viruses*

[Figure 16.6 — Structure of penicillins: Penicillins general structure (R—CONH—CH—CH with S, C(CH₃)₂, CO—N—CHCOOH ring); Benzylpenicillin (G), R = C₆H₅—CH₂—; Phenoxymethylpenicillin (V), C₆H₅—O—CH₂—; Phenethicillin, C₆H₅—O—CH(CH₃)—; Methicillin, 2,6-dimethoxyphenyl—; Oxacillin; Cloxacillin; Ampicillin, C₆H₅—CH(NH₂)—; Carbenicillin, C₆H₅—CH(COOH)—.]

FIG. 16.6. Structure of penicillins.

Fusobacteria, and *Actinomycetes* are also sensitive. The spirochaete of syphilis (*Treponema pallidum*) is extremely sensitive, and the introduction of benzylpenicillin revolutionized the treatment of syphilis.

Benzylpenicillin doses are still given in international units where 1 unit = 0·6 μg.; doses are usually in the range of 0·2–2 mega units (0·12–1·2 g.) per day. Penicillin absorption by the oral route is limited because penicillin is rapidly hydrolysed by the gastric acid, and it is not usually given by this route.

After subcutaneous injection the blood level reaches a peak at about 30 minutes but then falls very rapidly and after 3 hours the plasma concentration is about one tenth of the peak level. The rapid fall of concentration is due to the active secretion of benzylpenicillin into the urine by the proximal renal tubules; most of the penicillin can be recovered unchanged in the urine. The rapid excretion is a disadvantage, but since penicillin is cheap and virtually non-toxic, high doses may be given to avoid repetition of the dosage more often than every 6–8 hours. Alternatively, depot preparations may be used; procaine forms a water insoluble salt with penicillin (**procaine penicillin**) which is injected as a suspension and produces adequate blood levels for 18–36 hours. An even more insoluble salt is formed with dibenzyl ethylene diamine (**benzathine penicillin**) and the injection of an aqueous suspension of this salt leads to low blood levels persisting for a week or more. Penicillin penetrates the cerebrospinal fluid and serous cavities relatively poorly, but this is less important than originally considered because infected serous membranes are more permeable and hence for instance penicillin penetrates well into the CSF in meningitis. This is fortunate because it is poorly tolerated by injection into the subarachnoid space and is liable to produce convulsions.

Penicillin is an extraordinarily non-toxic drug and almost all the untoward reactions to the drug are due to hypersensitivity. These may appear as skin rashes of many kinds, angio-edema, serum sickness, and anaphylaxis. The high antigenicity of penicillin seems to be due to the readiness with which penicillin can acylate plasmaproteins to form penicilloyl or penicillenyl derivates which are excellent antigens. In such a situation it is to be expected that allergic reactions will be more common on the second or later course of treatment. Since the hypersensitivity reactions may be serious and indeed fatal, their presence is normally an indication to stop therapy and warn the patient against subsequent treatment.

The main disadvantages of benzylpenicillin are its susceptibility to hydrolysis by acid and penicillinase and a good deal of effort has been put into finding penicillins lacking these disadvantages. The addition of phenoxyacetic acid to the culture medium in place of phenylacetic acid leads to the formation of **phenoxymethylpenicillin** (Penicillin V) which is much more resistant to acid hydrolysis and can therefore be relied upon to give good blood levels when administered by mouth. Phenoxyethylpenicillin (**phenethicillin**) is very similar. Both have a range of activity and potency very similar to benzylpenicillin, but also share its susceptibility to penicillinase. Further advance came from the development of the semi-synthetic penicillins. These are made by direct acylation of 6-APA. These became possible after the discovery of a strain of penicillium which formed an amidase which splits the side chain of penicillin thus allowing the large-scale production of 6-APA. The first important semisynthetic penicillin was **methicillin** which is very resistant to penicillinase and so attacks strains resistant to benzylpenicillin, but it is not acid resistant and must be given by injection. Resistant staphylococci are highly susceptible to methicillin but it is less effective against other cocci, it is thus a narrow-spectrum antibacterial reserved for treating resistant staphylococcal infections. **Oxacillin** and **cloxacillin** are both acid and penicillinase resistant, they can thus be used as orally active drugs for sensitive and resistant strains; they have a broader spectrum than methicillin but are less active on sensitive strains than benzylpenicillin. **Acillinmpi** is surprisingly a broad-spectrum agent and is effective against many Gram-negative bacilli such as *E. coli*, *Shigella*, and *Salmonella*, notably *Salmonella typhi*. It is also very active against *Haemophilus influenzae* and is much used in respiratory infections. It is well absorbed by mouth but is hydrolysed by penicillinase. **Carbenicillin** has an even broader spectrum and is notably effective against *Pseudomonas* and *Aerobacter*. It is resistant to both penicillinase and acid but is poorly absorbed and must be given by injection. Unfortunately these semisynthetic penicillins are just as likely to cause hypersensitivity as benzylpenicillin. **Cephalosporins** are close relatives of the penicillins and have very similar actions. In structure they differ in having a six-membered ring, 7-amino cephalosporanic acid, compared with the five-membered ring in 6-APA. They are resistant to penicillinase, but resistant organisms form a related enzyme cephalosporinase. **Cephaloridine** and **cephalothin** [FIG. 16.7] are broad-spectrum antibiotics rather similar to carbenicillin and are not absorbed when given by mouth.

TETRACYCLINES

The tetracyclines are exceptionally broad-spectrum agents, and in addition to the ordinary range of bacteria they also inhibit rickettsia, amoebae, mycoplasma, and the agents of trachoma, lymphogranuloma venereum, and psittacosis and are marginally active in tuberculosis. They are not active against *Proteus*, *Pseudomonas aeruginosa*, or *Candida* and many strains of staphylococci are resistant; these organisms are a frequent source of annoying and even dangerous superinfection when tetracyclines are used. The development of resistance to tetracyclines is relatively slow and does not usually cross with other antibiotics.

There is little to choose between the various tetracyclines, which are rather poorly absorbed and rather slowly cleared unchanged in the urine. Toxicity is common; most frequently gastro-intestinal disturbances, nausea, vomiting, and diarrhoea. Tetracyclines are laid down in growing bone and teeth and may interfere with growth and are best avoided in

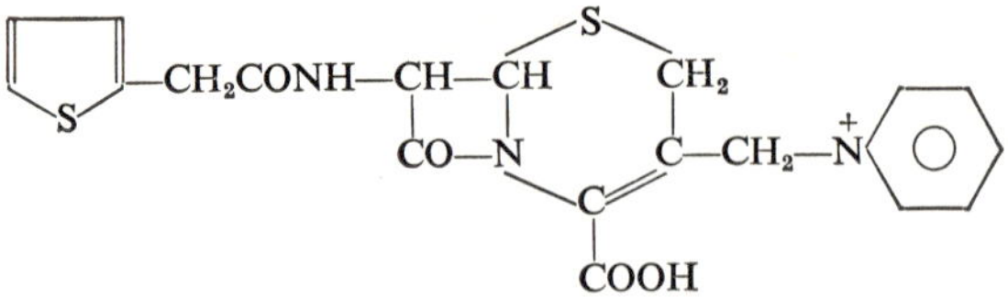

FIG. 16.7. Cephalosporins.

Cephaloridine

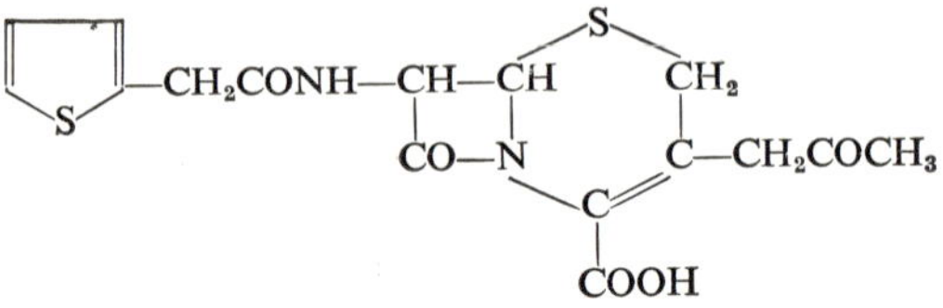

Cephalothin

pregnant women. Despite these defects, tetracyclines are valuable antibiotics and are widely used.

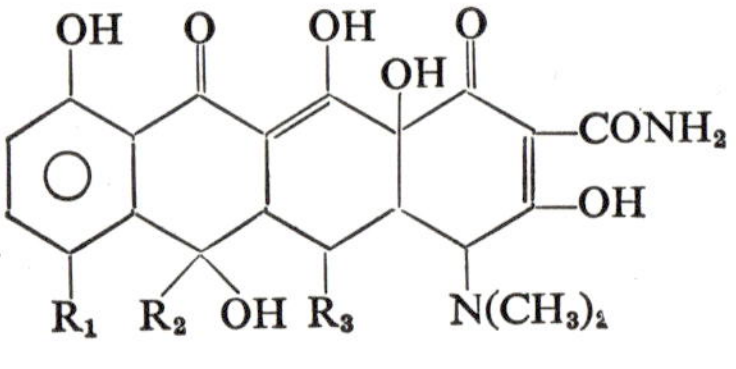

Tetracyclines

R_1	R_2	R_3	
H	CH$_3$	H	Tetracycline
Cl	CH$_3$	H	Chlortetracycline
H	CH$_3$	OH	Oxytetracycline
Cl	H	H	Demethylchlortetracycline

FIG. 16.8. Structures of tetracyclines.

SULPHONAMIDES

Despite being the first of the modern antibacterials, sulphonamides retain a substantial place in therapy and this has been extended by the recent introduction of a combined preparation of sulphonamide and trimethoprim (*Septrin*, *Bactrim*) which takes advantage of the synergistic actions of these two substances and the reduced likelihood of resistance occurring when the two are used in combination. Sulphonamides have a broad spectrum. Most streptococci are sensitive and pneumococci and meningococci especially sensitive, staphylococci in general are insensitive as are most currently isolated strains of gonococci. Many Gram-negative bacilli are sensitive, including most *E. coli*, *Shigella*, and some *Proteus*. They are also active in actinomycosis and toxoplasmosis.

The active sulphonamides all have a free amino group and differ in the amide substitution. The nature of this substituent has some effect on antibacterial activity but the objective in recent years has been to control solubility, protein binding, and rate of excretion. In the early sulphonamides crystal formation in the urinary tract was a hazard but many of the new sulphonamides such as sulphafurazole (sulfisoxazole) and sulphamethizole are very soluble. The sulphonamides are well absorbed from the gut and their duration of action depends mainly on the extent of protein binding. Sulphaphenazole and sulphamethoxypyridazine are strongly bound to plasma proteins and are long acting, hence only a single daily dose is needed, but they are not much in favour because of a high incidence of toxic effects. The sulphonamide in the *Septrin–Bactrim* combination, sulphamethoxazole, was chosen because its biological lifetime is similar to that of trimethoprim and hence the ratio of the two drugs stays approximately constant during dosage.

FIG. 16.9. Structure of sulphonamides.

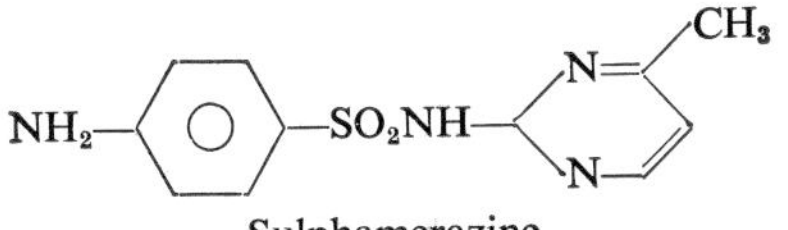

Sulphamerazine

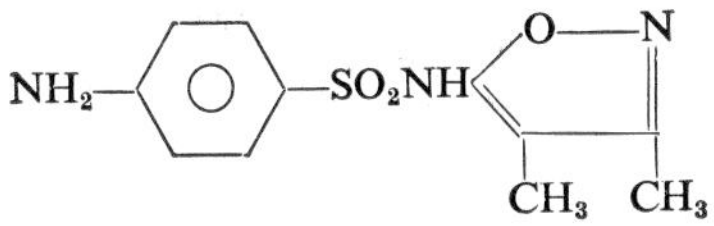

Sulfisoxazole

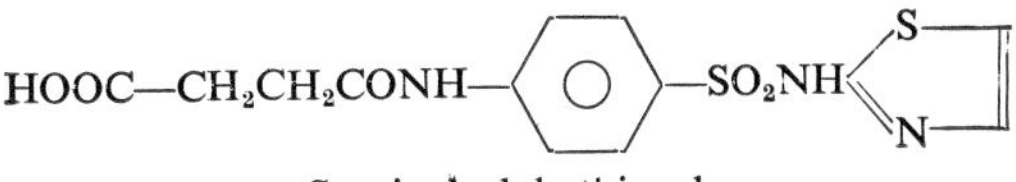

Succinylsulphathiazole

Sulphonamides are metabolized to N_4 acetylated derivatives that are inactive as antibacterials, which are excreted in the urine together with the unchanged sulphonamide. Sulphonamides with an acid group on N_4 (succinylsulphathiazole, phthalylsulphathiazole) are not absorbed from the small gut, but in the colon are hydrolysed by bacteria to free sulphathiazole which acts locally; free sulphathiazole is poorly absorbed in the large gut so that only a small fraction of the drug given is absorbed. These drugs are used in dysenteries and have the dual advantage of local action and minimum risk of crystalluria in a condition in which dehydration is important. Sulphasalazine (salicylazosulphapyridine) is a drug related to the original prontosil which is used in the treatment of colitis; it is not known how it acts.

Adverse effects to sulphonamides are not uncommon and frequently involve hypersensitivity. Skin rashes and bone marrow depression are the most important.

CHLORAMPHENICOL

Chloramphenicol was the first of the broad-spectrum antibacterials and has been very successful. Unfortunately, it may produce bone marrow aplasia which leads to death in about one case in 10,000. Modern chemotherapy is so safe that this risk is unacceptable except in severe illness where no other less hazardous agent is available. The risk can be minimized by limiting the total dose given, but in practice chloramphenicol is now used in typhoid, in severe infections with *H. influenzae* (meningitis), and rickettsial infections, although it has been largely displaced even from these uses by the broad-spectrum penicillins.

STREPTOMYCIN

Streptomycin is a glycoside formed from N-methyl glucosamine, streptose, and streptidine. It is a broad-spectrum agent, but as pointed out earlier, large jump resistance can occur extremely rapidly with streptomycin and organisms can then sometimes actually divide faster in the presence of the drug. The development of resistance can be substantially reduced by simultaneous administration of other antibiotics but this manœuvre is mainly used in the treatment of tuberculosis.

Streptomycin is a strong base and is not absorbed from the gut. Advantage is taken of this in the use of streptomycin or the closely related neomycin for sterilizing the gut before intestinal surgery or in hepatic cirrhosis. For systemic use it is injected intramuscularly and contact with the skin should be avoided

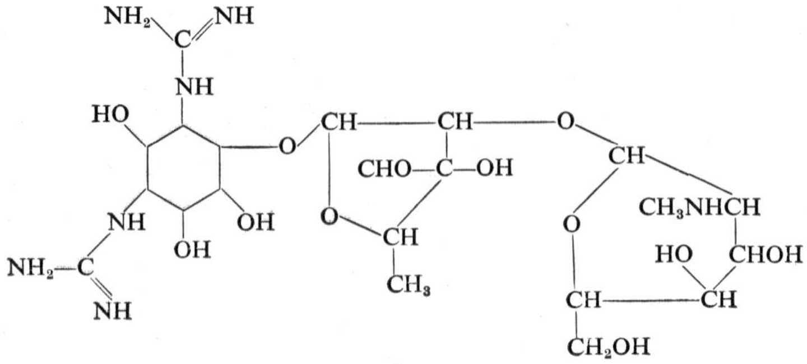

Streptomycin

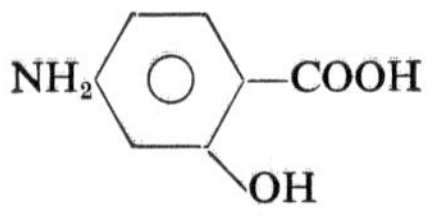

p-Aminosalicylic acid
(PAS)

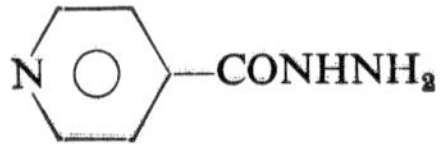

Isoniazid

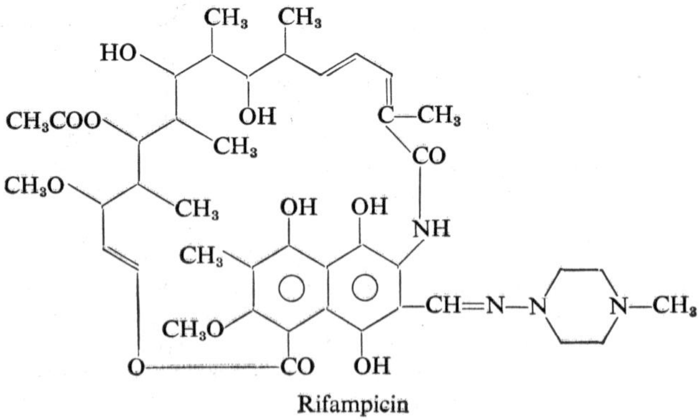

Rifampicin

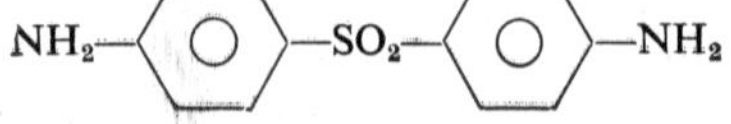

Dapsone

FIG. 16.10. Drugs used in the treatment of tuberculosis and leprosy.

because of the readiness with which contact dermatitis can be developed.

The main toxic effects of streptomycin are dose dependent and are exerted in the vestibular division of the eighth nerve. This manifests as dizziness, headache, nausea, and vomiting, and later ataxia. These effects are more likely to occur in older patients and may be irreversible. Less commonly the cochlear division of the eighth nerve is affected leading to deafness. Like most other antibacterials, streptomycin is largely excreted unchanged in the urine, and hence where renal impairment is present, excessive blood levels will occur in response to standard dosage with greater likelihood of eighth nerve lesions. The adjustment of the dose in these cases can be made according to the reduction in the glomerular filtration rate. **Kanamycin** and **paromomycin** are closely related drugs with similar antibacterial spectra and toxicity and there is a good deal of overlap of resistance.

CHEMOTHERAPY OF TUBERCULOSIS

The introduction of streptomycin for treatment of tuberculosis radically changed the handling and prognosis of patients with this disease. From a condition in which the mortality was high, with treatment by prolonged bed rest combined with drastic surgery, it has become amenable to simple treatment, much of it in the home or while ambulant, with a very high recovery rate. Chemotherapy in tuberculosis raises special problems because of the avascular nature of the lesions and the sluggish reproduction of the organism; in consequence therapy needs to be continued for about 2 years in most cases. Such prolonged treatment highlights problems of drug toxicity and of the development of resistance. Streptomycin is fairly toxic, but it has been found empirically that intermittent dosage, at first one dose a day and later twice a week, is adequate and is less toxic than when blood levels are maintained. However, resistance develops rapidly but can be greatly diminished by combination with **p-aminosalicylic acid (PAS)**. The substance is a feeble bacteriostatic, but greatly reduces the emergence of resistance. p-Aminosalicylic acid is given by mouth either as cachets or as effervescent granules taken in water. Either way it is very unpopular with patients because of the high incidence of gastro-intestinal upsets, nausea, vomiting, abdominal pain, and diarrhoea. **Isoniazid**, which was introduced in 1952, is an extremely effective antimycobacterial and is effective at concentrations less than $0.1 \mu g./ml$. Its mechanism of action is quite unknown. It is active by mouth and of relatively low toxicity. The most common toxic effect is a peripheral neuritis, although optic neuritis, ataxia, convulsions, and mental abnormalities may develop. A variety of other toxic effects occur less frequently. The main metabolic pathway of isoniazid is by N-acetylation. In about half the population of Europe and America the rate of acetylation is slow. This is an interesting case of genetically determined drug inactivation. The rapid inactivators are either homozygous or heterozygous dominants for the inactivating enzyme, the slow inactivators are autosomal homozygous recessives. Present evidence does not suggest that the effectiveness of isoniazid is reduced in the rapid inactivators, but the incidence of peripheral neuritis is lower.

Current therapy consists of the combination of streptomycin, PAS, and isoniazid. The number of resistant organisms is still relatively low but the therapy is not ideal. Streptomycin must be given by injection, which is unsatisfactory for home treatment and for larger-scale treatment in underdeveloped countries; the unpleasant side-effects of PAS lead many patients to avoid dosage; in comparison isoniazid is relatively trouble-free.

A new drug **rifampicin** (*Rifampin*) which inhibits DNA-directed RNA synthesis (a mechanism not discussed earlier) is as active against mycobacteria as isoniazid, is active by mouth, and is relatively non-toxic. Trials to date have been very successful and rifampicin is likely to replace streptomycin over the next few years particularly if the cost can be reduced. So far no acceptable substitute for PAS has been discovered. Where resistance or toxicity develop with these agents a number of second-line antimycobacterials are available of which ethambutol and ethionamide are the most useful but cycloserine, viomycin, and pyrazinamide are occasionally used. All these drugs are relatively toxic.

LEPROSY

This disease is caused by another mycobacterium, *M. leprae*, whose characteristics and sensitivity to chemotherapy are, however, very different from *M. tuberculosis*. The most active drugs are derivatives of **diaminodiphenylsulphone** (dapsone) and **thiacetazone** (amithiozone).

MISCELLANEOUS ANTIBACTERIALS

Erythromycin is a macrolide (large lactone) which inhibits protein synthesis on the ribosome. It is most effective against staphylococci, streptococci, and pneumococci, and is mainly used in staphylococcal infections where it is very effective. Erythromycin is absorbed from the gut, but is acid sensitive. This problem has been overcome by enteric coating or by administering as the stearate or estolate. Toxicity is low.

Related are **oleandomycin** and **spiramycin**. **Lincomycin** which is a hygrinic acid derivative has a similar range but is more toxic and frequently causes diarrhoea.

Fucidin is a steroid active against staphylococci, which, however, readily become resistant; it is orally effective and relatively non-toxic. **Novobiocin** has a similar range.

ANTIFUNGAL AGENTS

Griseofulvin is a systemic fungicide active against mycotic diseases of the skin, hair, and nails (ringworm, athletes' foot) due to *Epidermophyton*, *Trichophyton*, and *Microsporum*. The drug is very poorly absorbed by mouth but is, nevertheless, effective by this route. The main side-effects are headache and nausea and vomiting. Equally good effects can often be obtained by local application of a cream containing a synthetic compound **tolnaftate**, a compound that appears quite non-toxic.

Serious systemic infections with *Histoplasma, Coccidioides, Blastomyces,* and *Candida* can be treated with **amphotericin B** which acts on organisms whose cell membranes contain cholesterol. It is poorly absorbed from the gut and is therefore given by slow intravenous infusion. It is a very toxic drug and a large range of serious side-effects have been recorded but it is life-saving in these infections.

Nystatin is a related polyene that is used topically particularly for *Candida* infection of the vagina and gut (it is not absorbed).

ANTIVIRUS AGENTS

It can be seen from the foregoing account that so many good antibacterial agents are available that we can afford to be eclectic; in contrast is the poverty of effective antiviral agents. This is mainly because the available points of attack on viruses are so few—a virus is little more than a package of genes with a protective coat and penetrative apparatus that relies for its metabolic functions on the host cell. In order to be an effective parasite its metabolic needs must match what the host can provide. Nevertheless, there are several ways in which antiviral agents might act. Firstly they directly attack the free virus or prevent it adhering to or penetrating the host cell. There is some evidence that **amantadine** acts at this stage on some influenza viruses and a marginal effect has been demonstrated in man in A_2 influenza. **Phenoxymethylisoquinolines** appear to act as inhibitors of viral neuramidinase and interfere with attachment. Trials in human influenza are promising. They may also act on myxoviruses and enteroviruses but full trials have not yet been reported.

Actions on replication have been shown in the case of **idoxuridine**, which is incorporated into the virus DNA and may lead to coding errors. Idoxuridine has been successfully used in the treatment of corneal herpes by local application but is not practical for systemic use. **Methisazone** is a thiosemicarbazone of N-methylisatin and appears to inhibit the synthesis of the viral structural proteins necessary for assembly of completed pox viruses. Trials in India have established that methisazone is highly successful in reducing the incidence of smallpox among contacts but it is of no value in treating the established disease. **Interferons** are small proteins formed by many cells after infection with DNA or RNA viruses and which inhibit virus growth relatively unselectively. Great difficulties have been encountered in preparing interferon and effort has been concentrated more on methods of stimulating endogenous production. It has been found that a non-pathogenic virus DNA extracted from penicillium (statolon) and some synthetic polynucleotides are capable of stimulating interferon formation but they are unfortunately rather toxic.

ANTISEPTICS

A very large number of substances have been used for killing bacteria outside the body, unhampered as this process is by requirements of being harmless to the host. In fact, nearly all antiseptics are protein denaturants and act on enzymes, etc. in the bacteria and for the same reason the effectiveness of most antiseptics is considerably reduced in serum, blood, or pus. Antiseptics are used for the following purposes:

1. *Instrument and material sterilization*

Some instruments are too delicate to be boiled or autoclaved; suture material and implantable materials, e.g. plastic vascular grafts, middle-ear inserts, may also need other methods. The most effective sterilizing system used is **ethylene oxide** in gaseous form. A simple related method uses an aqueous solution of **glutaraldehyde**. Cationic agents (benzalkonium, cetyltrimethylammonium, cetrimide) and chlorinated phenols are also used for cold sterilization of instruments, thermometers, oxygen masks, etc.

2. *Cleaning of the skin before operations*

Cleaning of the skin is no easy matter because of the bacteria resident in sweat and sebaceous glands and in hair follicles. **Ethanol** and **isopropanol** are both used at 70 per cent. concentration and are effective but not persistent; they are improved by the addition of 0·5 per cent. **chlorhexidine,** a chlorinated phenyl-biguanide or of benzalkonium. The organic mercurial **thiomersal** (*Merthiolate*) is also very effective. Two per cent. iodine in isopropanol is a very efficient skin disinfectant but caution is needed since some individuals are sensitized to iodine.

3. *Coarse disinfection*

Disinfection of contaminated glassware, bed pans, benches, floors, etc. is most usually carried out with phenolics such as Lysol which is a mixture of cresols and soap, or Dettol, a chlorinated xylenol. Bath water is often made antiseptic by the addition of hexachlorophane.

4. *Water*

Drinking-water and swimming-baths are usually sterilized with gaseous chlorine or sodium hypochlorite.

FURTHER READING

BARBER, M., and GARROD, L. P. (1963) *Antibiotics and Chemotherapy*, Edinburgh.

BUSCH, H., and LEME, M. (1967) *Chemotherapy*, Chicago.

DOYLE, F. P., and NAYLER, J. H. C. (1964) Penicillins and related structures, *Advanc. Drug Res.*, **1**, 1.

GALE, E. F. (1963) Mechanism of antibiotic action, *Pharmacol. Rev.*, **15**, 481.

GOTTLIEB, D., and SHAW, P. D. (1967) *Antibiotics. Mechanism of Action*, Berlin.

MITSUHASHI, S. (1971) *Transferable Drug Resistance Factor R*, Baltimore.

NEWTON, B. A., and REYNOLDS, P. E. (1966) *Biochemical Studies of Antimicrobial Drugs*, Cambridge.

SCHNITZER, R. J., and HAWKING, F. (1963) *Experimental Chemotherapy*, New York.

WEISBLUM, B., and DAVIS, J. (1968) Antibiotic inhibitors of the bacterial ribosome, *Bact. Rev.*, **32**, 493.

17

CHEMOTHERAPY II: PROTOZOA AND WORMS

MALARIA

ALTHOUGH malaria has been eradicated or controlled in most parts of the world, this disease still affects about 200 million people and causes at least 1 million deaths each year.

The parasites responsible for the disease have a complex life cycle involving a human and an insect host and the susceptibility of the parasite to drugs depends on the stage which has been reached in the cycle, no single drug being effective against the parasite at all stages of its life cycle.

There are three common forms of malaria in man, each caused by a different protozoan parasite. *Plasmodium vivax* causes benign tertian malaria (B.T.) in which fever occurs every 48 hours. *Plasmodium falciparum* causes malignant tertian (subtertian) malaria (M.T.) which may cause death by invading the CNS. *Plasmodium malariae* is responsible for the rather rare quartan malaria in which fever occurs every 72 hours.

Life Cycle of the Malarial Parasite

The first stage of the development of the parasite in human red blood corpuscles is the trophozoite [FIG. 17.1], which appears as a ring which grows and develops amoeboid movements. The second stage is the development of the schizont in which the nucleus divides into about sixteen fragments. Eventually the blood cells burst and about sixteen merozoites are discharged into the plasma and it is this event, which involves the release of foreign proteins into the blood, which causes the fever of malaria. Some of the liberated merozoites invade fresh red cells and establish themselves as trophozoites so that the cycle is repeated.

Malaria is transmitted from one person to another by mosquitoes, but not in the form of schizonts. Special male and female parasites, known as gametocytes, are formed in the blood but do not develop until the blood is ingested by a female mosquito. When they are ingested by a mosquito they congregate in the stomach and develop through several stages to form sporozoites which are then injected by the mosquito into new human hosts.

These sporozoites disappear from the blood in about an hour and accumulate in macrophages and other reticulo-endothelial cells. During this pre-erythrocytic stage, which is symptomless, the sporozoites grow, segment, and sporulate to form merozoites. With the exception of *P. falciparum* a proportion of the parasites start an exo-erythrocytic cycle and this may continue for several years and eventually cause a relapse.

Drugs Producing Causal Prophylaxis

Drugs in this group prevent demonstrable infection by killing the parasites during their pre-erythrocytic stages and treatment must be maintained as long as the patient is at risk.

Pyrimethamine and **proguanil** are both effective prophylactic agents against *P. falciparum* but are less effective against *P. vivax* infections.

Pyrimethamine is active against the pre-erythrocytic forms of *P. falciparum* and kills the exo-erythrocytic parasites of *P. vivax*. It does not affect the infective sporozoites. The compound acts by interfering with folic–folinic acid systems, mainly when the nuclei are dividing, and so affects nucleoprotein metabolism. Pyrimethamine has little effect upon

196　Chemotherapy II: Protozoa and Worms

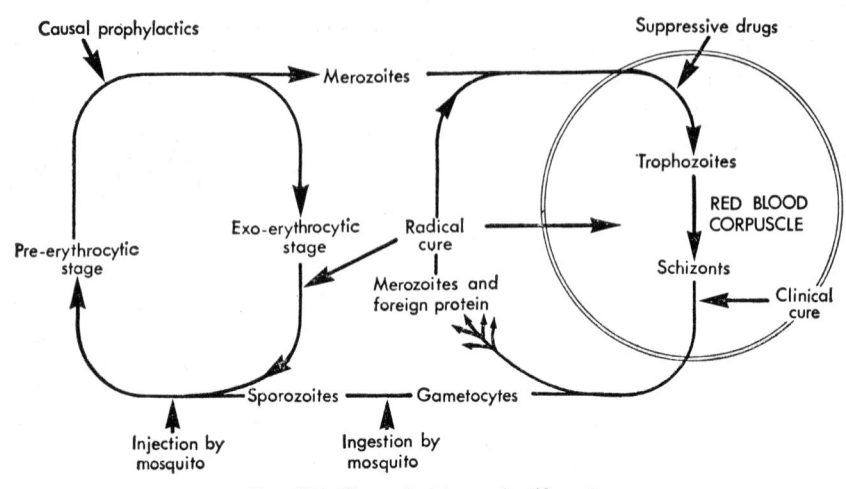

FIG. 17.1. The malarial parasite life cycle.

immature schizonts in the red cells and it is therefore slow to control a malarial attack. For this reason other drugs may be preferred for the treatment of acute attacks of malaria. The chief value of pyrimethamine is as a suppressant and, in the doses necessary for it to be effective, it has few toxic actions.

Proguanil (chloroguanide) is a biguanide which is an effective causal prophylactic and suppressive in sporozoite falciparum malaria. It is also effective in acute clinical attacks and usually eradicates the infection. It is not very effective against *P. vivax* although clinical attacks due to this organism can often be controlled.

Proguanil is absorbed only slowly from the gastro-intestinal tract and the drug itself has little antimalarial activity but is metabolized by the host to a triazine form, which is active.

Proguanil does not destroy gametocytes but prevents the development of gametes in the mosquito. It has been suggested that proguanil, or its active triazine metabolite, acts by inhibiting the reduction of folic acid resulting

TABLE 17.1. DRUGS USED IN THE TREATMENT OF MALARIA

FORM OF PARASITE	TYPE OF ACTION	*P. FALCIPARUM* (M.T. MALARIA)	*P. VIVAX* (B.T. MALARIA)
Pre-erythrocytic	Causal prophylactic (kills parasites)	Proguanil Pyrimethamine Primaquine	None known
Erythrocytic stage	Suppressive (inhibits erythrocytic stage)	Chloroquine Proguanil Pyrimethamine	Chloroquine Proguanil Pyrimethamine
Schizonts	Clinical cure (prevents schizogony)	Chloroquine Amodiaquine	Chloroquine Amodiaquine
Erythrocytic and exo-erythrocytic	Radical cure (kills all forms of parasites)	All above drugs (no exo-erythrocytic stage)	Primaquine (with chloroquine)

in the suppression of nucleic acid synthesis. This, together with the slow absorption of the drug and its conversion to an active metabolite, would explain the slow action of this drug in relieving the symptoms of acute malaria.

Suppressive Treatment

Suppressive drugs inhibit the erythrocytic stage of development of the malarial parasite and so prevent the onset of symptoms. The exo-erythrocytic stage is not destroyed and clinical attacks may occur on the cessation of treatment; this is particularly likely in the case of infections by *P. vivax*. Drugs used for this purpose include **chloroquine, amodiaquine, proguanil,** and **pyrimethamine.**

Chloroquine, which is a 4-aminoquinoline, is very effective against the asexual erythrocytic forms of *P. vivax* and *P. falciparum* and against the gametocytes of *P. vivax*.

It quickly controls acute clinical attacks of malaria and it usually completely eradicates falciparum infections, although it does not prevent relapses due to *P. vivax*. This is because the drug has little effect on the exo-erythrocytic stages of the parasite and this stage occurs in the life cycle of *P. vivax* but not in that of *P. falciparum*.

Chloroquine is well tolerated in normal doses and may safely be given to children and pregnant women. The occasional development of irreversible retinal damage (chloroquine retinopathy) is a serious toxic hazard of prolonged treatment with high doses.

Drugs Producing Clinical Cure

Drugs in this group prevent reproduction of the parasites within the erythrocytes and so terminate a malarial attack.

The drugs of choice are **chloroquine** and

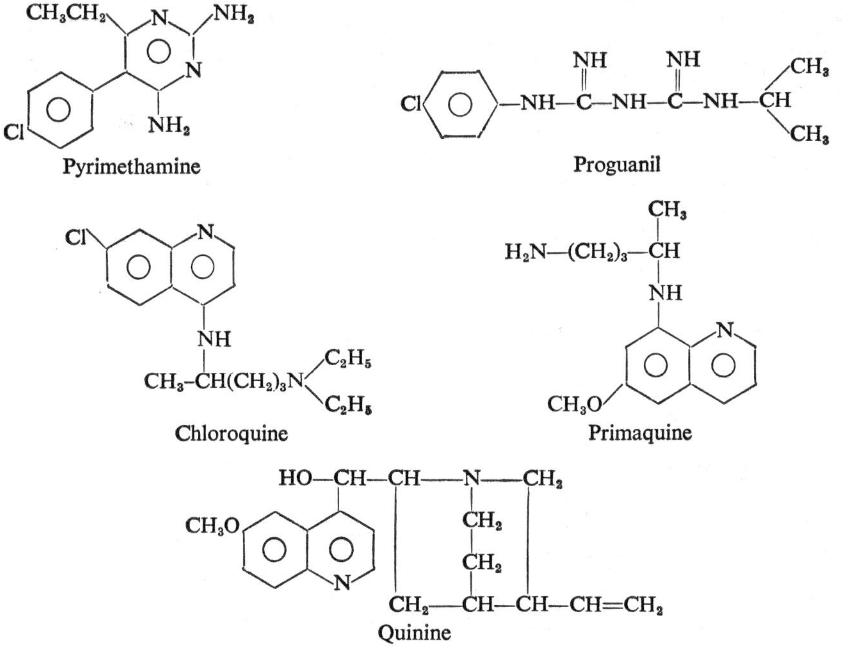

FIG. 17.2. The structures of drugs used in the treatment of malaria.

amodiaquine, both of which are derivatives of 4-aminoquinoline.

Radical Cure

Drugs which effect a radical cure eradicate both the erythrocytic and exo-erythrocytic parasites in an infected patient. In cases of *P. vivax* infection, primaquine is the only effective drug in current use. It is usually given together with chloroquine and in this combination it is particularly effective in producing a radical cure.

Radical cure following *P. falciparum* infection is relatively easy to secure and a number of drugs are effective [TABLE 17.1].

Primaquine is effective against the primary exo-erythrocytic forms of *P. vivax* and *P. falciparum* but has little effect on the asexual blood forms of *P. falciparum*, and a rather unpredictable action on these forms of *P. vivax*, but it is the most effective drug for the complete eradication of vivax malaria, especially if given with chloroquine.

Quinine is obtained from cinchona which contains a mixture of over twenty different alkaloids. At one time quinine was the only drug available for the specific treatment of malaria but experience during the Second World War demonstrated the superiority of **quinacrine** and other new compounds. Quinine is now used mainly for the treatment of malarial infections which are resistant to the action of more modern drugs.

Quinine does not kill sporozoites or pre-erythrocytic tissue forms of the parasite. Its main action is on the schizonts and it is effective as a suppressant and for the control of overt clinical attacks. The drug is readily absorbed from the small intestine and about half is destroyed in the liver while the rest is excreted in the urine.

Quinine has some toxic effects, particularly on the special senses. The first symptoms are ringing in the ears, deafness, and defects of vision which may be slight or which may lead to blindness. There may be headache, nausea, and vomiting and a few people show allergic reactions to the drug. Because quinine is more toxic and less effective than the more modern synthetic antimalarial drugs, it is now rarely used by itself.

Resistance to Antimalarials

Acquired resistance by the malarial parasites to the pyrimidines and biguanides is frequently observed. The mechanism of this resistance is not known but it may be that the drug acts selectively in killing only the susceptible parasites thus allowing the multiplication of resistant mutants. The malarial parasites rarely, if ever, become resistant to the cinchona alkaloids or to the 4 and 8-aminoquinolines.

AMOEBIC DYSENTERY

Amoebic dysentery is due to an infection of the mucous membrane of the large intestine with the organism *Entamoeba histolytica* and may include the invasion of the portal veins and the formation of abscesses in the liver.

The disease is widespread and many infected persons do not have dysentery, but only mild symptoms of amoebiasis. Such infected persons act as carriers of the disease and are a serious public health problem. Asymptomatic carriers may develop amoebic abscesses in the liver, brain, or lung.

No single drug is fully effective against amoebae in both the intestinal and extra-intestinal locations.

Emetine is an alkaloid obtained from ipecacuanha and is effective against the symptoms of amoebic dysentery but only eradicates the infection in 10–15 per cent. of patients. Even prolonged treatment does not eliminate the amoebic cysts and such patients may become carriers of the disease.

Emetine is usually given by deep subcutaneous or by intramuscular injection be-

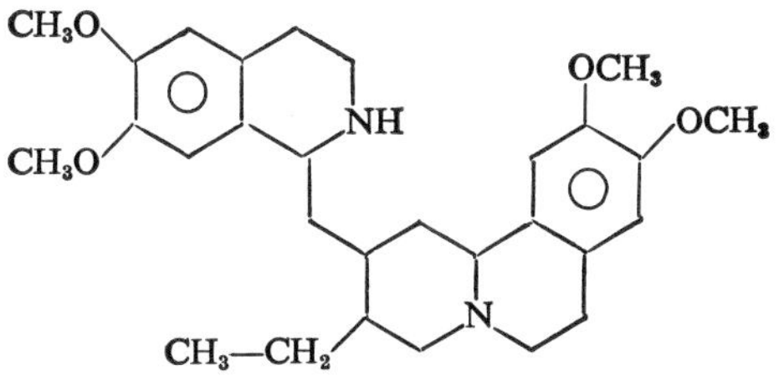

FIG. 17.3. Drugs used in the treatment of amoebic dysentery.

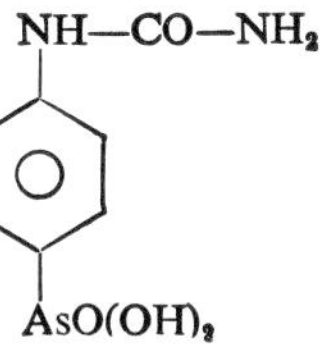

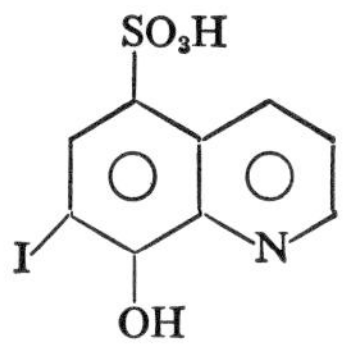

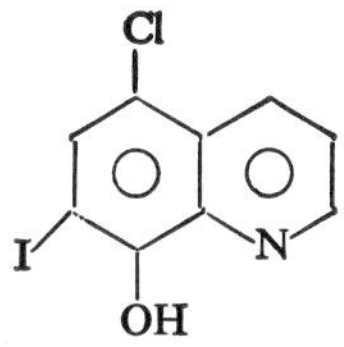

cause oral administration often causes vomiting. Excretion of the drug is erratic and may continue for several weeks. Cumulative effects are easily produced.

Emetine is thought to act by causing degeneration of the nucleus and reticulation of the amoebic cytoplasm. Repeated doses produce toxic effects of which heart damage is the most serious. **Emetine and bismuth iodide** has actions similar to those of emetine but it has the advantage of being effective when given orally.

Chloroquine is accumulated by the liver to a concentration several hundred times greater than that in the plasma. It is therefore extremely effective in hepatic amoebiasis and in other extra-intestinal amoebic infections.

The concentration of the drug in the intestinal wall is much lower than in the liver and it is almost completely absorbed from the small bowel. It is not very effective in treating colonic amoebiasis.

Carbarsone may be used in intestinal amoebiasis but the results of treatment with this drug have sometimes been poor.

The amoebicidal action of carbarsone is due to the arsenic which probably combines with thiol (—SH) groups in enzyme systems. It is of no value in the treatment of extra-intestinal forms of amoebiasis.

Chiniofon is effective against mobile and cystic amoebae but is ineffective against amoebic abscesses and hepatitis because it appears to act only on parasites in the intestinal tract.

The drug may be given orally, is practically non-toxic, and is usually regarded as the safest and most effective amoebicide.

Clioquinol (iodochlorhydroxyquin) has the same uses as chiniofon and is effective only against intestinal amoebiasis.

Other Drugs

Paromomycin is an antimicrobial which is useful in the treatment of acute and chronic amoebic dysentery and many types of bacterial enteritis.

Chlorphenoxamine and **diloxanide** are useful mainly in the treatment of chronic amoebiasis.

LEISHMANIA

Leishmaniasis is a disease produced by infection of the reticulo-endothelial system with *Leishmania donovani*, *L. brasiliensis*, and *L. tropica*.

Organic antimonials containing pentavalent antimony are the most effective and widely used drugs for the treatment of infections by *L. donovani* (kala-azar disease). Infection by *L. brasiliensis* and *L. tropica* is more difficult to treat but may respond to pentavalent antimonials or to pentamidine.

Stibamine is the sodium salt of a p-aminophenylstibonic acid. It is one of a large number of drugs containing pentavalent antimony. Others are **sodium stibogluconate**, **urea stibamine**, and **ethylstibamine**.

These drugs are all used to treat kala-azar.

Other Drugs

Pentamidine is used to treat leishmaniasis and is especially valuable in patients who do not respond to treatment with antimonial drugs.

TRYPANOSOMES

The trypanosomes belong to the genus *Trypanosoma* and, like the leishmanias, are mobile protozoan parasites which are injected by insects in tropical countries, into men and animals.

The parasites cause wasting diseases with intermittent fever, the best known of which is called sleeping-sickness and is caused by *T. gambiense* and *T. rhodesiense*. *T. cruzi* causes Chagas' disease which occurs in South America.

The Arsenicals

The pentavalent arsenicals which are active against trypanosomes are all reduced *in vivo* to a trivalent form. The vulnerability of different species of trypanosomes to these drugs varies, *T. gambiense* is sensitive but *T. cruzi* is unaffected.

An early theory of the mode of action of arsenicals was that the drug combined with thiol compounds such as cysteine and glutathione. It was suggested that this depressed cellular oxidation–reduction systems and produced death of the trypanosome. This suggestion is supported by the finding that the action of arsenicals is antagonized by glutathione, cysteine, and dimercaprol but it fails to explain why some trypanosomes are resistant to arsenicals and some are not. Non-resistant trypanosomes transport the arsenicals into their bodies, where the drug combines with vital —SH-containing enzymes. Hexokinase is thought to be inhibited and, since this enzyme catalyses the conversion of glucose to glucose-6-phosphate, the selective action of the arsenical may be due to the very high rate of metabolism in the trypanosome compared with that in the host.

Tryparsamide contains about 25 per cent. of pentavalent arsenic in organic combination. This compound penetrates the blood–brain barrier, is highly trypanocidal, and is therefore effective in advanced infections which have penetrated the CNS.

Tryparsamide is often employed in the early stages of disease as a supplement to pentamidine or suramin in order to ensure that early infections of the CNS do not escape attack.

Melarsoprol is a trivalent arsenical and is effective against parasites which have become resistant to tryparsamide. It is a valuable drug in the treatment of *T. gambiense* and *T. rhodesiense* but patients undergoing melarsoprol therapy should be treated in hospital and it is usually reserved for the treatment of advanced sleeping-sickness with the invasion of the CNS. Side-effects with the drug are common and may include encephalopathy, vomiting, and colic.

Other Drugs

Pentamidine is the least toxic of a number

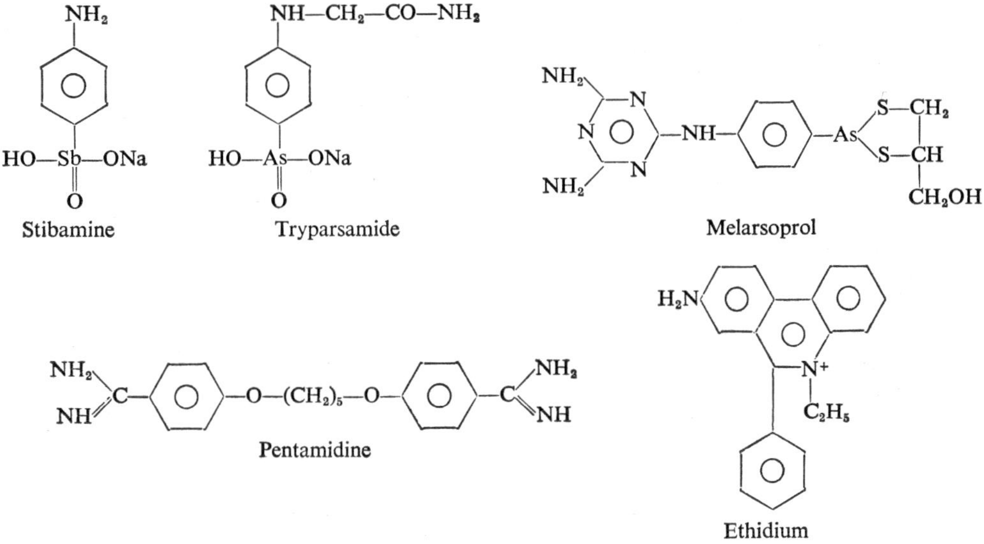

FIG. 17.4. The structures of drugs used to treat leishmaniasis and trypanosomiasis.

of diamidine compounds with trypanocidal actions. It is widely used as a prophylactic and for the treatment of early infection by *T. gambiense* and *T. rhodesiense*. It is not effective in treating the disease when the parasites have entered the CNS.

The mode of action of diamidines is unknown.

Suramin is effective in early infections due to *T. gambiense* and *T. rhodesiense* but is not able to pass the blood–brain barrier and so is inactive against parasites within the CNS. Suramin has a very prolonged action and is used prophylactically. Its mode of action is unknown.

Ethidium bromide is a phenanthridine which is irreversibly active against the growing trypanosome. In the presence of this drug the DNA content of the organisms quickly falls to half the normal value while the RNA levels remain unchanged. Protein and RNA synthesis are reduced after 2–3 hours and this inhibits the growth of the organism.

The drug has been used successfully against *T. vivax* infections in cattle.

Other compounds used to treat trypanosomiasis include **diminazene, aceturate,** and **nitrofurazone.**

HELMINTHES

Helminthiasis is a disease caused by infection with parasitic worms and it is estimated that the number infected in this way approaches 200 million.

Anthelminthics (vermifuges) are now broadly defined as drugs used in the treatment of any type of helminthiasis. During the last decade many drugs, which have been in use for a long period, have been superseded by more specific agents.

Many of the anthelminthic drugs are highly toxic and their use should always be preceded by an accurate diagnosis.

Most anthelminthics do not kill the parasites

Chemotherapy II: Protozoa and Worms

but merely weaken them so that they lose their grip on the intestinal wall and can be removed with a purgative.

NEMATHELMINTHES

Roundworms

The roundworm *Ascaris lumbricoides* is common in warm climates and lives in the intestine and lays eggs which may infect food. The larvae penetrate the wall of the intestine and migrate via the blood stream, the lung, the trachea, and the oesophagus, back again to the intestine where they develop into adult worms.

The drug of choice is **piperazine** which cures almost all cases of roundworm infection. Other effective drugs are **hexylresorcinol**, **diethylcarbamazine**, and **bephenium**.

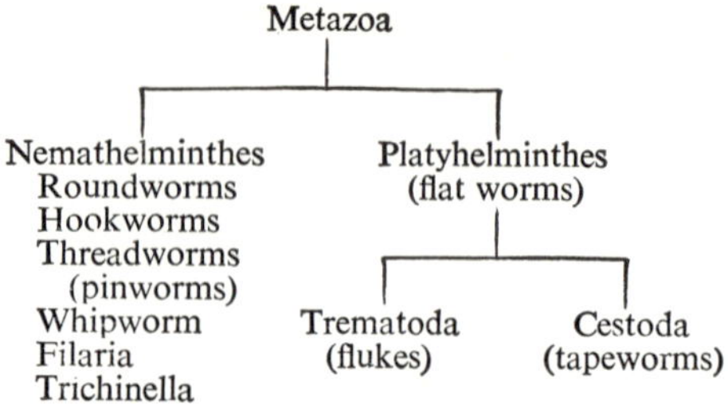

```
                    Metazoa
                       |
         ┌─────────────┴─────────────┐
   Nemathelminthes              Platyhelminthes
   Roundworms                   (flat worms)
   Hookworms                         |
   Threadworms                       |
   (pinworms)              ┌─────────┴─────────┐
   Whipworm            Trematoda            Cestoda
   Filaria              (flukes)           (tapeworms)
   Trichinella
```

FIG. 17.5. Classification of parasite worms.

Piperazine hyperpolarizes the muscle cells of *Ascaris* and abolishes their contractile response to acetylcholine. The hyperpolarized muscles are paralysed so that the worm becomes detached from the intestinal wall and may be expelled. Many piperazine derivatives have been investigated for anthelminthic

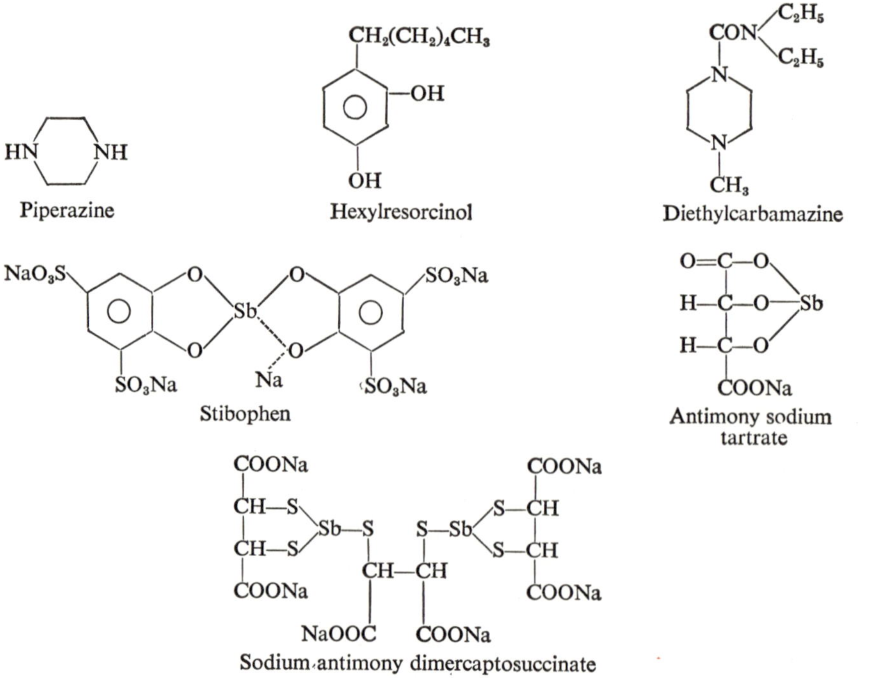

FIG. 17.6. The structures of drugs used in the treatment of helminthiasis.

activity but only **diethylcarbamazine** has proved to be of use. Piperazine is active when given by mouth and is almost non-toxic.

Hexylresorcinol is an effective anthelminthic for the expulsion of hookworms, roundworms, and threadworms, but for the treatment of the latter two infections it has been superseded by the piperazine salts. It is given orally and is usually followed by the administration of a saline purgative.

Hookworm

Necator americanus and *Ancylostoma duodenale* also live in the intestine and lay eggs which hatch in the soil. The larvae infect their host by boring through his skin, and then follow the same course as the larvae of *Ascaris*.

Bephenium is now the drug of choice for the treatment of infection by *Ancylostoma* and, in larger doses, it is effective against *Necator*. It is given orally and does not appear to have any serious side-effects although it may cause nausea and vomiting.

Whipworm

Infection by *Trichuris trichiura* is not normally a serious condition except in heavily infected young children. The parasite is resistant to most drugs except **dithiazanine** although **hexylresorcinol** has been extensively used. Because of the high toxicity of dithiazanine its use should be restricted to seriously infected patients.

Pinworm

Infection by *Enterobius (Oxyuris) vermicularis* usually produces only mild systemic symptoms. The parasite lives in the colon and does not normally invade the tissues, but causes itching by migrating out of the anus at night. Piperazine is the drug of choice but whatever method of treatment is used it is important to prevent reinfection from the anus to the mouth, or from one member of the family to another.

Filaria

Several genera of nematodes are classed together as the family Filariae. The adults live for years in the lymphatics and may cause elephantiasis by obstructing the flow of lymph. The embryos (microfilariae) are small enough to circulate in the blood without causing any symptoms. The most important kind (*Wuchereria bancrofti*) circulates by day and spends the night in the lungs. They are transmitted by mosquitoes.

Filaria infections can be treated with antimony compounds, but **diethylcarbamazine** is more effective and is the drug of choice. It removes the microfilariae from the blood so rapidly that most of them disappear within one minute and accumulate in the liver where they can be seen surrounded by phagocytes, which apparently destroy them. Diethylcarbamazine is relatively non-toxic and may be taken orally and is rapidly absorbed from the gastro-intestinal tract.

CESTODES (Tapeworms)

The adult worm lives in the intestine of a carnivorous animal and lays eggs which infect the food of herbivorous animals. The eggs grow into cysticerci and invade all the tissues of the herbivorous animal through the blood stream. When these tissues are eaten by a carnivorous animal, adult tapeworms appear in the intestine. Man is both carnivorous and herbivorous and may entertain different cestodes at either stage of their life cycle. There is no specific drug for killing the cysticerci, but they occur rarely in man, who is most frequently infected as a carnivore. The tapeworms in his intestines are removed by treatment with extracts of *filix mas* (**male fern, aspidium**).

The official drug is obtained from the rhizomes of the fern *Dryopteris filix-mas*. The extract from the rhizomes contains many biologically active compounds which are derivatives of phloroglucinol but the most important constituent is filicic acid.

Extract of male fern is an old and effective

drug in the treatment of tapeworms but it has toxic side-effects which include gastro-intestinal irritation, nausea, vomiting, headache, and liver damage. Over-dosage can cause death due to depression of the medulla with a subsequent depression of respiration and circulation.

Mepacrine (quinacrine) is also used for the expulsion of tapeworms. When given in high doses it is a safe and effective drug against infection by *Taenia saginata*, *T. solium*, *Hymenolepis nana*, and *Diphyllobothrium latum*.

TREMATODES (Flukes)

These parasites are related to tapeworms and exist mainly in the intestine although some may invade the tissues.

Most of them can only survive by spending a part of their life-cycle in a snail. Infestation with flukes produces the disease known as schistosomiasis or bilharziasis and in some parts of the world a large proportion of the population is infected. The disease is due to infection with *Schistosoma haematobium* or *S. mansoni* and drug treatment is the same for both species.

The trivalent arsenicals are the drugs of choice. **Antimony sodium tartrate**, which was widely used, has now been replaced by less toxic compounds such as **stibophen** and **sodium antimony dimercaptosuccinate**.

Stibophen is one of the most widely used drugs in the treatment of schistosomiasis. It is administered by intramuscular injection and, once exposed to the air, it becomes oxidized and must be discarded. It is less toxic, but also less effective than antimony sodium tartrate or antimony gluconate.

Antimony dimercaptosuccinate (stibocaptate) is less toxic but as effective as stibophen in the treatment of infections with *S. haematobium*. It is less active against *S. mansoni*.

Antimony sodium tartrate and **antimony potassium tartrate** are both effective in all types of schistosomiasis. They are given by intravenous injection and toxic effects may include vomiting, salivation, coughing, and collapse during injection. Following drug administration the side-effects may include liver damage, heart damage, haematuria, and skin rashes. Antimony potassium tartrate has been given orally and by this route both the toxic effects and the activity of the drug are reduced.

FURTHER READING

ADAMS, A. R. D. (1962) Amoebicides, *Practitioner*, **188**, 71.

BUEDING, E., and SWARTZWELDER, C. (1957) Anthelminthics, *Pharmacol. Rev.*, **9**, 329.

MANSOUR, T. E. (1964) The pharmacology and biochemistry of parasite helminthes, *Advanc. Pharmacol.*, **3**, 129.

ROLLO, I. M. (1964) Chemotherapy of malaria, in *Biochemistry and Physiology of Protozoa*, Vol. 3, New York.

SAZ, H. J., and BUEDING, E. (1966) Relationships between anthelminthic effects and biochemical and physiological mechanisms, *Pharmacol. Rev.*, **18**, 871.

STANDEN, O. D. (1963) Chemotherapy of helminthic infections, in *Experimental Chemotherapy*, Vol. 1, New York.

18

CHEMOTHERAPY III: CANCER

GENERAL PRINCIPLES OF CANCER CHEMOTHERAPY

The rational design of cancer chemotherapy really requires a full understanding of the way in which tumours differ from the host tissues. We have already pointed out in connexion with bacterial chemotherapy that the aim is, if possible, to find some unique metabolic difference between the invader and the host—this was well exemplified by the action of penicillin on cell wall synthesis—the cell walls of susceptible bacteria are built up from muramyl peptides which do not occur in animal tissues. Uniqueness in tumour cells is more elusive. Normal tissue cells divide and differentiate according to a predetermined genetic plan probably controlled by local growth-controlling substances. In tumour cells this control system has been abrogated either by mutation, by foreign nucleic acid of viral origin, or by interference by chemical carcinogens. The resulting tissue shows varying degrees of regression to a more undifferentiated state with defective organization and balance of growth. The extent of these changes varies with the type of tumour, and is rarely homogeneous, i.e. a tumour frequently contains areas of quite different orders of maturity. In many respects the regression of these cells is to a state comparable to that found in the embryo in which many enzyme systems are absent since the relevant operons are not activated till a later stage of development. Tumours also differ in the response induced in the surrounding tissues which may range from indifference to an active fibrotic, phagocytic response not dissimilar to that in inflammation. From this description it may be judged that metabolic differences in tumours may be largely deletive, i.e. restrictive of substrate utilization so that tumours are frequently at a natural disadvantage compared with normal cells and growth rate is limited by the turnover of particular metabolic pathways. In addition the cells are actively dividing whereas the majority of adult tissue cells show only the occasional mitoses. Obvious exceptions are the haemopoietic cells, skin, gut mucosa, and gonadal tissue all of which are involved in rather rapid turnover and have a partially differentiated stem cell population whose general characteristics are not very dissimilar to those of the tumour cells. It will be recalled that in bacterial chemotherapy there are two main classes of effective agents, those that kill, and those that control growth, the latter being effective mainly because the phagocytes are able to deal with restricted numbers of organisms. Since phagocytic destruction of tumour cells is less effective, growth control is less effective in tumours unless it can be kept up indefinitely. In a few cases this is so, for instance some mammary cancers retain the sensitivity to oestrogens of the parent cells and their growth can be depressed by lowering oestrogen levels by ovary or pituitary ablation, or by feedback control with androgens. Some prostatic cancers are correspondingly dependent on androgens and can be controlled by androgen suppression with oestrogens. In general the aim in tumour chemotherapy is therefore to kill the tumour cells, and to produce as complete a destruction as possible—this is the weakness. It is comparatively easy to kill 99 per cent. of cells, but owing to heterogeneity some resistant cells are nearly always present and from these recurrences can occur.

Up till the present the greatest promise has been shown by two general classes, the alkylating agents and the metabolic analogues. The alkylating agents are typically represented by the **nitrogen mustards,** and the chemically related ethyleneimines which have three-membered rings which are strained and hence unstable, and the alkylating esters of which the **methane sulphonates** are examples. Both groups selectively alkylate the N-7 position in guanine of both RNA and DNA. Since they will also attack normal cells equally well, they rely on the principle enunciated earlier of attacking a step which is rate limiting in tumour growth but is less so in most normal cells. The limitation to the use of these substances is primarily the susceptibility of rapidly dividing normal cells resulting in bone marrow depression and gut lesions, and this normally restricts the use of these agents to very susceptible tumours such as leukaemia and lymphomas; to some extent this disadvantage can be circumvented by local application of alkylating drugs by regional perfusion. In this case there is an advantage in using drugs with a very short half life to minimize the effects of escape into the general circulation.

The metabolic analogues affect either directly or indirectly the introduction of purines and pyrimidines into nucleic acid. Examples of direct actions are those of **6-mercaptopurine,** an analogue of adenine and hypoxanthine, **cytosine arabinoside,** a stereoisomer of cytidine, and **5-iododeoxyuridine,** an analogue of deoxyuridine. An example of indirect action is the antifolic **methotrexate** which inhibits the enzyme dihydrofolic reductase and so starves the cell of reduced folic coenzymes which are essential for the introduction of a one carbon moiety in the biosynthesis of purines and pyrimidines. For some reason that is not understood a radical cure of one rare type of cancer, chorionepithelioma, can be produced by antifolics, but this is the one shining light in the twilight of partial control with inevitable recurrence found with the other agents.

DRUGS USED IN THE CHEMOTHERAPY OF CANCER

THE BIOLOGICAL ALKYLATING AGENTS

Nitrogen Mustards

Mustine (mechlorethamine, mustargen) was the first nitrogen mustard to be used clinically and it has been more widely studied than other related compounds.

Mustine is made up immediately before use and is given intravenously. It causes a fall in the number of circulating leucocytes and platelets and, when used to treat generalized Hodgkin's disease, may provide periods of remission of up to 2 months or more. It is an extremely irritating substance and must be handled with care. Side-effects include anorexia, nausea, vomiting, and headache.

Mustine has been used to treat chronic myeloid leukaemia, bronchial carcinoma, and reticulosarcoma but its effects on these conditions are unpredictable.

Cyclophosphamide is a synthetic compound in which an alkylating agent has been phosphorylated. The compound is inert until it is dephosphorylated and since rapidly dividing cells contain more dephosphorylating activity than normal cells the cytotoxic agent tends to be released into the former cells. Because of this effect, cyclophosphamide is more selective than mustine in its action against malignant cells.

Most of the severe CNS side-effects associated with nitrogen mustards do not occur with cyclophosphamide although there may be nausea and vomiting. Because it is more selective than mustine there is less damage to megakaryocytes but the hair follicles, in which the cells are dividing rapidly, may be

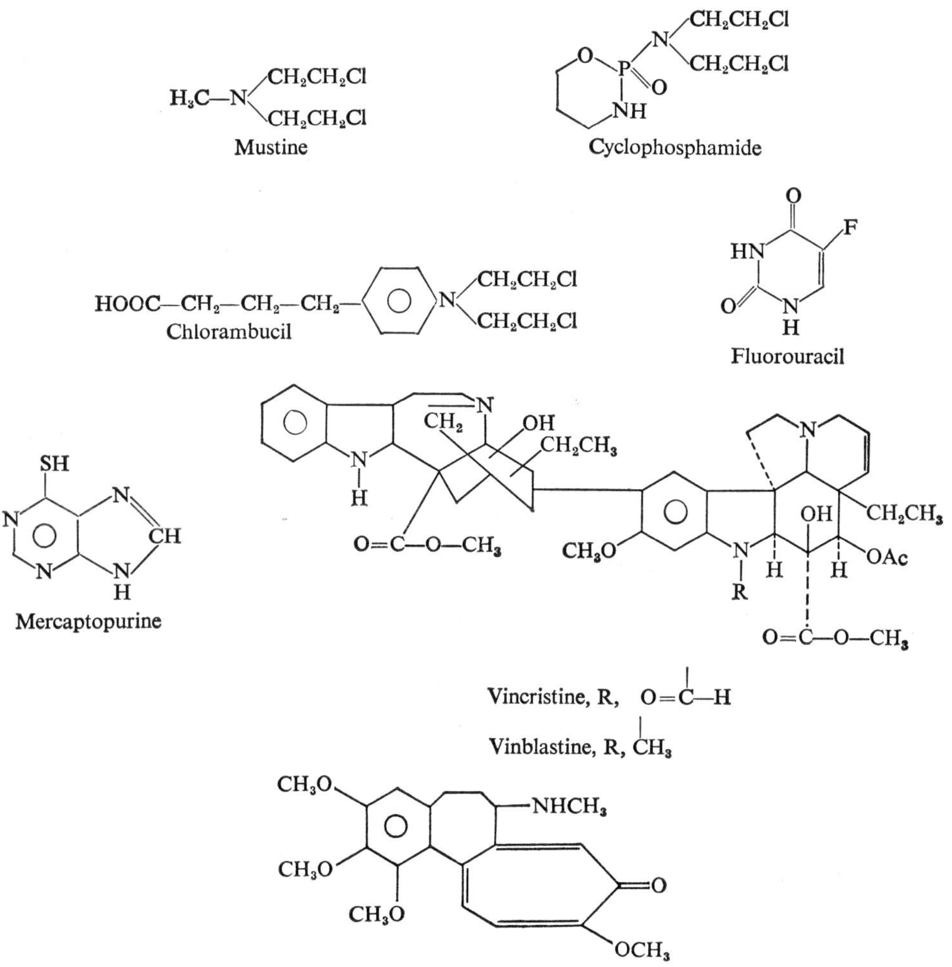

FIG. 18.1. The structures of drugs used in the treatment of cancer.

damaged by the drug. Unlike mustine, cyclophosphamide is not a local irritant.

The clinical uses of cyclophosphamide are similar to those of mustine but it has the advantage that it can be given orally and so can be used easily in divided doses over long periods.

Chlorambucil is an aromatic derivative of mustine which only affects the CNS in large doses although nausea and vomiting may occur with smaller doses.

Chlorambucil is the least toxic and slowest-acting nitrogen mustard and is the drug of choice for treating chronic lymphocytic leukaemia.

Ethyleneimines

Since it is known that the nitrogen mustards are converted into active ethyleneiminium compounds, a number of these substances have been synthesized and introduced into the treatment of cancer.

Triethylenemelamine has little local action on the gastro-intestinal tract and so causes less nausea and vomiting than the parenteral administration of mustine.

The therapeutic uses are the same as for mustine.

Alkyl Sulphonates

Busulphan exerts no pharmacological action except on the bone marrow. Cytotoxic effects do not affect lymphoid tissue or the gastro-intestinal tract.

The beneficial effects of busulphan in chronic granulocytic leukaemia are well established and remissions may be expected in most patients treated with this drug.

ANTIMETABOLITES

Antimetabolites of Folic Acid

Methotrexate, like other folic acid analogues, acts by competitive inhibition of folate reductase. Folic acid [see Chapters 12 and 13] is converted in the body, by folate reductase, to derivatives such as tetrahydrofolic acid which are necessary as co-factors in the synthesis of nucleic acid.

Methotrexate can be taken orally and is used in the treatment of acute leukaemia in children. It is used in the treatment of chorion-epithelioma in women and in carcinomas of the breast, tongue, pharynx, and testes.

In cases of acute leukaemia and chorion-epithelioma, it has often proved possible to provide extremely long periods of remission from the disease. The use of methotrexate to treat leukaemia in adults is of very limited value.

Methotrexate has to be used with extreme care so that serious toxic reactions do not occur. **Leucovorin,** which is an intermediate product of folic acid metabolism and is the active form into which that acid is converted, can be used as an antidote to methotrexate.

Occasionally treatment can be given without an associated leukopenia or aplasia of the bone marrow but in leukaemia it is usually necessary to produce an initial hypoplasia of the bone marrow.

Pyrimidine Analogues

Fluorouracil itself is probably not active in the body but is converted enzymatically to the corresponding ribonucleoside and ribonucleotide. Fluorouracil acts mainly on the bone marrow and gastro-intestinal tract and its effects on bone marrow constitute a toxic hazard. The compound is of palliative value in advanced carcinoma of the breast and gastro-intestinal tract and there are reports of its beneficial use in carcinoma of the ovary, bladder, and cervix. Toxic reactions to the drug are often delayed but usually begin with anorexia and nausea and are followed by stomatitis and diarrhoea. The most serious toxic effects result from bone marrow suppression and usually take the form of leukopenia.

Purine Analogues

Mercaptopurine (6-mercaptopurine, *Puri-nethol***)** is converted inside cells to the corresponding ribonucleotide. The main effects of this drug are on the bone marrow and gastro-intestinal mucosa. Large doses cause leukopenia, thrombocytopenia, and reticulocytopenia and there is destruction of the epithelium and congestion of the capillaries. These actions lead to toxic clinical reactions including anorexia, nausea, vomiting, and bloody diarrhoea.

Mercaptopurine is used to treat acute leukaemia in children and remissions are obtained in about 40 per cent. of cases.

ALKALOIDS

Vinca Alkaloids

Only two vinca alkaloids have been studied clinically: **vincristine** and **vinblastine**. The pharmacological and therapeutic properties of these substances are similar in most respects. The value of vinblastine as a chemotherapeutic agent has not yet been fully evaluated but it does seem effective in treating lymphomas even when the disease is refractory to alkylating agents. Toxic effects occur with this drug especially when high doses are used. These effects include leukopenia, thrombocytopenia, mental depression, paraesthesias and, sometimes, convulsions, psychoses, and disturbances of the autonomic nervous system. The therapeutic uses and toxicity of vincristine are similar to those of vinblastine but there is no cross-resistance between these agents. Vincristine is less effective in treating Hodgkin's disease than vinblastine but is more beneficial in cases of lymphocytic lymphosarcoma.

Although vinblastine does not help in cases of acute leukaemia in children, it has been found that vincristine secures similar remissions as do the antimetabolite and corticosteroid drugs.

Colchicine Derivatives

Colchicine and related alkaloids stop mitosis in early metaphase but colchicine is itself extremely unselective.

Demecolcine is more selective in its action in damaging granulocytes and is less toxic to the gastro-intestinal epithelium.

This compound has been used to treat chronic granulocytic leukaemia but it is not as reliable as busulphan which remains the drug of choice for this disease.

MISCELLANEOUS COMPOUNDS

There have been reports that, in high doses, **urethane** is of use in the treatment of multiple myeloma. Since high doses of urethane produce unpleasant side-effects including anorexia, nausea, and vomiting, the drug is no longer used for its possible antineoplastic action.

A drug known as **O,p'-DDD**, which is chemically similar to the insecticides DDT and DDD, is being investigated for use in the treatment of tumours of the adrenal cortex. Although the mechanism of action of O,p'-DDD is unknown, it appears to have a selective effect on adrenocortical cells whether they are normal or malignant. Apart from nausea and anorexia, side-effects with this drug seem to be rare.

ANTIBIOTICS

Actinomycin D

The **actinomycins** are the most potent antineoplastic drugs known and they owe this action to their ability to react with DNA and alter the properties of this compound. The drug inhibits cells which are dividing rapidly whether they are normal or of neoplastic origin and may, therefore, attack the hair follicles.

Because **actinomycin D** produces only temporary remissions and is toxic it has only a limited value in the chemotherapy of cancer. The toxic reactions associated with the use of this compound include anorexia, nausea, vomiting, bone marrow depression, diarrhoea, glossitis, and dermatological effects.

RADIOACTIVE ISOTOPES

Radioactive iodine (iodine^{131}, half-life 8 days, beta and gamma radiation) is readily taken up by the thyroid gland where the destructive action of the radiation may be effective in treating thyrotoxic goitre or carcinoma of the thyroid. The iodine is given orally and the treatment is extremely safe and uptake of significant amounts of radioactive iodine occurs only in the thyroid gland.

Radioactive phosphorus (phosphorus^{32}, half-life 14·3 days, beta radiation) in the form of sodium phosphate is useful in the treatment of polycythaemia vera because it inhibits the overproduction of red blood cells, platelets, and leucocytes.

Radioactive gold is a short-lived isotope (gold^{198}, half-life 2·7 days, beta and gamma radiation) and in the colloidal form may be injected into the pleural or peritoneal cavities. The colloidal particles are transported by phagocytic cells to the lymph nodes, bone marrow, liver, and spleen. Radioactive gold is used in the treatment of ascites and pleural effusion resulting from cancer. It has also been used to treat cancer of the prostate gland and the cervix.

The doses of radioactive gold used are high (40–150 millicuries) and so there is a significant risk to those attending the patient. The treatment is expensive and often has no advantage over the use of alkylating agents.

FURTHER READING

HARRIS, R. J. C. (ed.) (1961) *Biological Approaches to Cancer Chemotherapy*, London.

HENDERSON, J. F. (1963) Purine and pyrimidine antimetabolites in cancer chemotherapy, *Advanc. Pharmacol.*, 2, 297.

MANDEL, H. G. (1959) The physiological disposition of some anti-cancer agents, *Pharmacol. Rev.*, 11, 743.

PLATTNER, P. A. (ed.) (1964) *Chemotherapy of Cancer*, London.

SCHNITZER, R. J., and HAWKING, F. (eds.) (1966) *Experimental Chemotherapy*, Vol. iv, New York.

19

QUANTITATIVE AND HUMAN PHARMACOLOGY

BIOLOGICAL ASSAY

BIOLOGICAL methods of assay are used to detect, and measure the concentration of, substances by observing their pharmacological effects on living animals or tissues. They are usually more troublesome, and less accurate, than physical or chemical methods and are only used when there is no other reliable way, or when the physical or chemical methods are too insensitive. Most bacteriological products, such as toxins, antitoxins, and sera, can only be detected biologically. Some of the biological tests for hormones, chemical transmitters, and vitamins have been largely replaced by chemical and physical methods, and this process will doubtless continue; but it is probable that biological methods will always be necessary for some of the hormones, and few of the new methods are so well established that it is possible to dispense with the biological method altogether. When biological methods and chemical methods for the assay of a pharmacologically active substance disagree so widely that the disagreement cannot be due to the error of the tests, the biological method is, by definition, right and the chemical method is wrong. Biological methods are also applied for special reasons to various other substances such as digitalis and neoarsphenamine.

Biological assay is often very important, since drugs such as insulin could not be used unless it was possible to ensure a uniform product. If there was much variation between different supplies of the drug patients would die from overdosage or underdosage when they started to use a new supply. Accurate biological methods of testing insulin and other such substances have been developed in recent years, so that it is now theoretically possible, by using sufficiently large numbers of animals, to attain any required degree of accuracy; but this has only been achieved through the acceptance of certain general principles governing the design of the experiments.

Bioassays are also used in diagnosis and in clinical research. The concentration of gonadotrophins in the blood or urine may be estimated quantitatively by injecting these fluids into animals. Other hormones can also be estimated in the same sort of way, but chemical methods are generally preferred when these are available.

Manufacturers of hormones and vitamins sometimes state that their products are physiologically standardized, but give no information about the result of the standardization. It is as if a vendor of toffee stated on the label that he had tasted it but made no pretensions to having weighed it out and did not even say whether he liked the taste or not. An advance on this is made when the strength of a preparation is stated in animal units. For example, a Unit of insulin was originally defined as the quantity of insulin which reduced the blood sugar of a normal rabbit by a certain arbitrary amount. This depends, of course, on a number of factors such as the weight of the rabbit, its state of nutrition, and the room temperature, but even when all known causes of variation have been standardized, rabbits still vary in their response to insulin, and an animal unit must always be subject to large errors of unknown size, since a London rabbit is not necessarily the same as an American rabbit or a Cambridge rabbit or even as another London rabbit. The use of rabbit units or rat units has been compared with the convention, once adopted, that a cubit was the length of the king's forearm and was liable to vary with the size of the king.

These large and unknown errors have been reduced to reasonable and known proportions by the use of standard preparations, consisting of actual samples of various biological products, adopted and preserved by the 'Expert Committee on Biological Standardization' of the World Health Organization and issued to suitable persons for biological assay. A Unit is defined as a definite weight of one of these standard preparations, and assays involve comparisons of the tested preparations with the standard preparation. The error of the test still depends largely on the variability of the animals, but it is reduced because the variability involved is that between animals coming from the same stock and brought up together, instead of the general variability of animals of the same species. Even more important advantages of the use of a standard preparation are the facts that the error of the result can usually be calculated, and that it can be indefinitely reduced by the use of more animals. The methods of calculation are discussed below.

Accurate biological assays are only possible when the active principle of the standard preparation is identical with the active principle of the preparation compared with it. Methods of assay which did not fulfil this requirement have often been proposed in the past, but have never proved satisfactory. For example, it was found that posterior pituitary extracts and potassium salts both caused a contraction of the isolated uterus of a guinea-pig, and it was proposed that pituitary extracts should be compared with the potassium chloride on this preparation and that their activity should be expressed in terms of their potassium equivalent. It was found, however, that when the assay was repeated it did not give constant results because the sensitivity of uteri to potassium did not always vary in proportion to their sensitivity to pituitary extracts. The only satisfactory standard for the assay of the active principle of the pituitary which produces this effect is a stable preparation of the active principle itself.

So long as the standard preparation is suitable, there is no reason why the effects observed in an assay should be the same as those desired when the drug is used in therapeutics. Insulin can be assayed by its power to cause convulsions in mice, and the value of the result is not impaired by the fact that the production of convulsions will not be the usual purpose for which the insulin will be used in practice. In the same way vitamin C can be assayed by its power to reduce dichlorophenol indophenol, and the accuracy of the result is not affected by the fact that the vitamin C may later be used for other purposes than the reduction of this dye.

CALCULATION OF THE ERROR

Generally speaking, the best method of estimating the error of any measurement is to repeat the measurement several times, and to see how closely the results agree among themselves. When precision is important, and the experimenter is not content to accept the nearest round number as the result, repeated measurements of any kind always show a certain amount of variation, and the error can be calculated from the size of this variation. These principles are generally recognized by everyone who takes the trouble to make duplicate determinations of a measurement. Duplicate determinations are sufficient to show that the error of many simple physical measurements is small enough to be neglected, but the error of biological measurements is often so large that more attention must be paid to it. Duplicate determinations give only a very crude estimate of the error, since the actual size of the discrepancy between any particular pair of measurements is largely due to luck. At least a dozen parallel measurements or pairs of duplicate measurements are required for anything like a reliable estimate of the error. In the case of biological measurements this may involve a prodigious amount of work, and it is sometimes preferable to calculate the error in-

FIG. 19.1. Theoretical frequency distributions, in which the vertical scale denotes the frequency of the values shown on the horizontal scale. This figure can only be understood by reading the text. The curve on the right is a normal curve.

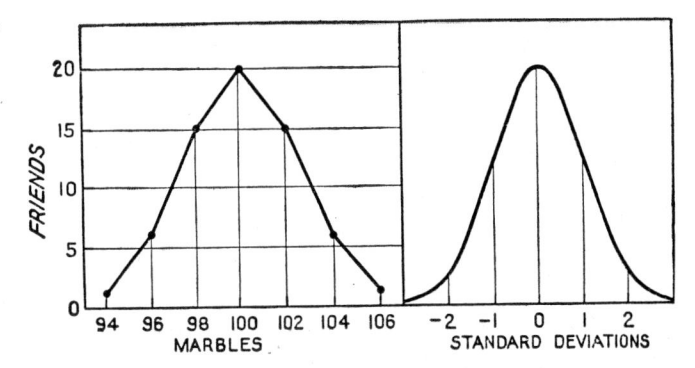

directly from the variability of the animals themselves. This variability is usually responsible for most of the error, which depends on which individual animals are chosen for any particular test. Such errors are called errors of sampling because they are due to the assumption that the animals chosen are a typical sample.

The mathematical methods used in calculating errors may appear arbitrary and unnecessarily complicated, but they fit the facts and can also be justified by theoretical arguments. The following argument is crude, but it illustrates the kind of principle involved.

A certain rich man had 64 friends and gave each of them 100 marbles. He then tossed a coin with each friend, and the loser of each toss paid one marble to the winner. Since the tossing was done fairly, half his friends lost and half of them won, so that after the first round of tossing 32 of his friends had 101 marbles and 32 of them had 99. They then tossed again and half of each group won again, so that there were 16 friends with 102 marbles, 32 with 100 marbles, and 16 with 98 marbles. The left part of FIGURE 19.1 shows the distribution of marbles that might be expected according to this argument after 6 rounds of tossing. The number of marbles is plotted on the horizontal scale against the number of friends that might be expected to have that number of marbles on the vertical scale. These calculations only give expectations, and in actual practice these expectations would not be exactly fulfilled, but that is another story.

This distribution is known as the binomial distribution, because the probability of each possible result (number of wins) is given by one of the terms of the binomial expansion of $(p+q)^n$, where p is the probability of a win and $q = 1-p$, and n is the number in a sample (the number of rounds of tossing). In the case of the rich man it is assumed that $p = q = 0.5$.

If the process is continued, the curve approximates more and more closely to a smooth curve whose shape can be calculated and which is known as the normal curve and is shown in the right part of FIGURE 19.1. The size of an animal (or any other measurement) may be considered to depend upon a large number of chances, each corresponding to a round of tossing, so that the distribution of sizes should, on this theory, be similar to the distribution of marbles among the friends of the rich man. The theory would, however, be worthless were it not for the fact that, if a large number of animals are measured and divided into groups so that all the animals in the same group are about the same size, and if the number in each group is plotted against the size, an approximately normal curve actually is obtained.

In biological measurements there is, however, a complication. The effect of each chance is likely to depend upon the size of the animal. A warm day which adds a hundredth of a ton to a 5-ton elephant will not add the same weight to a 5-milligram maggot; it is more likely to add a hundredth of a milligram. The effect of each chance on the weight of the animal is, in fact, likely to be proportional to the weight itself. Allowance can be made for this fact by calculating the weight of the animal in logarithms, since the difference between log 5 tons and log 5·01 tons is the same as the difference between log 5 mg. and log 5·01 mg.;

FIG. 19.2. Frequency distribution of systolic blood pressures. The vertical scale is proportional to the relative frequency with which different blood pressures occurred. The logarithmic scale of blood pressures gives a normal curve. The arithmetic scale does not. (From data by Alvarez (1923) *Arch. intern. Med.*, **32**, 17.)

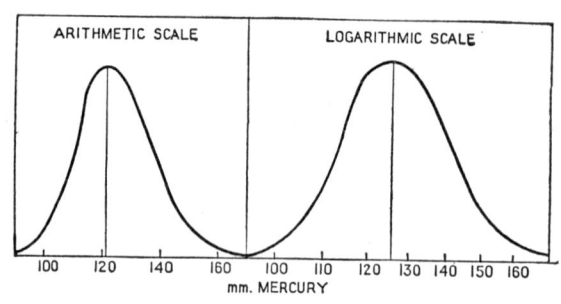

DISTRIBUTION OF BLOOD PRESSURE IN 1216 MALE AMERICAN STUDENTS (ALVAREZ 1923).

and this holds true whatever units of weight are used.

One of the advantages of this method of calculation is illustrated in FIGURE 19.2, which is based on measurements of the blood pressure of normal university freshmen. The curve on the left was obtained by dividing the scale of blood pressures into a number of small ranges at the points 80, 85, 90, 95, etc., mm. of mercury. The number of readings in each range was then plotted against the blood pressure. The curve on the right was obtained by converting each reading into a logarithm and repeating the same process. This second curve is more like a normal curve than the other one is. When the variations in biological data are large compared with the mean, the logarithmic method of calculation usually gives more nearly normal curves than the simpler method, but when the variations are small compared with the mean, both methods give equivalent results, and in these cases the use of logarithms is an unnecessary complication and only desirable for the sake of uniformity with the curves where the variation is large. It was found in these experiments that blood pressures over 180 and below 90 mm. of mercury were observed occasionally in healthy young men of 18 years of age. Such blood pressures are not necessarily an indication of disease, but may be merely due to the inevitable variability of all populations.

When an assay, or any other measurement, is repeated many times, the individual results vary in the same way as the weights of individual animals and are distributed in normal curves. It is therefore impossible to give the error in the form of a definite value which is never exceeded, but possible to estimate the value which is exceeded once in 100 times or once in 1,000 times.

The error is proportional to the breadth of the curve and is measured in terms of the standard deviation (σ). This can be estimated from a set of n observations by calculating first the mean of the observations ($\bar{x}$) and then the deviation (difference) of each observation from this mean (d). The expression $\sqrt{\left(\dfrac{\sum d^2}{n-1}\right)}$ then gives an estimate of the standard deviation. The square of the standard deviation is called the variance; the use of this term is sometimes convenient because it eliminates square-root signs from the formulae.

The standard deviation of the logarithms of the result (λ) is calculated by writing down the logarithms of the results, finding the mean logarithm, calculating and summing the squares of the deviations from this mean, dividing this sum by ($n-1$), and taking the square root.

When several sets of observations, distributed about different means, are available for calculating the standard deviation the appropriate formula is σ (or λ) $= \sqrt{\left(\dfrac{\sum d^2}{\sum (n-1)}\right)}$, and in applying this formula the summation is extended over all the values of d and n in all the different groups.

An example of the practical application of these formulae is given on page 216.

The standard deviation (σ) is a measure of the error of a single observation: the standard error of the mean of n observations is $\sigma/\sqrt{n}$; its variance is σ^2/n. The standard error of the sum or difference of two means is $\sqrt{\left(\dfrac{\sigma_1^2}{n_1}+\dfrac{\sigma_2^2}{n_2}\right)}$, where σ_1 and n_1 refer to one set of observations and σ_2 and n_2 refer to the other; the variance of the sum or difference is $\frac{\sigma_1^2}{n_1} + \frac{\sigma_2^2}{n_2}$, that is, the sum of the variances of the two means separately.

The main use of the standard deviation depends on the fact that the shape of the normal curve is known. The range of results between $\bar{x} - \sigma$ and $\bar{x} + \sigma$ includes about $\frac{2}{3}$ of all the results; the range $\bar{x} \pm 2\sigma$ includes about 95 per cent. and the range $\bar{x} \pm 2 \cdot 576\sigma$ includes 99 per cent. of the results. This fact was used in the British Pharmacopœia 1948, from which the following clear statement is taken by permission.

In expressing the limits of error of biological assays the term 'limits of error ($P = 0.99$)' is used. The statements of the errors of these assays are based on the convention that, for practical purposes, a probability of 0.99 is equivalent to certainty. In other words, it has been estimated that the result of the assay will be within the stated limits 99 times out of every 100 times that the assay is made. These limits are given as percentages of the true result. Thus, the statement 'limits of error ($P = 0.99$) 95 and 105 per cent.' means that it has been estimated that in 99 assays out of 100 the result will be greater than 95 per cent., and less than 105 per cent., of the true result.

If the error of the test, or its logarithm, is normally distributed, the stated limits of error correspond to the range covered by ± 2.576 times the standard deviation.

METHODS OF ASSAY

There are three methods of interpreting the result of a biological assay.

Method 1. Threshold Dose Measured on Each Animal

These assays are those in which a drug is administered slowly to an animal until some observable effect is produced. The assay of digitalis by means of cats is an example of such a test. The cat is anaesthetized with chloralose, its blood pressure is recorded, and a suitable extract of digitalis is allowed to run into a vein at a rate of about 1 ml. per minute. At the moment when the heart stops beating and the blood pressure falls to zero the volume of fluid which has run in is recorded. This volume contains the dose necessary to kill that particular cat under the conditions of the experiment. Two series of such experiments, using the standard preparation of digitalis and the unknown preparation respectively, are carried out and the potency calculated from the average results.

The results shown in TABLE 19.1 illustrate the best general method of calculating the result and its error.

The ratio of the potencies of the tinctures was estimated as antilog $(1.27 - 1)$ or 1.86. Since the standard tincture contained 1 unit per ml., the unknown tincture was estimated to contain 1.86 units per ml. Direct calculation without logarithms gives an estimate of 1.88 units per ml.

Since it is unlikely that the variability depends on which tincture is used, the standard deviation of the logarithm of the estimate for one cat (λ) is estimated from both sets of figures together from the expression $\sqrt{\left(\dfrac{\sum d^2}{\sum (n-1)}\right)}$ which is

$$\sqrt{\left(\frac{0.0059 + 0.0109}{5 + 5}\right)} \text{ or } 0.041.$$

This is equal to log 1.10, and is thus equivalent to a standard deviation of 10 per cent.

The standard error of the logarithm of the estimate of the ratio of the potencies is $\sqrt{\left(\dfrac{\lambda^2}{6} + \dfrac{\lambda^2}{6}\right)}$ or 0.0237. This is equal to log 1.056 and is thus equivalent to a standard error of 5.6 per cent. Direct calculation without logarithms gives an estimate of 5.9 per cent. In cases like this, where the standard deviation is not greater than 10 per cent., the two methods of calculation give practically identical results. When the error is large the method using logarithms is the only one which gives accurate results.

Method 2. Responses Recorded or Measured

Sometimes the effect of the drug can be observed repeatedly on the same tissue. The two samples of the drug are given alternately and the doses adjusted until they give equal effects. FIGURE 19.3 shows the result of an assay of this kind. This is a record of the contractions of a piece of guinea-pig's intestine which was

STANDARD TINCTURE				UNKNOWN TINCTURE				
LETHAL DOSE	LOG DOSE	D	D^2	LETHAL DOSE	LOG DOSE	D	D^2	
18·2	1·26	0·01	0·0001	12	1·08	0·08	0·0064	
19·6	1·29	0·02	0·0004	10	1·00	0·0	0·0	
17·0	1·23	0·04	0·0016	9·5	0·98	0·02	0·0004	
17·4	1·24	0·03	0·0009	8·7	0·94	0·06	0·0036	
19·7	1·29	0·02	0·0004	10·2	1·01	0·01	0·0001	
21·1	1·32	0·05	0·0025	9·6	0·98	0·02	0·0004	
	6⌡7·63	..	0·0059		6⌡5·99	..	0·0109	
Mean	1·27				1			

TABLE 19.1 SHOWING THE INDIVIDUAL LETHAL DOSE (ML. PER KG. OF CAT) OF TINCTURES OF DIGITALIS DILUTED 1/20 WITH SALINE

suspended in a bath of salt solution similar to that shown in FIGURE 1.1. When doses of a standard solution of histamine (1 in 5 millions) or of an extract of blood were added to the bath in small volumes of fluid they caused a contraction of the muscle which was recorded on the drum. When each contraction was complete the drum was stopped and the salt solution changed so that the muscle relaxed again. The effects labelled H were due

to the histamine solution, and the volumes of this solution are given in millilitres (ml.). The other effects whose summits are joined by a white line are all due to 0·1 ml. of the extract. It will be seen that the effect of this volume of the extract was less than that of 0·1 ml. H, and greater than that of 0·07 ml. H, and about equal to that of 0·09 ml. H. The concentration of histamine in the extract was therefore about 1 in 5·5 millions or 0·18 mg. per litre.

Since 2·5 ml. of extract had been made from 10 ml. of blood, the original concentration of histamine in the blood was 0·045 mg. or 45 μg. per litre. Such small quantities of histamine can only be detected by methods such as this.

Similar methods are used for the assay of the principle in the posterior lobe of the pituitary which causes a contraction of the uterus and for adrenaline, acetylcholine, and other substances.

Accurate estimates of the potency and the limits of error can be made by using methods of calculation originally designed for assays in which the standard and unknown preparations are tested on different animals. A simplified method of calculating the error in this case was described by Bliss.

Many of the vitamins and hormones can be assayed by methods of this class. One group of animals receives the standard preparation and a similar group receives the unknown preparation which is being tested. After a suitable interval of time the animals, or parts of the animals, are weighed and the result is cal-

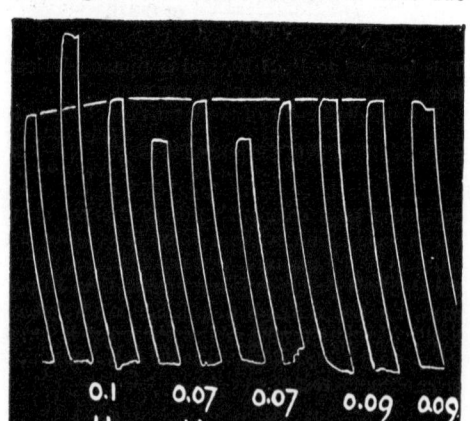

FIG. 19.3. Assay of histamine by its action on guinea-pig's intestine in a 2 ml. bath, showing ten independent contractions. The drum was stopped after each contraction and the solution changed. H = histamine. The figures denote ml. of a 1-in-5-million solution added to the bath. The alternate doses are 0·1 ml. of an extract, which was equivalent to 0·09 ml. of the histamine solution. (From Gaddum (1936) *Proc. roy. Soc. Med.*, **29**, 1373.)

culated from the average weights in the two groups.

The calculation of the results of such assays and their errors generally depends on a consideration of the relation between dose and effect. FIGURE 19.4 shows the results of a comparison between two steroid hormones found in extracts of adrenal cortex and known, for short, as compounds A and E (Kendall); compound E is cortisone. These two substances both have the effect of increasing the amount of glycogen in the liver. Groups of fasting adrenalectomized mice received various doses of each of them by subcutaneous injection and were killed after a suitable interval. The vertical scale shows the average amount of glycogen in the liver (mg. per 100 g. body weight) and the horizontal scale shows the total dose (mg.) given to each mouse (in a series of seven injections). On the left side of the figure the doses are plotted on an ordinary arithmetic scale, and on the right side they are plotted on a logarithmic scale. This means that the logarithm of each dose is plotted instead of the dose itself.

The use of logarithms has the following effects:

1. When each dose is double the preceding dose, they are plotted at equal intervals on the logarithmic scale. If the largest dose is many times as large as the smallest, the smaller doses are apt to be huddled too closely together on an arithmetic scale. The logarithmic scale avoids this trouble.

2. The two lines on the right side of the figure are parallel and the two curves on the left are not. In this case the result of the test is that E is about 3·5 times as active as A. This means that, for any given effect, the dose of A is about 3·5 times as large as the dose of E. On the arithmetic scale the distance from the vertical axis at any given height is 3·5 times as large for A as for E. On the logarithmic scale the horizontal distance between the two lines is about constant and equal to log 3·5.

3. The points can be fitted by straight lines when plotted on a logarithmic scale, but not when plotted on an arithmetic scale. These straight lines, of course, cannot be extended indefinitely in either direction, but it is commonly found that straight lines can be used to represent the middle part of the curve and that this device works best when logarithms are used. When necessary, the lines can sometimes be straightened by measuring the effect in some other way, or by using some function of the effect (such as its square or logarithm) instead of the effect itself.

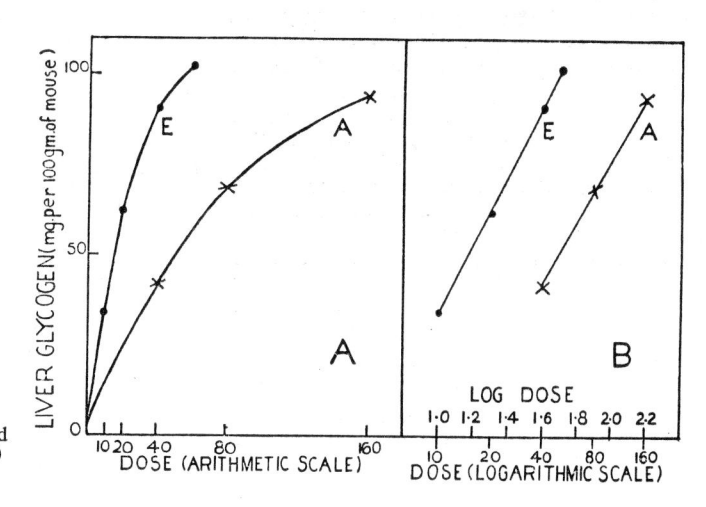

FIG. 19.4. The effects of 11-dehydrocorticosterone (A) and cortisone (E) on liver glycogen in mice. The dose–effect lines (*A*) are not parallel. The log-dose–effect lines (*B*) are nearly straight and parallel. (Venning *et al.* (1946) *Endocrinology*, **38**, 79.)

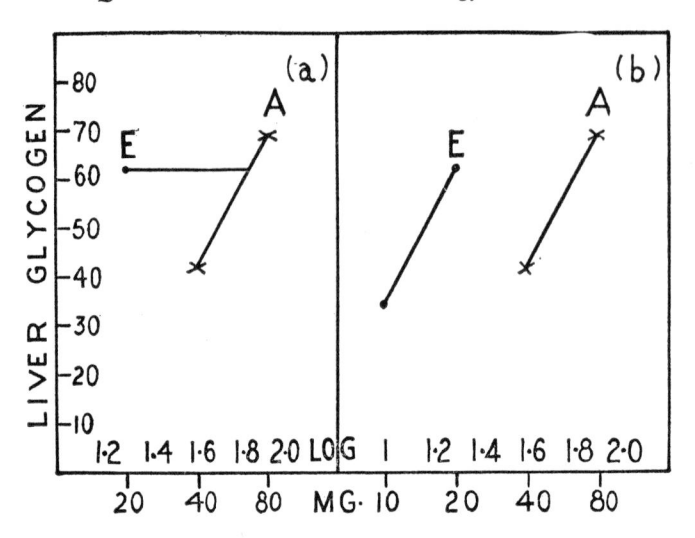

FIG. 19.5. Same data as Fig. 19.4 to show (a) a (2 and 1) dose assay, and (b) a (2 and 2) dose assay.

4. When arithmetic scales are used, the error of the test is generally not normally distributed, and increases as the dose increases. If logarithms are used the error is generally normally distributed and independent of the dose.

In all these ways the calculations are simplified by the use of logarithms, and this has been enough to induce those concerned with biological assays to overcome any initial distaste they may have felt, and to regard logarithms as a very useful tool.

Simpler Designs. The experiment whose results are shown in FIGURE 19.4A may be called a (4 and 3) dose assay. In routine testing it is generally more convenient to use fewer doses. The simplest satisfactory design is known as a (2 and 1) dose assay and is illustrated in FIGURE 19.5a which shows some of the same data as FIGURE 19.4. In this figure the effects of 40 and 80 mg. of A are plotted against log 40 and log 80 and the straight line through these points is taken as the dose–effect curve for A. A dose of 20 mg. of E caused an effect of 62 and the graph shows that this corresponds to 1·82 on the line. The antilog of 1·82 is 66·1 so that the ratio of the potencies is 66·1/20 or 3·3. Calculation from simple geometry gives the result as 3·336.

FIGURE 19.5b, which is taken from the same data, illustrates a (2 and 2) dose assay. In this case the two lines are very nearly parallel and the result can be obtained simply, and with reasonable accuracy, by actually drawing a horizontal line at some convenient place and measuring its length. This method gave the result as 3·34, but the actual figure depends on the place where the line is drawn, and on the skill of the draughtsman. It is really more satisfactory to calculate the result, and this raises difficulties because the lines are not exactly parallel even in FIGURES 19.4B and 19.5b, and are often much less nearly parallel than this. In such cases it is necessary to find lines which fit the results as well as possible. This can be done roughly on graph paper by drawing parallel curves which appear by eye to give the most satisfactory fit. This simple procedure is not ideal, since no two persons would fit exactly the same curves to a given set of results. In order to avoid this error, mathematical formulae are used for calculating the result. These formulae give not only the best possible estimate of the result of the assay and its error, but also the equations of the straight lines which provide the best fit for the observations as judged by the 'method of

FIG. 19.6. Theoretical log-dose–effect lines to illustrate the calculation of the result of a (2 and 2) dose assay (see text).

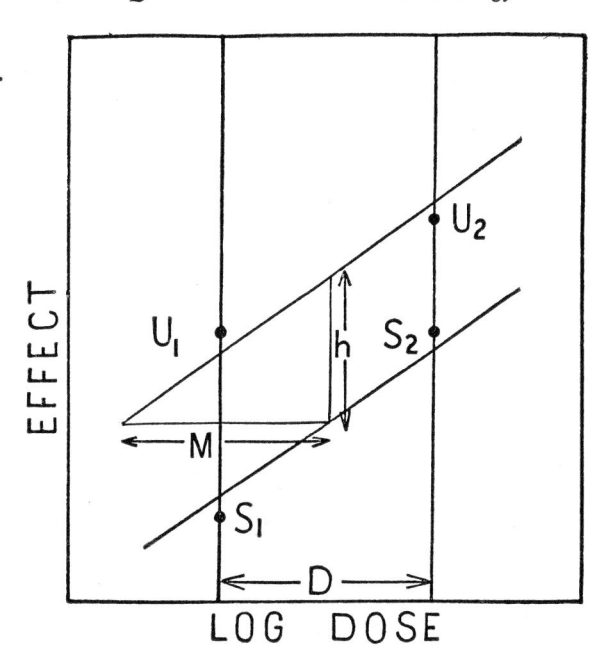

least squares'. When the number of doses is large the formulae are complicated, but they can be reduced to a simple form when (2 and 2) doses are used.

Consider an imaginary experiment to compare an unknown solution (U) with a standard solution (S). The design of the experiment depends on some assumption or other about the potency of U, based either on preliminary tests or previous experience. The solution U is adjusted so that it would be equal to S if these preliminary assumptions were exactly correct. Two groups of animals receive two different volumes of S and two other groups receive the same two volumes of U. The results are plotted in FIGURE 19.6 in which S_1 and S_2 are the effects of S, U_1 and U_2 are the effects of U, and D is the logarithm of the ratio of the two volumes used. The sloping lines show the log-dose–effect curves which fit the observed points as well as possible, while still remaining parallel to one another. The vertical distances of the observed results from these lines are all equal.

If the slope of a line is estimated as the tangent of the angle it makes with the base line, the slopes of the lines through the observed points are $(S_2-S_1)/D$ and $(U_2-U_1)/D$. The true slope (b) is taken as equal to the average of these figures, so that $b = (S_2-S_1+U_2-U_1)/2D$. The difference between the effects of the two preparations is estimated as either (U_1-S_1) or (U_2-S_2) and the average of these is taken as an estimate of this difference, which is equal to the distance h on the graph. The result of the test (M) is the logarithm of the ratio of the activities (U/S).

Now $b = h/M$.

$$\therefore M = h/b = \frac{U_1-S_1+U_2-S_2}{S_2-S_1+U_2-U_1}D.$$

This formula is the same as that given by the method of least squares.

The error of this estimate consists of two

parts since both the numerator and denominator are subject to error. It may be approximately estimated from the formula:

$$s_M^2 = \text{variance of } M = \frac{V}{b^2}\left(1 + \frac{M^2}{d^2}\right)$$

where V = the mean of the variances of the four estimates of the mean effect. The number 1 in the bracket represents that part of the error due to the estimate of the difference of the mean effects of U and S, and the M^2/d^2 represents that part due to the error of the estimate of the slope.

When the animals are few, or very variable, this formula becomes unreliable and it is then necessary to calculate the 'fiducial limits' by means of a more elaborate formula.

The term is not easy to explain, but if the fiducial limits ($P = 0.95$) are calculated for each assay, the true result should be within these limits in 95 per cent. of assays. If, for example, the fiducial limits are 80 and 125 per cent., it is reasonable to assume that the true result lies in this range. Such an assumption should be correct 95 times out of 100.

In microbiological assays the dose–effect curve is sometimes straight without the use of logarithms and in this case different methods of calculation are used.

Cross-over Test. When the effect of a drug can be observed and measured more than once in the same animal, the accuracy may be very greatly increased by arranging the experiment as a cross-over test, which is carried out in two stages. On the first day one group of animals receives the standard drug and another similar group receives the unknown preparation and the effects are measured; on another day the drugs are crossed over, so that the first group receives the unknown preparation and the second group receives the standard. The average effect of each preparation, for both stages of the experiment together, is then calculated and the result interpreted by the methods discussed above using a dose–effect curve. The advantage of this arrangement is that it eliminates errors due to the difference between one animal and another, since both drugs are tested on the same animals. The effect of the difference between one day and another disappears in the calculation of the mean response of each dose-group. Cross-over tests were introduced by Marks, who used them for the assay of insulin on rabbits.

The experimental design actually used in Britain for assays of insulin on rabbits is known as the twin cross-over test. It combines the advantages of a cross-over test with those of a (2 and 2) dose assay.

Method 3. Percentage of Positive Effects Measured

The most familiar example of a test of this class is a toxicity test, in which a poison is injected into a group of animals and the percentage mortality determined. FIGURE 19.7 shows the type of curve obtained when the percentage mortality is plotted against the dose given; the same methods of calculation can be used when the observed effect is not death, but some other effect such as oestrus, or hypoglycaemic symptoms.

The curve shown in FIGURE 19.7 is sigmoid (S-shaped). The doses are given as percentages of the dose causing a mortality of 50 per cent. This dose is usually called the LD 50, in which the letters stand for 'lethal dose'. This term is not applicable when the observed effect is not death, but oestrus, and it has been

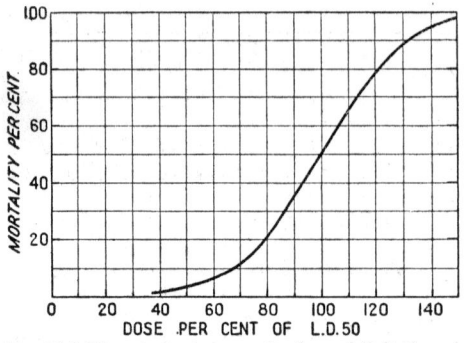

FIG. 19.7. The relation between the dose of digitalis and the percentage mortality among frogs. The curve is based on data given in the *British Pharmacopœia 1932*.

Fig. 19.8. The curve on the left is a normal frequency distribution like those shown in Figures 19.1 and 19.2. The curve on the right is a dose–mortality curve like that shown in Figure 19.7. The diagram illustrates the theoretical discussion of the relation of these two curves to one another. (From Gaddum (1933) *Spec. Rep. Ser. med. Res. Coun.* (Lond.), No. 183.)

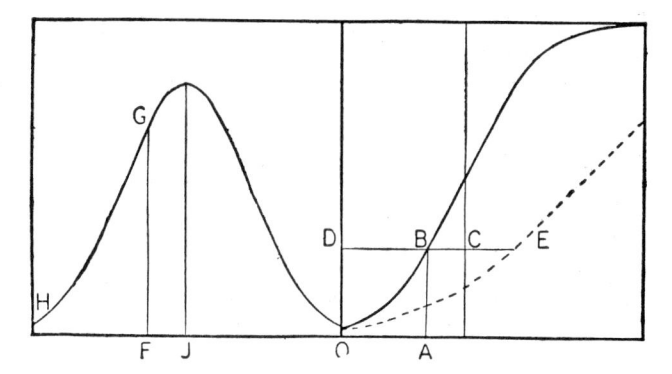

suggested that in this case the dose should be called the OD 50, but it would really be better to use the term ED 50 in all cases except when the observed effect is death and to explain that the letters meant 'effective dose'.

In the interpretation of an assay of this type each percentage is converted into a probit by means of special tables. If these probits are plotted against the logarithm of the dose the results can be fitted with straight lines and the results can then be interpreted as described above for method 2. In this case the error is calculated from theoretical considerations. The logical basis of the probit is outlined below.

If all the facts were known about each animal, the distribution of individual effective doses (I.E.D.) could be plotted as a frequency curve similar to those shown in Figures 19.1 and 19.2. This has been done on the left of Figure 19.8, in which the horizontal scale is a scale of doses and the vertical scale is a scale of frequencies. If any given dose is injected into a group of animals it will be effective in all those animals whose I.E.D. is equal to, or less than, the given dose. The percentage of responses (*AB*) will therefore be proportional to the area of the frequency curve to the left of a vertical line through the point corresponding to the given dose (the area *FGH*). In mathematical language the dose-percentage curve is the integral of the frequency distribution. This means that the exact theoretical shape of the sigmoid dose–percentage curve can be calculated, on the assumption that the distribution is normal. It is found that theory agrees with practice so long as the doses are plotted on a logarithmic scale.

This conclusion has been reached by plotting the results in a special way which has the effect of straightening the sigmoid curve. For this purpose, not only are the doses plotted on a logarithmic scale, but the percentages are plotted on a probability scale. The simplest way of doing this is to use logarithmic probability paper such as is shown in Figure 19.9. The results of a test can be plotted on this paper and then interpreted as in method 2.

If logarithmic probability paper is not available it is necessary to convert the doses into logarithms and the percentages into probits, and then to plot the logarithms against the probits.

The probit is best defined in terms of the normal equivalent deviation (N.E.D.). The N.E.D. corresponding to any given percentage is calculated from the shape of a normal curve whose standard deviation is one. The N.E.D. is the deviation (from the mean) equivalent to the given percentage of the area of the curve. The probit is equal to the N.E.D. plus 5.

The relationship between percentages and probits is shown in Figure 19.10. This curve is an integrated normal frequency curve. An interval of one unit on the scale of probits corresponds to one standard deviation, and the midpoint of the curve, corresponding to a mortality of 50 per cent. is arbitrarily taken as 5. If the distribution of individual lethal doses is normal, the relation of the dose to the observed mortality (as shown in Figure 19.7) will be the same as the relation of the probit to the mortality [Figure 19.10]. Both these quantities (dose and probit) are thus related to the mortality in the same complex way, and

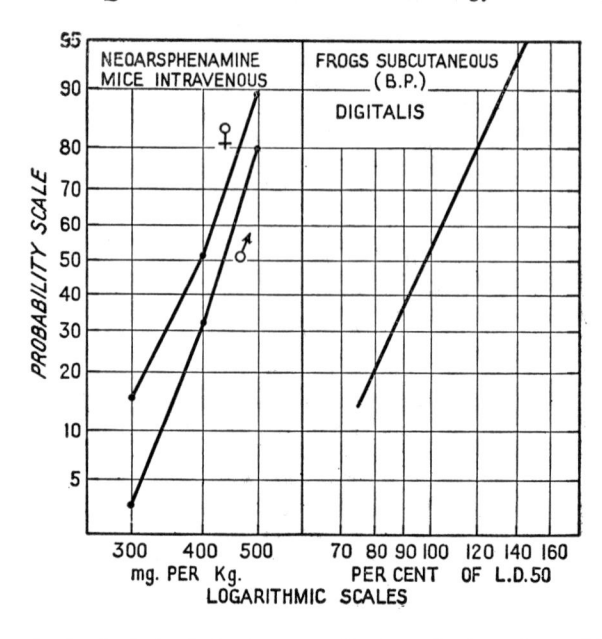

FIG. 19.9. Logarithmic probability paper. The horizontal scale is a logarithmic scale of doses. The vertical scale denotes percentage mortality and the lines are spaced in a way that depends on the shape of a normal curve. The distances are proportional to the corresponding probits. The right-hand figure portrays the same data as FIGURE 19.7. The effect of using this paper is that the results lie approximately on straight lines.

that is why their relation to one another is so simple that it can be expressed as a straight line [FIGURE 19.9], about which the actual observations are distributed with deviations due to the sampling error.

Straight lines are only obtained by the above method when the I.E.D. is normally distributed, but a similar argument applies to the more usual case where the log of the I.E.D. is normally distributed instead of the I.E.D. itself so that log I.E.D. gives a straight line when plotted against the probit. In practice the value of the probit is obtained from tables instead of from FIGURE 19.10.

The whole relationship of dose to percentage is completely defined in terms of two quantities that can easily be estimated. One of these quantities is the ED 50, and the other is the standard deviation of the logarithms of the individual effective doses, which is known as λ and is approximately equal to the difference between the logarithms of the ED 69 and the ED 31. Its reciprocal is known as

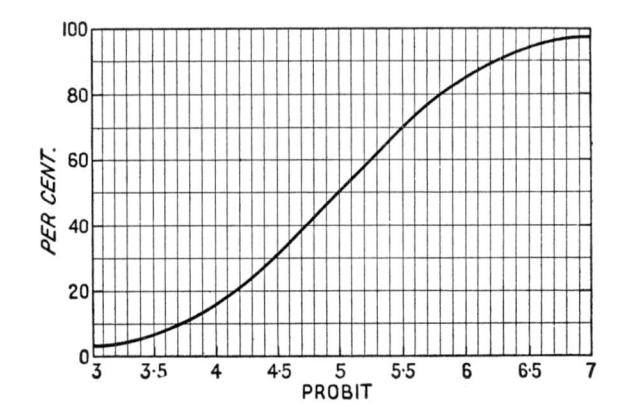

FIG. 19.10. Curve showing the relation between probits and mortality. The main object of this diagram is to clarify the explanation of probits given in the text. It can be used to determine roughly the probit corresponding to any given mortality. If mortalities are converted to probits and doses to logarithms the results can be plotted on ordinary graph paper, and the result is the same as if they had been plotted on the special paper shown in FIGURE 19.9.

b and is equal to the slope of the curve. Those who determine the shapes of these curves should always estimate and state the values of these two quantities.

The error of a test of this kind can be calculated from theoretical considerations which will not be discussed here. It depends on the fact that the percentages observed with small groups vary widely owing to the chances associated with choosing animals for the experiment.

QUALITATIVE PHARMACOLOGICAL ANALYSIS

The quantitative methods of biological assay have been discussed first because qualitative identification depends on quantitative methods. The quantitative results are, however, meaningless unless it is known that the observed effects of the solutions under test are actually due to the substance which is used as a standard of comparison. If an extract of intestine is injected into a cat it causes a fall of blood pressure, and there are at least five substances in the extract which collaborate in the production of this effect—histamine, choline, acetylcholine, adenosine compounds, and substance P. A quantitative assay of the extract by this method using any one of the substances as a standard would obviously be meaningless, but the test can easily be made more specific. If the extract is boiled with strong acid the pharmacological activities of adenosine and substance P are destroyed and that of acetylcholine is greatly diminished. If atropine is injected the cat may be made insensitive to choline and acetylcholine, but histamine survives the treatment with acid and its action survives the injection of atropine. If, therefore, the extract is boiled with acid its histamine content can be measured by comparing its action on an atropinized cat with that of pure histamine.

This example illustrates the ways in which specific tests may be discovered. In the first place, the extract can be submitted to physical or chemical methods which eliminate pharmacologically active substances other than that under study. It may be boiled, treated with acids, alkalis, or enzymes, dialysed, fractionated with solvents, chromatographed, or treated in numerous other ways. In the second place, the actual test itself may be modified by the use of appropriate drugs, as atropine was used in the above example. If a tissue can be found which is very sensitive to one of the substances in an extract and quite insensitive to the others these precautions may be unnecessary. For example, the acetylcholine in an extract of intestine can be assayed by its effect on the rectus abdominis isolated from a frog, which is not affected by histamine, adenosine, or substance P, and is only affected by high concentrations of choline. It can also be assayed by its action on leech muscle, but in this case it is necessary to use eserine to sensitize the muscle.

It is, of course, very important in all such work to make certain that the method finally decided upon really is a specific test for the substance studied. For this purpose it is not enough to eliminate interference from all the substances which are known to be present in extracts, since new unknown substances may be present.

This possibility must always be borne in mind and statements, such as that made above, that the effect of extracts of intestine, boiled with acid, on the blood pressure of an atropinized cat is entirely due to histamine must not be lightly made. The surest method of demonstrating the specificity of the methods used is to devise several quite different specific tests for the same substance and to carry out a quantitative assay by each test. If these assays agree there can be little doubt that all the tests really were specific. It has already been mentioned [p. 212] that the attempt to use potassium as a standard for the assay of posterior pituitary extracts on guinea-pig's uterus was unsuccessful because the test did not always give the same result even when it was repeated under exactly the same conditions.

If it was not already known that this action of pituitary extracts was not due to potassium such experiments would establish this fact. If a series of quite different pharmacological tests are used it is extremely unlikely that their results will agree quantitatively with one another unless the effects of the extracts are really due to the substance used as a standard. This method of parallel quantitative tests has been used to show that the substance liberated at cholinergic nerve endings is acetylcholine and not some other choline ester; it showed that the substance liberated by adrenergic nerves is not adrenaline; it showed that the vitamin D_3 in fish-liver oils was different from calciferol, which is obtained by irradiating ergosterol, since, when calciferol was used as a standard, the results of tests of oils on rats did not agree with the results of tests on chickens; it can be used to distinguish testosterone and androsterone by testing extracts on the capon's comb and the rat's prostate. The statement about histamine and the cat's blood pressure was based on quantitative agreement between assays on the guinea-pig's uterus, the guinea-pig's intestine, the cat's blood pressure, the rabbit's blood pressure, and the human skin which gave values of 8·4, 7·3, 6·8, 8·3, and 7 μg. of histamine per g. of tissue from which the extract was made.

The ratio of the results of two parallel assays is called the 'index of discrimination'. When the two solutions contain the same active principle the index is about 1; when it is 10 or more the active principles must be different. The value of two tests for distinguishing two substances is measured by the index of discrimination. Their value for identifying a substance depends on the indices found when this substance is compared with closely allied substances.

When parallel quantitative tests do not agree with one another the disagreement may foreshadow the discovery of a new active substance, but it may also be due to the presence in the extract of substances which are not themselves active, but nevertheless modify the effects of the active principle itself. Extracts of urine, for example, contain such substances which interfere with assays by increasing the action of oestrogens, but are not themselves oestrogenic.

Evidence for, or against, the identification of substances in extracts can often be obtained in various other ways. If the effects of the active substance are modified by the action of drugs such as atropine, eserine, or ergotoxine, the effects of the extracts should be modified in the same way. The discovery of substance P arose from an attempt to assay acetylcholine by applying extracts to a piece of rabbit's intestine, which was used because it is comparatively insensitive to histamine and choline and is inhibited by adenosine. Extracts of intestine cause a contraction of rabbit's intestine, but it was found that this effect was not abolished, like that of acetylcholine, by atropine. This effect could not be attributed to any known substance, and it was therefore necessary to postulate a new one. Such tests can be regarded as a special case of the method of parallel quantitative tests, since the extract was compared with acetylcholine twice, before and after atropine.

The extracts can also be tested before and after they have been subjected to various chemical and physical processes in order to see whether these processes eliminate the active substance. They can, for example, be subjected to heat, various chemicals, dialysis, solvents, or enzymes. They can be fractionated by chromatographic methods. In carrying out such tests it must be remembered that the properties of the active substance may be modified by other substances in the extract. A control experiment should therefore be carried out in which the pure active principle is added to the extract in order to see whether it is affected by the treatment in the same way as the active substance in the extract.

The methods used for identifying substances like adrenaline, acetylcholine, and histamine in tissue fluids may seem complicated, but it is only when elaborate precautions have been taken that it is justifiable, for example, to speak of 'acetylcholine' instead of 'the vagus stuff'.

THE DISCOVERY OF NEW DRUGS

The original drugs in our pharmacopoeia were of mainly vegetable origin and were discovered because certain plants were found to be unsuitable for foods owing to toxic properties; of some of these toxic properties it was readily recognized that they had medicinal virtues, an obvious example being the tranquillizing and analgesic actions of opium. Most had to await the isolation of active principles which began with the development of chemistry in the early nineteenth century. Today, plant products have become a diminishing source of new drugs as the flora of the more remote regions of the world have been examined. An exception has been the chemotherapeutic drugs of bacterial or fungal origin that were found as a result of extensive searches following the successful use of penicillin and streptomycin. By far the greatest number of chemotherapeutic drugs in use have been found in this way and often they have been of entirely novel chemical types.

However, the major effort in finding new drugs has been, for many years, by the deliberate synthesis of new compounds, and the principles used in this search are of several kinds. The one having the greatest chance of success is to use some model compound which either shows a feeble action of the type desired, or has the right kind of action in full but suffers from disadvantages due to side-actions, toxicity, or is poorly absorbed or metabolized at an unsuitable rate, and to modify it in the hope of improving its qualities. This may involve a simple approach of introducing or removing groups or it may involve a more sophisticated approach in which, by the comparison of the structure of available active compounds, the part of the structure essential for activity is preserved and new drugs are built around this skeleton. Good examples of this are the development of gallamine and other neuromuscular blocking drugs from curare or of the newer morphinone analgesics from morphine. In rare cases the nature of the drug actions required is known sufficiently precisely so that completely rational design is possible. The classic example of this is pralidoxime which is used to reverse the inhibition of cholinesterase by organophosphorus anticholinesterases [p. 62]. Another approach frequently used is to attempt to discover antagonists for known drugs by structural modifications; this has a rather good chance of success and recent examples are propranolol, an anti-adrenergic substance modelled on isoprenaline, nalorphine in which the N-methyl group of morphine has been replaced by an allyl group, aminopterin in which replacement of the 4-hydroxy group of folic acid by an amino group leads to a potent inhibitor of folic reductase.

It is unlikely that the methods described will lead intentionally to the discovery of entirely novel classes of drugs and these have usually been found by accident in using drugs for an entirely different purpose, for instance the very important group of phenothiazine tranquillizers resulted from their use as anti-emetics when it was noted clinically that there was a striking improvement in the psychiatric state of a mentally disturbed patient, or the discovery that chloroquine caused improvement of lupus erythematosus in patients being treated for malaria. Because it is so hard to anticipate useful drug actions it is customary for all new drugs to be screened for numerous actions. This means in practice setting up a battery of simple animal tests that are capable of detecting as wide a variety of drug actions as possible. The synthesis of the new compounds may then be directed either to an attempt to find a drug of a particular type, usually dictated by an estimate of the available market, or to the synthesis of novel chemical structures in the hope that they may show new types of action—a good example of the latter are the adamantine antiviral agents. It is an interesting fact that when a new series of drugs is examined, if any useful activity is to be found there is a high probability of it being found in the first few members of the series and extension of the series is more frequently undertaken to ensure patent coverage than to find a better member of the series—Ehrlich's prolonged search of organic arsenicals in which the 606th member was arsphenamine and the 912th neoarsphenamine is not the usual pattern.

It is always somewhat dismaying to consider how much new discovery in pharmacology (as in other sciences) is due to chance, but if we could foresee all there would be less excitement in discovery.

THE DEVELOPMENT OF NEW DRUGS

When a promising new drug action has been found, there follows an intensive study of its pharmacology in animals designed to explore both the characteristic action and any additional pharmacological actions in a variety of species. It is usual at the same time to examine the alterations produced by different routes of administration both on actions and on the acute toxicity; in most cases chemical methods will need to be developed for detecting the drug and its major metabolites so that duration of action and comparison of metabolism in several species can be carried out.

A preliminary study of chronic toxicity is usually carried out at this stage. The drug is given at just sublethal dose for several weeks, usually in rats and dogs, and the effects on behaviour, growth, and on some simple biochemical parameters such as haemoglobin, blood sugar, and urine composition, examined together with histological examination of the major tissues. If the drug passes these hurdles consideration must now be given to what potential uses the drug may have in man and whether these merit a preliminary trial. This should be a joint evaluation of all the evidence by the developers of the drug and the clinical pharmacologists. If it is agreed to proceed there follows a careful study in single individuals starting with very cautious dosage to assess how well the drug is tolerated after single doses and, if the drug is of the kind that produces direct physiological effects, whether the effects are similar in character and magnitude to those already revealed in animals. If this is all right, it is then usual to proceed to a limited therapeutic evaluation in man, at the same time extending the examination of chronic toxicity over a longer time and a wider range of situations; in particular, since the thalidomide disaster, a manufacturer would be unwise not to administer the drug both to young animals and to mating pairs continuing through pregnancy and some would even require that administration be continued until the progeny have reproduced.

It is as well to be clear about what is attempted in designing and carrying out animal toxicity tests. Ideally animal tests should predict toxic effects occurring in man; this presupposes that the same type of toxic effects do occur, but in fact there are several rather curious human toxic effects for which no animal tests are known. These are blood dyscrasias, skin effects, allergy, and most central nervous effects. Excluding these one can make a comparison and in TABLE 19.2 is shown a retrospective evaluation of six drugs that went to a full-scale clinical trial. It can be seen that toxicity in the rat was a poor indicator of toxicity in man and that the dog was a good deal better but still only detected a little over half the toxic effects found in man. What is more disturbing is that in both species toxic effects were found that did not arise in man. These results indicate first that study of animal toxicity is only a rough indicator of toxicity in man and further that some poten-

TABLE 19.2

Detectable toxic signs (6 drugs)	234
Found in man	53
Rat { toxic effects also found in man	18
{ toxic effects not found in man	19
Dog { toxic effects also found in man	29
{ toxic effects not found in man	24
Toxic effects in man detected in neither dog nor rat	23

tially valuable drugs may be damned for toxicity that would never appear. The classic case here is penicillin which has an extremely low toxicity in man and most other species but produces a lethal haemorrhagic enteritis in guinea-pigs. Fortunately this was not known when penicillin was introduced into therapeutics. The present position is therefore that animal testing will normally reveal gross toxicity precluding use of a drug in man, and experienced toxicologists develop a feeling for the animal data which can be a valuable guide in deciding whether to proceed. The clinical pharmacologist is now ready to proceed with a carefully planned trial to establish therapeutic usefulness under conditions in which the patients can be kept under close surveillance so that unexpected toxic effect or unexpected therapeutic effect can be picked up quickly. The kind of action exerted by the drug will determine the character and duration of the assessment at this time. It is usual to use some sort of sequential trial in which the effects of the drug can be compared with a placebo or with some established treatment so that a decision on effectiveness can be reached as early as possible. This initial trial may be broadened out into a multicentre trial so that sufficient experience is obtained and the probability of encountering the less common drug hazards is increased. Most of the toxic effects of drugs are relatively uncommon and will only become apparent when a considerable population is at risk. For instance, chloramphenicol will produce serious blood dyscrasias in about 1 patient in 10,000 and this has made it unsuitable for general use as a chemotherapeutic. Before preparations of a new drug are released for use by the medical profession or the public the assent of the Committee on Safety of Drugs is required. This body has, in fact, no statutory powers, but it examines both clinical and animal data on new drugs and gives advice on toxicity and therapeutic efficacy to the manufacturers.

FURTHER READING

BURN, J. H., FINNEY, D. J., and GOODWIN, L. G. (1950) *Biological Standardization*, 2nd ed., London.

FINNEY, D. J. (1964) *Statistical Methods in Biological Assay*, 2nd ed., London.

FISHER, R. A. (1941) *Statistical Methods for Research Workers*, Edinburgh.

GADDUM, J. H. (1933) *Spec. Rep. Ser. med. Res. Coun. (Lond.)*, No. 183, London, H.M.S.O.

GOLDSTEIN, A. (1964) *Biostatistics*, London.

HILL, A. B. (1967) *Principles of Medical Statistics*, 8th ed., London.

HILL, A. B. (ed.) (1965) *Controlled Clinical Trials*, Oxford.

LAURENCE, D. R. (ed.) (1959) *Quantitative Methods in Human Pharmacology*, Oxford.

LAURENCE, D. R., and BACHARACH, A. L. (eds) (1964) *Evaluation of Drug Activities: Pharmacometrics*, New York.

WAIFE, S. O., and SHAPIRO, A. P. (eds) (1959) *The Clinical Evaluation of New Drugs*, New York.

ZAIMIS, E. (ed.) (1965) *Evaluation of New Drugs in Man*, Oxford.

ADDITIONAL GENERAL READING IN PHARMACOLOGY

ALBERT, A. (1968) *Selective Toxicity*, 4th ed., London.

ARIËNS, E. J., and ROSSUM, J. M. VAN (1964) *Molecular Pharmacology*, London.

BARLOW, R. B. (1964) *Chemical Pharmacology*, 2nd ed., London.

BOVET, D., and BOVET-NITTI, F. (1948) *Médicaments du système nerveux végétatifs*, Basle.

BURGER, A. (ed.) (1970) *Medicinal Chemistry*, 3rd ed., New York.

GOLDSTEIN, A., ARONOW, L., and KALMAN, S. M. (1969) *Principles of Drug Action*, New York.

GOODMAN, L. S., and GILMAN, A. (1970) *The Pharmacological Basis of Therapeutics*, 4th ed., London.

GORDON, M. (ed.) (1964) *Psychopharmacological Agents*, Vol. 1; (1967) Vol. 2, New York.

HEFFTER, A. *Handbuch der experimentellen Pharmakologie*. An encyclopaedia of pharmacology with advanced authoritative specialist volumes mostly written in English.

HENRY, T. A. (1949) *The Plant Alkaloids*, 4th ed., London.

KOROLKOVAS, A. (1970) *Essentials of Molecular Pharmacology*, New York.

LAURENCE, D. R. (1966) *Clinical Pharmacology*, 3rd ed., London.

LAURENCE, D. R., and BACHARACH, A. L. (eds.) (1964) *Evaluation of Drug Activities*, New York.

MARLEY, E. (1966) *Pharmacological and Chemical Synonyms*, Amsterdam.

MODELL, W. (ed.) (1970–71) *Drugs of Choice*, St. Louis.

ROOT, W. S., and HOFMANN, F. G. (eds.) (1963–8) *Physiological Pharmacology*, New York.

SCHNITZER, R. J., and HAWKING, F. (1963–7) *Experimental Chemotherapy*, London.

SOLLMANN, T. (1957) *Manual of Pharmacology*, 8th ed., Philadelphia.

Review articles on pharmacology

Recent Advances in Pharmacology (1968) ed. Robson, J. M., and Stacey, R. S., 4th ed., London.
Pharmacological Reviews.
Advances in Pharmacology.
Advances in Drug Research.
Progress in Medicinal Chemistry.
Annual Review of Pharmacology.

Pharmacopoeias

Pharmacopoeias are official or semi-official publications giving accounts of preparations of drugs used therapeutically.
British Pharmacopœia (1968).
British Pharmaceutical Codex (1968).
British Veterinary Codex (1965).
British National Formulary.
United States Dispensatory.
The Extra Pharmacopœia (Martindale).
New and Non-Official Remedies.

UNITS OF MEASUREMENT

mega (M) 10^6 micro (μ) 10^{-6}
kilo (k) 10^3 nano (n) 10^{-9}
centi (c) 10^{-2} pico (p) 10^{-12}
milli (m) 10^{-3} femto (f) 10^{-15}

WEIGHTS

	ng.	μg.	mg.	g.	kg.
1 nanogram (ng.) =	1	10^{-3}	10^{-6}	10^{-9}	10^{-12}
1 microgram (μg.) =	10^3	1	10^{-3}	10^{-6}	10^{-9}
1 milligram (mg.) =	10^6	10^3	1	10^{-3}	10^{-6}
1 gram (g.) =	10^9	10^6	10^3	1	10^{-3}
1 kilogram (kg.) =	10^{12}	10^9	10^6	10^3	1

VOLUME

	Å^3	μm.^{3}	mm.^{3}	cm.^{3}	m.^{3}
Å^3 =	1	10^{-12}	10^{-21}	10^{-24}	10^{-30}
μm.^{3} =	10^{12}	1	10^{-9}	10^{-12}	10^{-18}
mm.^{3} =	10^{21}	10^9	1	10^{-3}	10^{-9}
cm.^{3} =	10^{24}	10^{12}	10^3	1	10^{-6}
m.^{3} =	10^{30}	10^{18}	10^9	10^6	1

	μl.	ml.	l.
μl. =	1	10^{-3}	10^{-6}
ml. =	10^3	1	10^{-3}
l. =	10^6	10^3	1

CHEMICAL UNITS OF MEASUREMENT

Mole (mol) ≡ molecular weight × grams.
Molarity (mol/l.) ≡ Moles of substance in 1 litre of solution (0·1 M, 0·01 M, etc.).
Volume per cent. (vol. %) ≡ ml. of solute in 100 ml. of solution.
Grams per cent. weight/volume ≡ grams per cent. w/v = grams in 100 ml. solution.

AQUEOUS SOLUTIONS

The following salts and glucose are dissolved in water to produce 100 ml. of solution. Weights in grams.

	NaCl	KCl	CaCl$_2$ (anhyd.)	MgCl$_2$ (anhyd.)	NaH$_2$PO$_4$ (anhyd.)	Na$_2$CO$_3$	NaHCO$_3$	Glucose
Ringer (frog)	0·65	0·014	0·012	··	0·001	··	0·02	0·2
Ringer (mammalian)	0·9	0·042	0·024	··	··	··	0·02	0·2
de Jalon	0·9	0·042	0·006	0·0005	··	··	0·05	0·05
Tyrode	0·8	0·02	0·02	0·01	0·005	··	0·1	0·1
Sea water	3·0	0·09	0·11	0·51†	0·006	0·003	0·02	0·025
Krebs–Henseleit original Ringer bicarbonate*	0·68	0·035	0·028	0·029†	0·016‡	··	0·21	··
Krebs original Ringer phosphate	0·68	0·035	0·028	0·029†	§	··	··	··

* Gassed with 5% CO$_2$ in gas phase.
† MgSO$_4$.7H$_2$O.
‡ KH$_2$PO$_4$.
§ Use 16·4 ml. of 0·1 M phosphate buffer (17·8 g. Na$_2$HPO$_4$.2H$_2$O + 20 ml. N-HCl diluted to 1 litre).

INDEX OF CHEMICAL RINGS

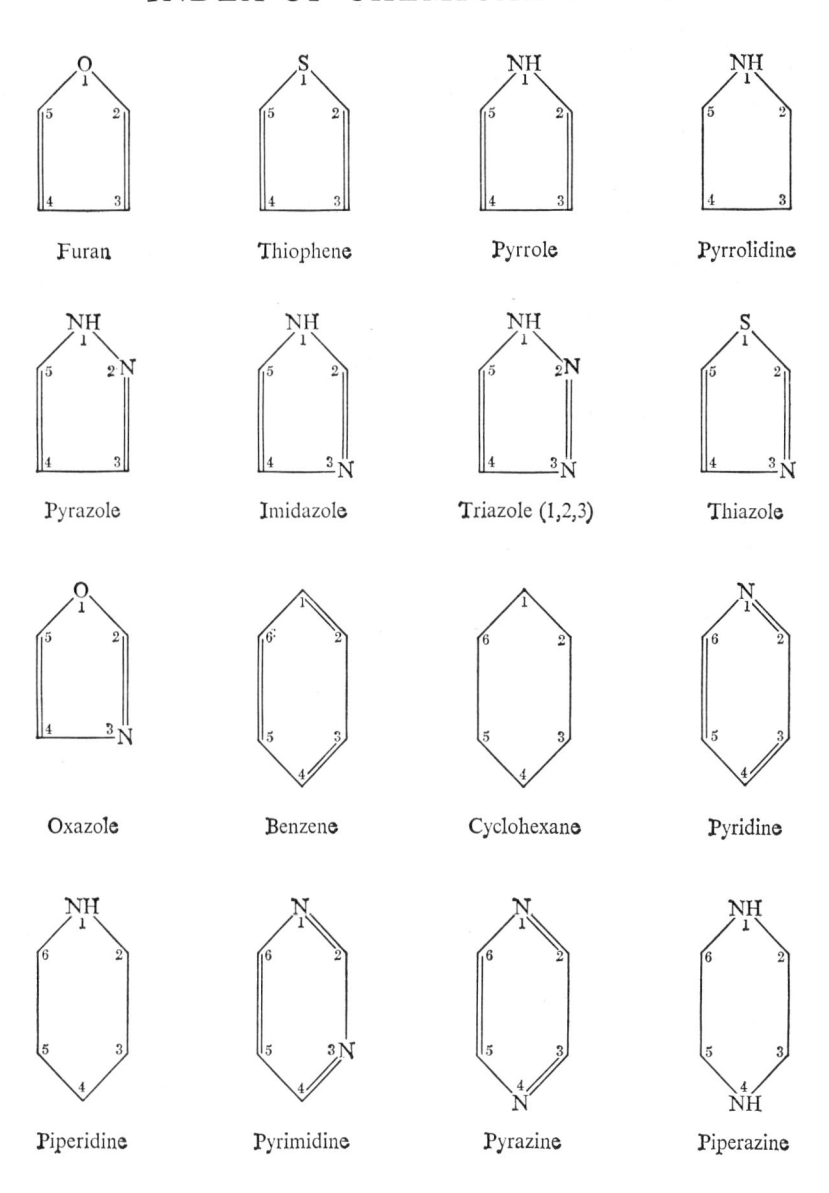

Furan · Thiophene · Pyrrole · Pyrrolidine

Pyrazole · Imidazole · Triazole (1,2,3) · Thiazole

Oxazole · Benzene · Cyclohexane · Pyridine

Piperidine · Pyrimidine · Pyrazine · Piperazine

Index of Chemical Rings

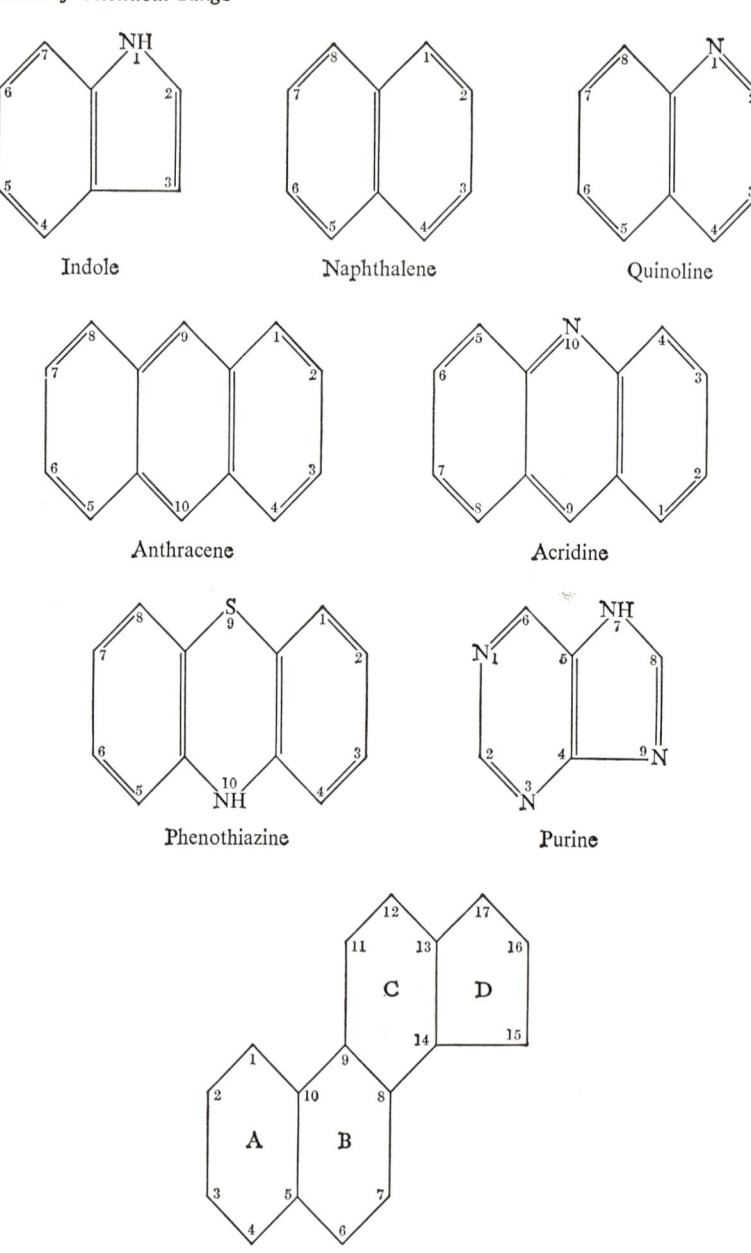

Indole

Naphthalene

Quinoline

Anthracene

Acridine

Phenothiazine

Purine

Steroid ring system

INDEX

48/80, 92.

Å³, 229.
ACTH, *see* Corticotrophin.
ADH, *see* Antidiuretic hormone.
ADP (Adenosine diphosphate), 113.
3'5' AMP (Adenosine monophosphate), 86, 100.
—, cyclic, 85.
ATP, *see also* Adenosine triphosphate, 85, 86, 113.
ATPase, 108.
Absorption of drugs from suspensions, 11.
— — — — tissues, 10–12.
Acacia, 123.
Acenocoumarol, *see* Nicoumalone.
Acetaminophen, *see* Paracetamol.
Acetanilide, 113, 115.
—, structure, 114.
Acetate, 153, 154.
Acetazolamide, 170–1.
— and gout, 173.
Aceturate, 201.
Acetylcholine, 1–4, 7, 9, 54 et seq., 71, 74–5, 84.
— and ascaris, 202.
— — atropine, 5, 6.
— — autonomic ganglia, 62–3.
— — choline, 130.
— — cholinergic nerve endings, 224.
— — cholinesterase, 82.
— — eserine, 72.
— — ether, 23.
— — gastrin, 117.
— — general anaesthesia, 18.
— — heart, 8.
— — mixed receptor sites, 68–70.
— — morphine, 36.
— — muscarinic receptors, 64, 65, 74–5.
— — nicotine, 64, 70.
— — nicotinic receptors, 70, 74.
— — striated muscle, 7.
— — synapses, 78.
—, assay of, 55, 216.
—, drugs which preserve, 61–2.
— in qualitative analysis, 223–4.
—, metabolism of, 13.
—, structure, 3.
Acetylcholine esterase, 75.
N-acetyl-dopamine, 142.

N-acetylglucosamine, 182.
N-acetylhistamine, 93.
Acetyl-β-methylcholine, 68.
—, structure, 76.
N-acetylmuramic acid, 182.
Acetylnorcholine, 74.
Acetylphenylhydrazine, 138.
Acetylsalicylic acid (aspirin), 99, 113, 115–16.
— —, structure, 114.
Acidosis, 119, 169–71.
Acridine ring, 232.
Acromegaly, 143.
Actinomycin, 142, 209.
Action potential, 57, 65, 85, 105.
α-actions, 85 et seq., 103.
β-actions, 85 et seq., 103.
Acyl enzyme, 62.
Acylcholines, 7.
Adamantine antiviral agents, 225.
Addiction, *see also* Dependence.
— to amphetamine, 39.
— — cocaine, 52.
— — glutethimide, 28.
— — meprobamate, 32.
— — methadone, 37.
— — morphine, 36.
— — nicotine, 64.
— — pethidine, 37.
— — tobacco, 64.
Addison's disease, 152, 155, 158.
— — and ACTH, 144.
— — — aldosterone, 172.
Adenine, 206.
Adenohypophysis, 143.
Adenosine, 224.
— compounds in qualitative analysis, 223.
— diphosphate, *see* ADP.
3'5' adenosine monophosphate, *see* 3'5' AMP, 86.
Adenosine triphosphate (ATP, Adenosine 3'5' phosphate), 85, 86, 108, 113, 128.
Adenylcyclase, 86, 99.
3'5' adenylic acid, 100.
Adermine, *see* Vitamin B₆.
Administration of drugs by mouth, 12.
— — — inhalation, 12.
Adrenal cortex, 86.
— — and aldosterone, 172.
— — — androgens, 165.
— — — oestrogens, 159.

— —, assay of, 217.
— insufficiency, 158.
— steroids, 107, 152 et seq., 169.
— — and insulin, 150.
— — — kidney, 169.
— —, biosynthesis of, 153.
Adrenaline, 78 et seq.
— and adrenergic nerves, 224.
— — antihistamines, 94.
— — blood sugar, 151.
— — circulation, 103.
— — cocaine, 52.
— — nicotine, 63.
— — peristalsis, 121.
— — phaeochromocytoma, 88.
— — prostaglandins, 99.
— — salicylates, 115.
— — temperature, 113.
—, assay of, 216.
—, biosynthesis, 80.
—, metabolism, 82.
—, structure, 80, 86.
Adrenergic nerves and adrenaline, 224.
— — — cocaine, 52.
— receptors, distribution of, 84.
Adrenocorticoids, 153 et seq.
Adrenocortictrophic hormone, 150, 152–3, *see also* Corticotrophin.
Adsorbents, 123.
Adsorption of drugs in the mouth, 12.
Agar, 121.
Aglycone, 107.
Agonist, 5–9.
— receptor complexes, 7.
— response, 6, 7.
Agranulocytosis, 30.
D-alanine, 183.
Alcohol, 33–4.
— and meprobamate, 32.
— — temperature, 113.
— as anaesthetic, 17.
— poisoning, 34.
Alcoholic neuritis, 34.
Alcoholics, vitamin B deficiency in, 129.
Alcoholism and pellagra, 129.
Aldocorten, 156.
18-aldocorticosterone (*see* Aldosterone), 153.
Aldosterone, 153–4, 156, 172.
— and angiotensin, 96.
— — kidney, 169.

Index

Aldosterone and triamterene, 172.
—, structure, 154.
Alflorone acetate, 156.
Alkaline phosphate, 144.
Alkaloids, 123, **208**.
Alkalosis, 117–19.
— and diuretics, 169, 170.
Alkyl sulphonates, 208.
Alkylating agents, 206–8, 209, 210.
Allantoin, 173.
Allergic reactions, *see also* Allergy.
— — and iron, 136.
— — — organic mercurials, 170.
— rhinitis, 94.
— states, vitamin P and, 128.
Allergy, *see also* Allergic reactions.
— and antihistamines, 94.
— — corticosteroids, 156.
— — salicylates, 116.
— — sulphonylureas, 152.
— in toxicity tests, 226.
Allobarbitone, 26.
Allopurinol, 174.
Allostery, 6.
Aloes, 122–3.
Aluminium hydroxide, 119.
— salts, 123.
Amantadine, 192.
Amenorrhoea, 159.
Amethocaine, 51.
Amidines, 96.
Amiloride, 172.
Amines, sympathomimetic, structures, 86.
4-aminobenzoic acid (*see also*, Para-aminobenzoic acid), 178, 180.
γ-amino-butyric acid, *see* GABA.
Aminocephalosporanic acid, 187.
6-aminopenicillanic acid, 185.
p-aminophenylstibonic acid, 200.
Aminophylline, 100.
Aminopterin, discovery of, 225.
4-aminoquinoline, 197.
8-aminoquinoline, 198.
p-aminosalicylic acid (PAS), 191.
— —, structure, 190.
Amiphenazole, 46.
—, structure, 43.
Amithiozone, *see* Thiacetazone.
Amitriptyline, 41.
— and noradrenaline, 90.
—, structure, 40.
Ammonium chloride, 170.
— — and urine pH, 175.
Amobarbital, *see* Amylobarbitone.
Amodiaquine, 196, **197–8**.
Amoebic dysentery, 198–9.
— —, structure of drugs used for, 199.

Amphenone B, **153**, 155.
—, structure, 155.
Amphetamine, **39**, 41.
— and phenobarbitone, 29.
— — temperature, 113.
— — urine pH, 175.
—, structure, **40**, 86.
—, sympathomimetic action, **88**.
Amphotericin B, 182, **192**.
Ampicillin, 181, 185, **187**.
—, structure, 186.
Amyl nitrite, 106.
Amylobarbitone, 26, 27.
— and dexamphetamine, 39.
—, duration of action of, 26.
—, metabolism of, 13.
Amylopectin sulphate, 118.
Amytal, 26.
Anabolism, protein, and androgens, 167.
Anaemia, megaloblastic, 130.
—, pernicious, 126, 137.
—, — and liver extracts, 130.
Anaesthesia, block, 51, 52.
—, general, **17** et seq.
—, — and electroencephalogram, 20–1.
—, — — temperature, 113.
—, —, signs of, **19**.
—, —, stages of, 19–20.
—, infiltration, 52.
—, local, **49** et seq.
—, regional, 52.
—, spinal, 51, 52.
—, theories of, 17–19.
Anaesthetic solutions, **24**.
Anaesthetics, local, and bretylium, 83.
—, — — central nervous system, 50.
—, — — noradrenaline, 90.
—, —, as antiarrhythmics, 110.
—, —, effect of pH on, 49.
—, —, metabolism of, 50.
—, —, structures, 51.
—, mode of action, 17.
—, volatile and gaseous, **21–4**.
Analeptics, **42** et seq.
—, structures, 43.
Analgesia, local, 23.
Analgesics, **34–7**.
— and temperature, 113.
Analysis, qualitative, 223–4.
Anaphylaxis and penicillin, 186.
Ancylostoma duodenale, 203.
Androgen-like properties, structures of drugs with, 166.
Androgens, 144, 158, 160, **165–7**.
— and adrenal cortex, 153.
— as anti-oestrogens, 160.

Androstenedione, 165.
Androsterone, **165**, 167, 224.
Androteston, *see* Testosterone propionate.
Aneurine, *see also* Vitamin B₁, 126, **128**.
— and chronic alcoholism, 34.
Angina pectoris, 106–7.
Angiotensin, 96.
— and aldosterone, 172.
— I and II, 155.
Angiotensinogen, 96.
Anovlar, 164.
Antabuse, *see* Disulphiram.
Antacids, 118–19.
Antagonist actions, **7**.
Antazoline, 120.
Anthelminthics, **201** et seq.
— and purgatives, 122.
Anthracene purgatives, 123.
— ring, 232.
Anthraquinone, 123.
Anti-adrenergic drugs and glucagon, 152.
Antiarrhythmic drugs, 90, **110**.
Antibacterials, **177** et seq.
Antibiotics, *see also* Antibacterials, 177 et seq.
— as anti-neoplastics, 209.
Antibodies, 5.
Antibody formation and corticosteroids, 153, 158.
Anticholinergic drugs and gastric secretion, 118.
Anticholinesterase, 7, 55, 59, **61–2**, 70, 72 et seq.
— and acetylcholine, 14, 74.
— — benzoquinonium, 72.
— — mixed receptor sites, 68.
— — muscarinic receptors, **64–5**, 75.
— — procaine, 53.
Anticholinesterases, structures, 73.
Anticoagulant therapy, **139–41**.
Anticonvulsants, 29–30.
Antidepressants, **39–42**.
Antidiuretic hormone, 64, 143, **145**, 169.
Antifolics, 206.
Antifungal agents, 192.
Antigens, 5.
Antihistamines, **93–4**.
— as anti-emetics, 119.
Antimalarials, discovery of, 177.
—, resistance to, 198.
—, structures, 197.
Antimetabolites, **208–10**.
Antimonials, organic, 200.
Antimony compounds as anthelminthics, 202.

Index

— dimercaptosuccinate, 204.
— gluconate, 204.
—, pentavalent, 200.
— potassium tartrate, 204.
— sodium tartrate, 204.
— — —, structure, 202.
Antimuscarines, 65–7, 93.
Anti-oestrogens, 160–2.
Antipyretic-analgesic group, 113.
— — —, structures, 114.
Antipyrine, *see* Phenazone.
Antiseptics, **193**.
Antistin, *see* Antazoline.
Antithyroid drugs, 145–6.
Antitoxins, assay of, 211.
Antitrypanosome drugs, 184.
Antitumour drugs, **206** et seq.
— — and vomiting, 119.
Antivirus agents, **192–3**.
Aplastic anaemia and phenylbutazone, 116.
— — — troxidone, 30.
Apnoea and succinylcholine, 70.
Apoferritin, 135.
Apomorphine and vomiting, 119.
Arachidonic acid, 99.
Arecoline, 4, 65–6, 75.
—, structure, 4, 76.
Argentaffin cells, 94.
Arginine, *see* Vasopressin.
Ariboflavinosis, 126.
Arsanilic acid, *see* Atoxyl.
Arsenicals, **200–1**.
—, organic, 177.
—, pentavalent, 200.
—, trivalent, 204.
Arsenoxides, 177.
Arsphenamine, 177.
—, discovery of, 226.
Arterenol, 78.
'Artificial hibernation', 32.
Arylsulphonal ureas, 151–2.
Ascaris lumbricoides, 202–3.
Ascites and radioactive gold, 210.
Ascorbic acid, *see also* Vitamin C, **125–6**.
— — and corticotrophin, 144.
— —, structure, 127.
Aspidium, 203.
Aspirin (Acetylsalicylic acid), 113, 114, **115–16**.
— and bradykinin, 97.
— — thyroid, 146.
Assay, biological, **211** et seq.
— —, methods of, **215** et seq.
Asthma and aminophylline, 100.
— — antihistamines, 99.
— — ephedrine, 87.
Astringents, 123–4.
Atoxyl, 177.

Atrial fibrillation, 110.
— — and digitalis, 108.
— flutter, 110.
Atropa belladonna, 67.
Atropine, 7, 66–7, 77.
— and acetylcholine, 5, 6, 64.
— — anticholinesterases, 62.
— — cardiac glycosides, 108.
— — central nervous system, 67.
— — histamine release, 92.
— — muscarinic actions, 54, 55, 65, 74–6.
— — neostigmine, 72.
— — peristalsis, 120.
— — premedication, 21.
— — prostigmin, 72.
— in qualitative analysis, 223–4.
— methonitrate, 9.
— poisoning, 67, 113.
—, structure, 76.
Atropine-like actions and antihistamines, 93.
— compounds and muscarinic receptors, 66.
Auerbach's plexus, 36, 45, 120–1.
'Autocatalytic reaction', 138.
Autonomic ganglion, 60, **62** et seq.
— — and acetylcholine, 74.
— ganglia, drugs blocking transmission at, 73.
— nervous system and vinblastine, 209.
Autoradiographs, 17.
Avidin, 130.
Azapetine, 88.
Azide and nitrites, 106.
Aziridine of phenoxybenzamine, 89.

BOL, *see* Bromo-lysergic acid diethylamide.
BW 545 C64, 96.
— structure, 95.
Bacitracin, 182.
Bacteria, resistant strains, 184–5.
Bacterial cell walls, 181–2.
Bactericidal agents, **180** et seq.
Bacteriostatic agents, 180.
Bactrim, 188.
Banthine, *see* Methantheline.
Barbitone and urine pH, 175.
—, duration of action of, 26.
Barbiturate poisoning, 173.
— — and bemegride, 46.
— — — ethamivan, 46.
Barbiturates, **25–7**.
—, absorption of, 12.
— and dexamphetamine, 39.
— — strychnine poisoning, 45.
—, duration of action of, 26.

—, effects of overdosage, 27, 42.
—, for premedication, 21.
—, in general anaesthesia, 24.
—, tolerance to, 27.
Basedow's disease, 148.
Basophil cells, 92.
— — and heparin, 138.
Bemegride, 27, **46**.
—, structure, 43.
Benadryl, *see* Diphenhydramine.
Bendrofluazide, 171.
—, structure, 170.
Bendroflumethiazide, *see* Bendrofluazide.
Benzalkonium, as antiseptic, 193.
Benzathine benzylpenicillin, 11.
— penicillin, 186.
Benzene ring, 231.
Benzhexol, 9.
Benzidine-azo dyes, 177.
Benzilic acid, 6.
Benzilylcholine mustard, 67, **75**, 77.
— —, structure, 76.
Benzocaine, structure, 51.
Benzodiazepines, 31, **33**.
Benzoquinonium, 61, **72**.
Benzthiadiazines, 171.
Benzylpenicillin, 181, **185–7**.
Bephenium, 202, **203**.
Beriberi, 126, 128.
Beta rays, 148, 209.
Betamethasone, 156.
—, structure, 157.
Betel nut, 4, 75.
Bethanidine, 84, **90**.
— and hypotension, 104.
—, structure, 83.
Bezold receptors, 105.
— reflex, 95.
Bicarbonate ions and kidney, 168.
Bicuculline, 45–6.
—, structure, 43.
Biguanides, 151, **152**, 196, 198.
Bile, 120.
Bilein, 120.
Bilharziasis, 204.
Biliary colic and morphine, 36, 37.
— — — pethidine, 37.
Binomial distribution, 213.
Biological assay, 55, **211** et seq.
— — of acetylcholine, 55.
Biotin, *see also* Vitamin H, 126, 128, **130**.
Bisacodyl, 122.
Bisonium compounds, 65.
Black widow spider venom, 58.
Bladder and atropine, 67.
— — muscarinic actions, 65, 67.
Bleeding time, 139.

Index

Block anaesthesia, 51, 52.
α-blockers, 85–6, **88–9**, 104–5.
—, structures, 89.
β-blockers, 85 et seq, **89–90**, 104.
—, structures, 91.
Blood–brain barrier, 68.
— — and arsenicals, 200.
— — serotonin, 96.
— — suramin, 201.
Blood coagulation, **138–41**.
— — and corticosteroids, 158.
— — factors, 139, 140.
— dyscrasia and chloramphenicol, 227.
— — — sulphonyl ureas, 152.
— — — toxicity tests, 226.
— flow in various organs, 10.
— — limited access, 9.
— platelets and thiouracil, 146.
— pressure and anaesthesia, 20.
— — — corticosteroids, 158.
— — — ganglion blocks, 65.
— — — histamine, 92.
— — — nicotine, 64.
— — — nikethamide, 45.
— — — vasopressin, 97.
—, red cells of, 135.
— sugar and ACTH, 144.
— — — insulin, **149–51**.
— —, factors controlling, **149–50**.
— vessels and muscarinic actions, 65.
— — — xanthines, 100.
— volume and corticosteroids, 158.
Bone and parathyroid, 149.
— — rickets, 133.
— — tetracyclines, 187.
— marrow, 208.
— — and actinomycin D, 209.
— — — anti-neoplastics, 206.
— — — chloramphenicol, 189.
Botulinum toxin, 58.
— — and acetylcholine, 63.
Bradycardia and anaesthesia, 21.
— — veratrine, 105.
Bradykinin, **96–7**.
— and salicylates, 115.
Brain and cocaine, 52.
— serotonin, 96.
— xanthines, 42.
—, blood flow in, 10.
Bran, 121.
Bretylium, 84.
—, structure, 83.
Brevital, 26.
Bromides, 28–9.
Bromo-lysergic acid diethylamide, 47.
— — — and serotonin, 96.

Bronchi and atropine, 67.
— — histamine, 92.
— — prostaglandins, 99.
Bronchial carcinoma and nitrogen mustards, 206.
— irritation and tobacco, 64.
Bronchioles and serotonin, 95.
Buccal mucosa, absorption by, 12.
Bundle of His, 110.
Busulphan, **208**, 209.
Butazolidine (Phenylbutazone), 113.
Butobarbitone, 26.
Butoxamine, 90.
—, structure, 91.
Butyrylcholine, 3, 4, 7, 74.

C 10, see Decamethonium.
C^{14}, 79.
COMT, see also Catechol-O-methyl transferase, 80–1, 87.
cm.^{3}, 229.
Caffeine, **41–2**, 86.
— and aspirin, 115.
— — smooth muscle, 100.
Calciferol, see also Vitamin D_2, 133, 224.
Calcium, 108.
— and acetylcholine, 63.
— — adrenergic system, 78.
— — androgens, 165.
— — cardiac glycosides, 108.
— — digitalis, 109.
— — hyperthyroidism, 147.
— — liquid paraffin, 121.
— — parathyroid, 148–9.
— — prothrombin, 138.
— — vitamin D, 133.
— carbonate, 118.
— permeability, 85.
Calomel, see Mercurous chloride.
Cancer chemotherapy, **205** et seq.
Candida, 192.
Cannabis, 47.
— sativa, 47.
Carbachol, **65–6**, 71, 75.
Carbasone, 199.
Carbenicillin, 181, **187**.
—, structure, 186.
Carbenoxalone, 118.
Carbimazole, 146.
Carbolic, 177.
Carbonic anhydrase, 8, 168.
— — inhibitors, **170–1**.
Carboxypeptidase, 7.
Carbutamide, 146.
Carcinogens, 205.
Carcinoma of breast and oestrogens, 160.
— — lung, 63.

— — prostate and oestrogens, 160.
Cardiac arrhythmia and halothane, 22.
— failure and aminophylline, 100.
— — — frusemide, 171.
— — — organic mercurials, 170.
— glycosides, **107** et seq.
— — and thiazides, 171.
— — — thyroid, 145.
— — — vomiting, 119.
Cardiovascular system and corticosteroids, 155, 158.
— — — serotonin, 94–5.
— —, drugs acting on, **103** et seq.
β-carotene, 132.
Carotene and liquid paraffin, 121.
Carotid-aortic pressor receptors, 102.
Cascara, 122–3.
Castor oil, 122.
Catechol-O-methyl transferase, 81–2.
Catecholamines, 63, **85–6**.
— and adrenergic system, 78, 81.
— — anaesthesia, 21, 22.
— — antidepressants, 39, **41**.
— — β-blockers, 89–90.
— — circulation, 101.
— — cocaine, 52.
— — halothane, 22.
Celestone, 156.
Cell membranes, bacterial, 181.
— — and chemotherapeutic agents, 182, 183.
— — — general anaesthesia, 19.
— — — insulin, 149.
— — — urine pH, 174.
— potentials, 65.
— walls, bacterial, **181–3**, 205.
— — and penicillin, 182, 205.
Cellular metabolism and xanthines, 42.
Cellulose, 121.
— acetate phthallate, 12.
Central nervous system and anti-trypanosomal drugs, 200–1.
— — — — imipramine, 41.
— — — — iproniazid, 40.
— — — — local anaesthetics, 50.
— — — — nitrogen mustards, 206, 207.
— — effects in toxicity tests, 226.
Centrally acting drugs, **15** et seq.
Cephaloridine, 187, 188.
Cephalosporins, 187, 188.
Cephalothin, 187, 188.
Cerebral cortex and cocaine, 50.
Cestodes, 202, **203–4**.
Cetrimide, 193.
Cetyltrimethylammonium, 193.

Index

Chagas' disease, 200.
Chalk, 123.
Ch'an su, 107.
Charcoal, activated, 123.
Chelators, 135.
Chemical rings, index of, 231–2.
— transmitters, assay of, 211.
— units of measurement, 229.
Chemotherapeutic action, principles of, 178 et seq.
— spectra, 185.
Chiniofon, 199.
Chloral hydrate, 27.
Chloraluric acid, 27.
Chlorambucil, 207.
Chloramphenicol, 184, 185, **189**.
—, resistance to, 185.
—, toxicity, 227.
Chlorcyclizine, 120.
Chlordiazepoxide, 31, **33**.
—, structure, 28.
Chlorhexidine, 193.
Chloride ions and adrenal steroids, 152.
— — — androgens, 165.
— — — kidney, 168.
Chlorinated phenols, 193.
Chlorine as antiseptic, 193.
Chlormadinone, 162, 163.
Chloroform, 17.
—, partition coefficient of, 22.
Chloroguanide, 196.
Chloroquine, 225.
— for amoebic dysentery, **199**.
— — malaria, 196, **197**.
Chlorothiazide, 171.
— and digitalis, 110.
—, structure, 170.
Chlorotrianisene, 160–2.
Chlorphenoxamine, 199.
Chlorpromazine, 31, **32**, 34, 37.
— and alcohol, 34.
— — LSD, 47.
— — temperature, 113.
— as anti-emetic, 119.
Chlorpropamide, 151–2.
Chlortetracycline, 188.
8-chlortheophylline, 86.
Chocolate, laxative, 122.
Cholagogues, 120.
Cholecystokinin, 120.
Choleretics, 120.
Cholesterol, 120, 154.
— and adrenal steroids, 152–3.
— — cell membranes, 183.
— — corticotrophin, 144.
— — thyroid, 147.
Choline, 58, 63, 71, **75**.
— and smooth muscle, 100.

— as vitamin, 126, 128, **130**, 132.
— in qualitative analysis, 223–4.
Choline acetyltransferase, 58, 63.
— ethylether, 4.
Cholinergic drugs, **70–2**.
— —, antagonists to, 70–2.
— nerves, 1, **54** et seq., 224.
— system, 70, 78.
Cholinesterase, 8, **56** et seq., 71.
— 'ageing of', 62.
— and acetylcholine, 74, 82.
— — local anaesthetics, 50.
— — nicotine, 70.
— — pralidoxime, 225.
Chorionepithelioma, 206, 208.
Chorionic gonadotrophins, 144–5.
Chromaffin cells, 78.
Chronotropic action, 103.
— effect, 107, 108.
— — and adrenaline, 104.
Chrysophanic acid, 123.
Cinchocaine, 52.
—, structure, 51.
Cinchona, 198.
— alkaloids, 177.
Cis-vitamin A, 132.
— aldehyde, see Retinene.
Citric acid cycle, 18, 33.
Citrin, see Vitamin P.
Clathrates, 18.
Claviceps purpurea, 97.
Clinical trials, 226–7.
Clioquinol, 199.
Clomiphene, 160–2.
Clotting time, 139.
Cloxacillin, 181, **187**.
—, structure, 186.
Cobalamin, see also Vitamin B_{12}, 126, **136–7**.
—, structure, 136.
Cobamide, 130.
Cocaine, 49, 50, 51, **52**, 83.
— and cerebral cortex, 50.
— — 'contact purgatives', 122.
— — noradrenaline, 82, 90.
— — temperature, 113.
— poisoning, 52.
—, structure, 51.
Cod-liver oil, 133.
Codeine, 35, **37**.
— and aspirin, 115.
—, structure, 35.
Coeliac disease, 137.
Coenzyme A, 129.
Coenzyme B_{12}, 135, 137.
Colchicine, 8, **209**.
— derivatives, 209.
Colic and arsenicals, 200.
Coma, diabetic, 150.
—, hypoglycaemic, 151.

Competitive inhibition, 178, 208.
Conjugation of drugs, 13.
Consciousness, 19.
Constipation and morphine, 36.
— — strychnine, 45.
'Contact purgative', 122.
Contraceptives, oral, 164–5.
Convulsants, **42** et seq.
—, structures, 43.
Convulsions, epileptic, 29.
— and amiphenazole, 46.
— — atropine, 67.
— — central nervous stimulants, 42.
— — cocaine, 52.
— — local anaesthetics, 50.
— — pethidine, 37.
— — strychnine, 45.
— — temperature, 113.
— — vinblastine, 209.
— — xanthines, 42.
Copper salts as astringents, 123.
— sulphate, 119.
Corpus luteum, 162.
— — and contraceptives, 164.
— — — menstrual cycle, 159.
Cortexolone, 172.
Corticosteroids, see also Adrenal steroids, **152** et seq., 209.
—, action of, **155** et seq.,
—, side-effects of, 158.
Corticosterone, 144, 153.
—, structure, 154.
Corticotrophin, 86, 143, **144**, 152–3, 155.
— and prostaglandins, 99.
Cortisol, see also 17-hydroxycorticosterone, 144, 153, 156.
Cortisone, 156.
—, assay of, 217.
—, structure, 154.
Cortisone acetate, see also 11-dehydro-17-hydroxycorticosterone, 153, 156.
Corydalis, 45.
Coumarin group, 139–41.
Coupled beats and digitalis, 108.
Cretins, 147.
Cromoglycate, 13, 94.
Cross-over test, 220.
C-terminal dipeptide, 96.
Cumulative action of barbiturates 27.
Curare, **61**, 65, 225.
— and nicotinic receptors, 54.
Curare-like compounds and acetylcholine, 59.
— — — anticholinesterases, 62, 72.
— — — ether, 23.
— — — halothane, 22.

Index

Cushing's disease, 152, 155, 158.
Cyanide and nitrites, 106.
Cyanocobalamin, *see also* Vitamin B₁₂, 126, 128, **130**.
— and macrocytic anaemia, 137.
Cyclic AMP (adenosine monophosphate), 42, **85–6**, 99.
Cyclizine, 93.
Cyclobarbitone, 26.
Cyclohexane ring, 231.
Cyclophosphamide, 206–7.
Cyclopropane, 7, 21, **23–4**.
— and procaine, 53.
—, partition coefficient of, 22.
D-cycloserine, **182**, 183, 192.
Cyproheptadine and serotonin, 96.
—, structure, **95**.
Cysteine, 200.
Cysticercus, 203.
Cytidine, 206.
Cytochrome C, 125.
— oxidase, 106, 125.
Cytosine arabinoside, 206.

DBI, *see* Phenformin.
DCI, *see* Dichloroisoprenaline.
DDD, 209.
O,p'-DDD, 209.
DDT, 10, 209.
DFP, *see* Dyflos and Diisopropylfluorophosphonate.
DHE, *see* Dihydro-β-erythroidine.
DMPP, *see* Dimethyl-4-phenylpiperazium.
DNA, 201, 206, 209.
DNOC, *see* 3,5,dinitro-orthocresol.
DOCA, *see also* 11-deoxycorticosterone, 153, 156.
—, structure, 154.
DOPA, *see also* Dihydroxyphenylalanine, 3-hydroxytyrosine, **78–81**, 142.
—, structure, 80.
DOPA decarboxylase, **78–81**, 94.
Dapsone, 192.
—, structure, 190.
Dark adaptation, 133.
Darmstoff, 99.
Deadly nightshade, 66.
Deafness and quinine, 198.
Debrisoquine, 84.
—, structure, 83.
Decamethonium, **60**, **70–1**.
—, structure, 71.
Decarboxylases and pyridoxine, 129.
Dehydroascorbic acid, 125.
— —, structure, 127.

7-dehydrocholesterol (Vitamin D₃), 133, 224.
Dehydrocholic acid, 120.
11-dehydrocorticosterone, 153, 217.
11-dehydro-17-hydroxycorticosterone, 153.
de Jalon's solution, 230.
Delatestryl, *see* Testosterone enanthate.
Delirium tremens, 34.
— — and chloral hydrate, 27.
Deltahydrocortisone, 156.
—, structure, 207.
Demecolcine, 209.
Demethylation of drugs, 13.
Demethylchlortetracycline, 188.
Demulcents, **123–4**.
11-deoxycorticoids (mineralocorticoids), 153.
11-deoxycorticosterone, 153.
Deoxycortone acetate, *see also* 11-deoxycorticosterone, 153, 156.
Deoxyhydrocortisone, 153, 154.
Deoxyuridine, 206.
Dependence, *see also* Addiction.
— on barbiturates, 27.
— — morphine, 36.
— — pethidine, 37.
Depolarizing block, 59.
Depot penicillin, 186.
Derazil, *see* Chlorcyclizine.
Dermatitis, seborrhoeic and vitamin B₂, 129.
Desferrioxamine, 136.
Desipramine and noradrenaline, 82, 90.
Desmethylimipramine, 41.
Desoxycorticosterone acetate, *see also* 11-deoxycorticosterone, 153, 156.
Dettol, 193.
Development of new drugs, **226–7**.
Deviation, normal equivalent, 221.
—, standard, 221.
Dexamphetamine, 39.
Dextran, 92.
Dextro amphetamine, *see* Dexamphetamine.
Dexytal, *see* Drinamyl.
Diabetes and salicylates, 115.
— insipidus and thiazides, 171.
— mellitus, **149**, 173.
— — and thiazides, 171.
Diabetic coma, 150.
Dial, 26.
Diamidine compounds, 201.
Diamine oxidase, 93.
Diaminodiphenylsulphone, 192.

Diamorphine (heroin), 37.
—, structure, 35.
Diaralkylamines, 93.
Diarrhoea and actinomycin D, 209.
— — antimetabolites, 208.
— — fluorouracil, 208.
— — iron salts, 136.
— — mercaptopurine, 208.
'Diastolic drift', 110.
Diatrizoate, 174.
Diazepam, 31, **33**.
—, structure, 28.
Dibenamine, 77, **88**.
—, structure, 89.
Dibenzazepine derivatives, 41.
Dibenzylethylenediamine, 186.
Dibotin, *see* Phenformin.
Dibozane, 88–9.
Dibucaine, *see* Cinchocaine.
Dibutoline, 67, **75**.
—, structure, 76.
Dibutyryl cyclic AMP, 86.
Dichloral phenazone, 27.
Dichloroisoprenaline, 85, **89**.
—, structure, 91.
Dichlorophenol indophenol, 212.
Dichlorphenamide, 170.
Dicophane, 10.
Dicoumarol, **140–1**.
—, metabolism of, 14.
Dienoestrol, 162.
—, structure, 161.
Diethyl ether, 23.
— —, partition coefficient of, 22.
Diethylaminoethanol, 53.
Diethylcarbamazine, 202, **203**.
Diethylstilboestrol, 162.
Digitalis, **107** et seq.
—, assay of, 211, 215, 220.
— lanata, 109.
— leaf, 107.
— poisoning, **108–10**.
— purpurea, 109.
Digitoxigenin, 107.
Digitoxin, 107, **109**.
Digitoxose, 109.
Digoxin, 109.
Dihydro-β-erythroidine, 61, 68, **71**.
Dihydrofolate, 130.
Dihydrofolic acid, 180.
— —, structure, 179.
— reductase, 8, 206.
Dihydromorphinone, 37.
—, structure, 35.
Dihydropteroic acid, 180.
— —, structure, 179.
2,5,dihydroxybenzoic acid, 115.
Dihydroxydihydroisoquinolines, 78.

Index

3,4,dihydroxymandelic acid, 81, 82.
3,4,dihydroxyphenylalanine, 3-hydroxytyrosine, see also DOPA, 78.
Diiodotyrosine, 146.
Diisopropylfluorophosphonate, 62, 72, 73.
Dilantin, 110.
Diloxanide, 199.
Dimenhydrinate, 120.
Dimercaprol (BAL), 200.
Dimethyl-4-phenylpiperazium, 64.
Dimethyl xanthines, 100.
Diminazene, 201.
3,5,dinitro-orthocresol, 113.
2,4,dinitrophenol, 113.
Dioctyl sodium sulphosuccinate, 121.
Diodrast, 174.
Di-paralene, see Chlorcyclizine.
Diphenhydramine, 120.
—, structure, 93.
Diphenylhydantoin, see Phenytoin.
Diphenylisatin, 121.
Diphosphopyridine nucleotide, 129.
Diphyllobothrium latum, 204.
Dipyridamole, 107.
Discovery of new drugs, 225-6.
Discrimination, index of, 224.
Distribution of drugs in tissues, 9 et seq.
Disulfiram, 34, 81.
Dithiazanine, 203.
Diuresis and alcohol, 34.
— — posterior pituitary extract, 97.
Diuretics, 169 et seq.
Dopacetamide, 81.
Dopamine, (3-hydroxytyramine), 78, 81.
—, structure, 80.
Dopamine-β-hydroxylase, 77, 81.
Dopamine-β-oxidase, 78, 87.
Dose assay, 218–19.
— effect curve, 220.
— effective, see also ED 50, 221, 222.
—, individual effective, see also IED, 221.
—, lethal, see also LD, 220.
— mortality curve, 221.
— response curve, 1.
— — —, graph of, 3.
Dramamine, see Dimenhydrinate.
Drinamyl, 39.
Dropsy and digitalis, 107.
Drug action, 1 et seq.
— combinations, 184.

— excretion, 13.
— inactivation, 191.
— interaction, 14.
— metabolism, 13–14.
— receptors, 4–9.
Drug-combining sites, 5.
Drug-receptor complex, 7.
Drugs, delay of absorption, 11, 12.
Dryopteris filix-mas, 203.
'Dual block', 70.
Durabolin, see Nandrolone phenylpropionate.
Dydrogesterone, 162.
Dyes and chemotherapy, 177.
Dyflos, 72.
Dysentery, amoebic, 198–9.

ED 50, 221, 222.
Ecdysone, 142.
Edrophonium, anticholinesterase action, 61.
— and nicotine receptors, 72.
—, structure, 73.
Ehrlich, 177.
Eighth nerve and streptomycin, 191.
Electroencephalogram, 29.
— and alcohol, 33.
— — anaesthesia, 20–1.
— — benzodiazepines, 33.
— — leptazol, 45.
Electrolyte excretion, 168 et seq.
Electrolytes and corticosteroids, 158.
Electro-shock therapy and phenytoin, 29.
Electron-spin resonance, 19.
Emetics, 119.
Emetine, 198–9.
— and bismuth iodide, 199.
Emodin, 123.
Enavid (Enovid), 164.
Encephalopathy and arsenicals, 200.
End-plate potentials, 61.
Enemas, 121.
Entamoeba histolytica, 198.
— — and tetracyclines, 187.
Enteramine, 94.
'Enteric' coating, 12.
— — and erythromycin, 192.
Enterobius vermicularis, 203.
Enterochromaffin cells, 94.
Enzyme system and general anaesthesia, 18.
Enzymes, 6.
— in drug metabolism, 13.
Ephedrine, 87.
—, structure, 86.
Epilepsy, 29.

— and acetazolamide, 171.
— — bemegride, 46.
— — leptazol, 45.
Epinephrine, see also Adrenaline, 78, 103.
Ergometrine, 97, 98.
Ergonovine, see Ergometrine.
Ergosterol, 133, 224.
— and calciferol, 133.
Ergot, 88, 97–8.
— alkaloids, 88, 97–8.
— and histamine, 92.
Ergotamine, 85.
Ergotoxine, 224.
Error in biological assay, 212 et seq.
—, limits of, 215, 216.
Erythrocytic stage of malaria parasite, 196–8.
Erythromycin, 192.
Erythropoietin, 135.
Erythroxylon coca, 52.
Eserine, see also Physostigmine, 72, 224.
— and peristalsis, 120.
— in qualitative analysis, 223–4.
Ethacrynic acid, 171–2.
Ethambutol, 192.
Ethamivan, 46.
—, structure, 43.
Ethamoxytriphetol, 160–2.
Ethanol, 12.
— as antiseptic, 193.
Ether, anaesthetic, see Diethyl ether.
Ethidium bromide, 201.
Ethinyl estradiol, 162.
Ethinyloestradiol, 162, 164.
—, structure, 161.
Ethionamide, 192.
Ethisterone, 162.
—, structure, 163.
Ethyl chloride, 23.
N-ethyl noradrenaline, 84.
Ethylene diamine, 100.
— oxide as antiseptic, 193.
Ethyleneimines, 206, 208.
Ethyleneiminium, 77, 88.
Ethylstibamine, 200.
Ethynodiol diacetate, 164.
— —, structure, 163.
Etiocholanolone, 165, 167.
Etorphine, 37.
Evipan, 26.
Exfoliative dermatitis and phenytoin, 30.
Exocrine glands and muscarinic actions, 65.
Exo-erythrocytic stage of malaria parasite, 195–8.

Index

Exophthalmos, 147–8.
— -producing substance, 143.
Eye and anticholinesterase, 62.
— — atropine, 67.
— — castor oil, 122.
— — chloroquine, 197.
— — cocaine, 52.
— — homatropine, 75.
— — muscarinic actions, 65.
— — pilocarpine, 65.

FSH, *see* Follicle-stimulating hormone.
Fat, blood flow in, 10.
Fat-soluble vitamins, **132** et seq.
— —, structures of, 131.
Fatigue and xanthines, 42.
Fehling's solution and chloral hydrate, 27.
Ferric ammonium citrate, 136.
Ferritin, 135.
Ferrous fumarate, 136.
— gluconate, 136.
— sulphate, 136.
Fever, 113.
Fibrin, 138.
Fibrinogen, 138, 139.
Fibrinopeptide, 138.
Fick method, 103.
Fiducial limits, 220.
Field of vision and strychnine, **45.**
Filaria, 202–3.
Filicic acid, 203.
Filipin, 182.
Filix mas, 203–4.
Filling pressure, 101.
Fish-liver oils, 224.
Flavine adenine dinucleotide, **128.**
Flavonoids, 126.
Fludrocortisone, 172.
— acetate, 156.
—, structure, 157.
Flufenamic acid, 116.
Flukes, *see* Trematodes.
9α-fluorohydrocortisone, 172.
Fluorouracil, 208.
—, structure, 207.
Fluoroxene, 23.
Fluoxymesterone, 166, 167.
Folate reductase, 179, 180.
— — inhibitors, 184.
Folates, 136, 180.
Folic acid, 14, **130,** 180, 196.
— — and aminopterin, 225.
— — — erythrocyte formation, 137–8.
— — — gluten, 137.
— — — vitamin B complex, 128, **130.**
— —, antimetabolites of, 208.

— — deficiency, 126.
— —, structure, 127, **138.**
— — coenzymes, 206.
Folic-folinic acid system, 195.
Folic reductase, 137, 180, 208, 225.
Folinic acid, 138.
Follicle-stimulating hormone, 143, **144.**
— — and contraception, 164.
— — — menstrual cycle, 159.
Formaldehyde, 14.
Formylcholine, 3, 4.
N[5] formyltetrahydrofolinic acid, *see* Folinic acid.
Foxglove, 107.
Frusemide, 171.
—, structure, 170.
Fucidin, 192.
Fuller's earth, 123.
Fungi and antibiotics, 183, 192.
Furan ring, 231.

GABA, 44, 46.
Gall-bladder, 120.
— and muscarinic actions, 65.
Gallamine, 8, 61, **72.**
—, discovery of, 225.
—, excretion of, 13.
—, structure, 71.
Gametocytes, 195–7.
Gamma globulins, 143.
— rays, 148, 209.
Ganglion blockers, 9, 64–5, 75, **104** et seq.
Gastric acid and penicillin, 186.
— motility and propantheline, 77.
— secretion, **117–18.**
— — and heparin, 139.
— — — histamine, 93, 94.
— — — insulin, 151.
— — — propantheline, 77.
Gastrin, 117.
—, I and II, 117.
Gastro-intestinal tract and serotonin, 95.
Gentamicin, 184.
Gentisic acid, 115.
Gigantism and pituitary, 143–4.
Glaucoma, 72.
— and acetazolamide, 170–1.
— — pilocarpine, 75.
Globin zinc insulin injection, 151.
Globulin, 155.
Glossitis and vitamin B$_2$, 128.
Glucagon, 152.
— and insulin, 150.
Glucocorticoids, **152** et seq, 156.
Gluconeogenesis, 152, 156.
— and corticosteroids, 155.
Glucose and acetylcholine, 63.

— — adrenal steroids, 152, 155.
— — diuresis, 173.
— — growth hormone, 144.
— — hexokinase, 200.
— — insulin, **149–51.**
Glucose-6-phosphate, 200.
Glucose-1-phosphate, 86.
Glucuronic acid and thyroxine, 147.
Glutamate, 130, 179.
Glutamic acid, 130, 180.
— —, structure, 127.
Glutaraldehyde, 193.
Glutathione, 125, 200.
Gluten and folic acid, 137.
Glutethimide, 27–8.
Glycerin, 123.
Glyceryl trinitrate, 106, **107.**
— —, absorption of, 12.
Glycine, 13, 44.
Glycogen, 86, 100.
— and cortisone assay, 217.
— — glucagon, 152.
— — insulin, 149.
— — salicylates, 115.
Glycoside, 189.
Glycosides, anthracene, 123.
—, cardiac, **107–10.**
Glycuronic acid, 13.
Glycuronides, 115.
Goitre, 145, 147.
—, exophthalmic, 147–8.
Gold[198], 209.
Gonadotrophins, 143, **144–5,** 160.
— and contraceptives, 164.
—, assay of, 211.
Gout, 173–4.
— and ethacrynic acid, 172.
— — thiazides, 171.
Gram, 229.
Gramicidin, 183.
Grand mal, 29.
Graves' disease, 148.
Griseofulvin, 185, **192.**
Growth and testosterone, 167.
— — tetracyclines, 187.
— — thyroid, 147.
— — vitamin A, 132.
— — — B$_{12}$, 128.
— hormone, 142, **143–4.**
Guanethidine, 84, **90.**
— and hypotension, 104.
—, structure, 83.
Guanochlor, 90.
Guanoxan, 90.
Gull's disease, 147.
Gums, 123.

HC-3, *see* Hemicholinium.
5-HT, *see* Serotonin.

5-HTP, see 5-hydroxytryptophan.
— decarboxylase, 94.
Haematuria and antimony, 204.
Haemenzymes, 135.
Haemoglobin, 7, 135.
Hair follicles, 206.
— — and actinomycin D, 209.
Haldrone, 156.
Half life of drugs, 206, 209.
Halibut-liver oil, 133.
Hallucinogens, **46** et seq.
Haloalkylamines, 94.
β-haloalkylamines, 75, **88.**
Halotestin, 167.
Halothane, 10, 21, **22–3.**
—, partition coefficient of, 22.
Hashish, 17.
Hay fever and antihistamines, 94.
Heart and anticholinesterases, 75.
— — antimony, 204.
— — digitalis, **107** et seq.
— — emetine, 199.
— — muscarinic actions, 65.
— — physostigmine, 75.
—, blood flow in, 10.
— disease and thiazides, 171.
Heat regulating mechanisms, **112** et seq.
Heavy metals and tannic acid, 124.
Hellebore, 107.
Helminthes, **201** et seq.
Helminthiasis, structure of drugs used for, 202.
Hemicholinium, **58, 63.**
Hemp, 47.
Heparin, 92, **138–9.**
Hepatic cirrhosis and neomycin, 189.
Heroin, see Diamorphine.
Herpes, corneal, and idoxuridine, 193.
Hesperidin, see Vitamin P.
Hexachlorophane, 193.
Hexadimethrine, 139.
Hexamethonium, 55, 65, 68, **104.**
—, absorption of, 12.
— and anticholinesterases, 62.
—, excretion of, 13.
—, structure, 74.
Hexitol, 173.
Hexobarbitone, 26.
Hexokinase, 200.
Hexylresorcinol, 202, **203.**
Hippurate, 174.
Histamine, **92–3,** 95, 99.
— and antihistamines, 94.
— — corticosteroids, 158.
— — gastric secretion, 117.
— — heparin, 139.
— — plain muscle, **7.**

—, assay of, 216, 223–4.
—, in qualitative analysis, 223–4.
— receptors, 88.
—, structure, 93.
Histantin, see Chlorcyclizine.
Histidine, 92, 93.
— decarboxylase, 92, 93.
Histostab, see Antazoline.
Hodgkin's disease, 206.
— — and vinblastine, 209.
Homatropine, 67, **75.**
—, structure, 76.
Homologous series, 1, 4.
Hookworms, 202–3.
'Hormone-releasing factors', 143.
Hormones, assay of, 211, 216.
Hydralazine, 105.
Hydrazines, **40, 81.**
Hydrochloric acid, 118, 175.
Hydrochlorothiazide, 171.
—, structure, 170.
Hydrocortisone, see also 17-hydroxycorticosterone, 142, **153–8.**
—, structure, 154.
Hydrolysis of drugs, 13.
Hydroxocobalamin, 137.
2-hydroxy-4-amino-6-hydroxymethyl dihydropterin, 179.
17-hydroxycorticosteroids, 155.
17-hydroxycorticosterone, 153.
17-hydroxy-11-deoxycorticosterone, 153.
6-hydroxydopamine, 82.
5-hydroxy indole acetic acid, 94.
β-hydroxylase, 153.
17-α-hydroxypregnenolone, 154.
17-α-hydroxyprogesterone, 154.
11-β-hydroxyprogesterone, 154.
5-hydroxytryptamine, see also Serotonin, 31, 47, **94–6.**
— and morphine, 36.
5-hydroxytryptophan, 94, 96.
3-hydroxytyrosine, see DOPA.
Hymenolepis nana, 204.
Hyoscine, 67, **75,** 94.
— and anaesthesia, 21.
— for motion sickness, 119–20.
—, structure, 76.
Hyoscyamine, 67.
Hypercalcaemia, 149.
— and adrenals, 158.
— — corticosteroids, 158.
Hypercalciuria, 149.
Hyperchlorhydria, 118.
Hyperglycaemia and adrenal steroids, 155.
— — insulin, **149** et seq.
— — thiazides, 171.
Hypersensitivity reaction, see also Allergy, 92.

— to methyldopa, 105.
— — penicillin, 186–7.
— — quinidine, 110.
— — sulphonamides, 189.
Hypertension, 65, 73.
— and corticosteroids, 158.
— — ganglionic blocks, 64–5.
— — iproniazid, 41.
— — reserpine, 90.
Hyperthyroidism and β-blockers, 90.
— — iodine, 148.
Hypervitaminosis D, 133.
Hypnotics, **25** et seq.
—, non-barbiturate, 27–9.
Hypocalcaemia and adrenals, 158.
Hypoglycaemia, 150–1.
Hypoglycaemic agents, oral, 151–2.
Hypokalaemia, 170, 171.
— and chlorothiazide, 110.
Hypoparathyroidism, 149.
Hypotension and noradrenaline, 104.
—, postural, 65.
Hypotensive drugs, 90, **104** et seq.
Hypothalamus and pituitary, 143.
Hypoxanthine, 206.
— and gout, 174.
Hypoxia and nitrous oxide, 23.

I[131], 148.
IED, 221, 222.
IgE, 94.
IPSP, see Inhibitory postsynaptic potential, 46.
IUR, see Idoxuridine.
Idoxuridine, see also 5-iododeoxyuridine, 192, 193, 206.
Imidazole carboxylic acid, 93.
— ring, 231.
Imidazolines, 88.
Imipramine, 41.
— and noradrenaline, 90.
—, structure, 40.
Immune reactions and corticosteroids, 158.
'Index of discrimination', 224.
Indole ring, 232.
Indomethacin, 116.
Infertility, 162.
Inflammation and adrenal steroids, 153, 158.
Inhalation of drugs, 13.
Inhibitors, ionic, of thyroid, 148.
Inhibitory postsynaptic potential, 44–6.
Inotropic action, 103, 107, 108.
Insecticides, 61, 72.

Index

Insulin, 86, 142, **149–51.**
—, absorption of, 11.
— and adrenal steroids, 155.
— — biguanides, 152.
— — cross-over test, 220.
— antagonists, 150.
—, assay of, 211, 212, 220.
— preparations, **151.**
Intal, 94.
Interferons, 193.
Intestinal colic and atropine, 67.
Intestines and anticholinesterases, 62, 75.
— — histamine, 92.
— — morphine, 36.
— — muscarinic action, 65.
— — physostigmine, 75.
— — prostaglandins, 99.
— — strychnine, 45.
— — vitamin K, 134.
Intoxication, alcoholic, 33.
Intra-ocular tension and acetazolamide, 170.
— — dyflos, 72.
— — — physostigmine, 75.
— — — pilocarpine, 75.
Intravascular clotting and contraceptives, 165.
'Intrinsic factor', 137.
Iodine[131], see Radioactive iodine.
Iodine and thyroid, 148.
—, antibacterial action, 177.
— as antiseptic, 193.
—, radioactive, 148.
Iodochlorhydroxyquin, 199.
5-iododeoxyuridine, 192, 193, 206.
Iodothyronines, 146.
Iodotyrosine, 80, 145.
Ionic inhibitors of thyroid, 148.
Iopanoic acid, 174.
Ipecacuanha, 198.
Iproniazid, 40–1.
Iproveratrine, 85.
Irin, 99.
Iron, 135, 138.
— and polycythaemia vera, 138.
—, body requirement of, 135.
— deficiency, 135.
— dextran, 136.
— dextrin, 136.
— preparations, 136.
— salts, 136.
— — as astringents, 123.
— sorbitol, 136.
Islets of Langerhans, 149.
Isocarboxazid, 40.
Isoniazid, 185, **191.**
—, structure, 190.
Isonicotinic acid hydrazide, see also Isoniazid, 129.

Isophane, 151.
Isoprenaline, 12, 84, 85, **87–90.**
—, absorption of, 13.
— and circulation, 103.
— — propanolol, 225.
—, structure, 86.
Isopropanol, 193.
N-isopropyl noradrenaline, see also Isoprenaline, 84.
Isopropylamine, 87.
Isoproterenol, see also Isoprenaline, 84, 103.
Isoricinoleic acid, 122.
Isotopes, radioactive, 209–10.
Isoxsuprine, 87.
—, structure, 86.
Itching and morphine, 36.

Kala-azar, 200.
Kallidin, 96.
Kallikrein, 96, 97.
Kanamycin, 184, **191.**
Kaolin, 123.
Kemithal, 26.
Kenacort, 156.
α-keto-glutaric acid, 128.
Ketonuria, 150.
4-ketopentyl trimethylammonium, 4.
Ketosis and adrenal steroids, 155.
17-ketosteroids, 155.
— and ACTH, 144, 155.
Kidney, 97.
— machines, 139.
Kidneys and vasopressin, 145.
—, blood flow in, 10.
Kieselguhr, 123.
Kilogram, 229.
Kinase, 86.
Krebs–Henseleit solution, 230.
Krebs–Ringer phosphate solution, 230.

l., 229.
μl., 229.
LD 50, 220.
LH, see also Luteinizing hormone, 165.
LSD, see also Lysergic acid diethylamide, 47, **48.**
Lachesine, 9, 67, **75.**
—, structure, 76.
β-lactam ring, 185.
Lactic acid, 128.
Lactobacillus casei, 130.
— lactis, 137.
Lactoflavin, see Vitamin B$_2$.
Lanatocide C, 109.
Largactil, see Chlorpromazine.
Laxative chocolate, 122.

Lead salts as astringents, 123.
Lecithin, 120.
Leishmaniasis, 200.
—, structures of drugs used for, 201.
Leprosy, 192.
Leptazol, 45.
—, structure, 43.
Lethal dose, 216.
Leucovorin, 208.
Leukaemia, drugs used in, 206–10.
Leukopenia and antimetabolites, 208.
— — antithyroids, 146.
— — phenindione, 141.
— — purine analogues, 208.
— — vinblastine, 209.
Levallorphan, 38.
— structure, 35.
Levorphanol, 37.
—, structure, 35.
Lidocaine, see Lignocaine.
Lignocaine, 50, **52,** 90.
— as antiarrhythmic, 110.
—, structure, 51.
Lincomycin, 192.
Lipid barriers and local anaesthetics, 49–50.
— metabolism, 84.
— solubility, 10, 18.
Lipolysis and prostaglandins, 99.
Lipopolysaccharides, 113.
Lipoprotein lipase, 139.
Liquid paraffin, 121.
— — and vitamin K, 134.
Liquorice, 118.
Liver, blood flow in, 10.
— damage and antimony, 204.
— — — filix mas, 204.
— — — iproniazid, 41.
Lobelia, 46.
Lobeline, **46,** 64.
—, structure, 43.
Log-dose–effect lines, 217, 219.
Log-dose–response curve, 2, 6.
Logarithmic probability paper, 221.
— scale, 2, 3, 214, 217, 221–3.
Long-acting thyroid stimulator, 143.
Loop of Henle, 168, 169, 171.
Lumiflavine, 128.
Luminal, 26.
Lung infections and ampicillin, 187.
Luteinizing hormone, 99, 143, **144.**
— — and contraceptives, 164.
— — — menstrual cycle, 159.
Lymphoma, 206, 209.
Lymphosarcoma, 209.

Index

Lysergic acid, 97.
— — diethylamide, 47, **48**, 98.
— propanolamide, 97.
Lysine, 139.
Lysol, 193.

ml., 229.
m.³, 229.
mm.³, 229.
μm.³, 229.
MAO, *see also* Monoamine oxidase, 40–1, **80–3**, 87.
MAO inhibitors, 39, **40** et seq., 87.
MER 25 (Ethamoxytriphetol), 160.
Macrocytic anaemias, 136–8.
Magnesium and acetylcholine, 63.
— carbonate, 118, **121.**
— hydroxide, 118.
— oxide, 118, 121.
— salts as purgatives, **121.**
— sulphate, 121.
— trisilicate, **118**, 123.
Malaria 177, **195** et seq.
—, clinical cure of, 197–8.
—, drugs used for, 196.
—, radical cure of, 198.
Male fern, 203.
Maleic anhydride, 171.
Malonic acid, 25.
Malonylurea, 25.
Mammary carcinoma and oestrogens, 160, 205.
— — — progesterones, 162.
Mannitol, 173.
Mast cells, 92, 94.
— — and heparin, 138.
— — — histamine, 92.
Measurement, units of, 229.
Mecamylamine and autonomic ganglia, 65, 73.
— — urine pH, 175.
— as hypotensive, 104.
—, excretion of, 13.
—, structure, 74.
Mechlorethamine, *see* Mustine.
Medrol, 156.
Medroxyprogesterone acetate, 162, 164.
— —, structure, 163.
Medulla and anaesthesia, 20.
— — filix mas, 204.
— — strychnine, 45.
—, stimulants of, 42.
Mefenamic acid, 116.
Megakaryocytes, 206.
Megaloblastic anaemia, 126.
— — and phenytoin, 30.
Megestrol, 162.
Melanophore-stimulating hormone, 145.

Melarsoprol, 200.
—, structure, 201.
Membrane permeability, 66.
— — and local anaesthetics, 49.
Menadiol diphosphate, 141.
— —, structure, 140.
Menadione, *see* Menaphthone.
Menaphthone, 134.
—, structure, 131, 140.
Meningococci and sulphonamides, 188.
Menstruation, 159.
— and progesterone, 162.
Mepacrine and cestodes, 204.
Meperidine, *see* Pethidine.
Mephenesin, **32–3.**
— and strychnine poisoning, 45.
— carbamate, 33.
Mepps, 57, 58, 62.
Meprobamate, 31, **32.**
—, structure, 28.
Mepyramine, 7.
—, structure, 93.
Meralluride, 169.
Mercaptopurine, **206–8.**
Mercurials, organic, 169–70.
Mercuric chloride, 177.
— — as emetic, 119.
Mercurophylline, 169.
Mercurous chloride, **122.**
Merozoites, 195–6.
Mersalyl, 174.
—, structure, 169.
Merthiolate, 193.
Mescaline, 47.
Messenger-RNA, 142.
Mestranol, 162, 164.
Metabolic analogues, 206.
Metabolism and corticosteroids, 155, 158.
— — sympathetic nerve stimulation, 79 et seq.
— — temperature, 113.
— — thyroid, 147.
—, sugar, 150.
Metals, heavy, as antibacterials, 177.
Metanephrine, 81, 82.
Metaraminol, 87.
— and circulation, 104.
—, structure, 86.
Methacholine, **65–6, 75.**
Methadone, 37.
Methaemoglobin and nitrites, 106.
Methallenoestril, 162.
—, structure, 161.
Methamphetamine, 88.
—, structure, 86.
Methane sulphonates, 206.
Methanol, metabolism of, **14.**

Methantheline, 67, **77.**
Methiacil, *see* Methylthiouracil.
Methicillin, 186.
Methimazole, 146.
Methionine, 130, 132.
Methisazone, 193.
'Method of least squares', 218–19.
Methohexitone, duration of action of, 26.
Methotrexate, 14, 206, **208.**
— and folic acid, 180, 184.
—, structure, 181.
Methoxamine, 87, 103.
—, structure, 86.
Methoxyflurane, 23.
3-methoxy-4-hydroxy mandelic acid, 81, 82.
Methoxyphenamine, 87.
—, structure, 86.
p-methoxyphenylethylmethylamine, 92.
Methyl dilvasene, **4.**
— furmethide, 4.
N-methyl glucosamine, 189.
— lysergic butanolamide, 97.
Methyl reserpate, 31.
β-methyl xylocholine, 83.
Methyldopa, 80, **90.**
— as hypotensive, 104–5.
—, structure, 81.
α-methyldopamine, 81.
3,3-methylene-bis-4-hydroxycoumarin, 140.
l-methylhistamine, 93.
Methylmorphine, 35.
α-methylnoradrenaline, 90.
—, structure, 81.
n-methylphenobarbitone, 30.
Methylprednisolone, 156.
—, structure, 157.
Methyltestosterone, 167.
—, structure, 166.
Methylthiouracil, 146.
α-methyltyrosine, 80.
β-methylxylocholine, 83.
Methyprylone, 28.
Methysergide, 97, 98.
— and serotonin, 96.
—, structure, 95.
Metopon, 35.
Metrulen, 164.
Metyrapone, **153**, 155.
Microcrystals of ice, 18.
Micro-electrophoresis, 15–16, 44, 68–9.
Microfilaria, 203.
Microgram, 229.
Migraine, 98.
Milligram, 229.
Mineral oil, *see* Liquid paraffin.

Index

Mineralocorticoid action and cortexolone, 172.
Mineralocorticoids, **152** et seq.
— and spironolactone, 173.
Miniature end-plate potentials (mepps), **57**, 58, 62.
Mipafox, 72.
—, structure, **73**.
Mists, 13.
Mitosis, 205.
— and colchicine, 209.
Molarity, 229.
Mole, 229.
Moniodotyrosine, 146.
Monoamine oxidase, **40–1**, 80, 81.
— — and serotonin, 94.
— — inhibitors, 39, **40** et seq, 80, 83, 87.
— — — and serotonin, 96.
Monosodium urate, 173.
'Moon face', 158.
Morphine, **35–6**, 225.
— and central nervous stimulants, 45.
— — histamine release, 92.
— — serotonin, 96.
— — temperature, 113.
— antagonists, **38**.
— dependence and methadone, 37.
— for premedication, 21.
—, overdoses of, 42.
Morphine-like compounds, 36.
Morphinone analgesics, discovery of, 225.
Mosquitoes, 195–6.
Motion sickness, 94, **119–20**.
— — and hyoscine, 75.
Mucilages, 123.
Mucin, 120.
Mucopeptide, 182.
Muramyl peptides, 205.
Muscarine, 7, **65–6**, 68, 74.
— and nicotine, 63.
—, structure, 4, **76**.
Muscarine-like drugs and atropine, 67.
Muscarinic action, 54, 55, 70, 71.
— — and gall-bladder, 120.
— — — gastric secretion, 117.
— — — peristalsis, 120.
— — of acetylcholine, 8.
— receptors, 54, 65–7, 72, 88.
— —, agonists at, 74.
— —, —, structures, 76.
— —, antagonists at, 75.
— —, —, structures, 76.
— — in Renshaw cells, 68.
Muscle action potential, 66.
—, blood flow in, 10.

Mustargen, *see* Mustine.
Mustine, 206.
—, structure, **207**.
Mutation, 205.
Myasthenia gravis, 58.
— — and anticholinesterases, 62.
— — — edrophonium, 72.
— — — neostigmine, 72.
— — — tubocurarine, 61.
Mycobacteria, 191, 192.
Myocardium and local anaesthetics, 50.
— — nikethamide, 45.
— — xanthines, 42.
Myoglobin, 135.
— and xenon, 7.
Mytolon, *see* Benzoquinonium.
Myxoedema, 147–8.

NAD, *see also* Diphosphopyridine nucleotide, 129.
NADP, *see* Triphosphopyridine nucleotide.
NAG, *see* N-acetylglucosamine.
NAM, *see* N-acetylmuramic acid.
N.E.D., *see* Normal equivalent deviation.
Nalorphine, 37, **38**.
—, discovery of, 225.
— in morphine dependence, 36.
—, structure, 35.
Nandrolone phenylpropionate, 167.
Nanogram, 229.
Naphthalene ring, 232.
Naphthoquinone, 134.
Narceine, 35.
Narcotine, 35.
Necator americanus, 203.
Nemathelminthes, 202–3.
Nembutal, 26.
Neoarsphenamine, assay of, 211.
—, discovery of, 226.
Neomercazole, *see* Carbimazole.
Neomycin, 184, **189–91**.
Neopyrithiamine, 128.
Neostigmine, 7, 59, 62, **72**.
—, structure, 73.
Nephritis and phenacetin, 116.
Nerve fibres, differential sensitivity of, 49.
'Nerve gases', 61, 72.
Nerve growth factor, 84.
Neuraminidase, 192.
Neuritis and vitamin B, 128.
—, peripheral and isoniazid, 191.
Neurohypophysis, 143, **145**.
Neuromuscular blocking drugs, 60, **70 et seq.**
— junction and acetylcholine, 74.

— transmission, **54** et seq., **56** et seq.
Niacin, *see* Nicotinamide.
Nialamide, 40.
Nicotinamide, 126, 128, **129**.
Nicotine, 7, 62, **63–4**, 70.
—, structure, 71.
Nicotinic acid, *see* Nicotinamide.
— action, 71.
— — of acetylcholine, 8.
— receptors, 54, 55, **56** et seq.
— — and acetylcholine, 74.
— — in Renshaw cells, 68.
Nicoumalone, 141.
—, structure, 140.
Nictitating membrane, 63.
Nikethamide, **45**, 46.
—, structure, 43.
Nilevar, *see* Norethandrolone.
Nitrates, 105–6.
Nitrites, 105–6.
Nitrofurazone, 201.
Nitrogen and ACTH, 144.
— — androgens, 165.
— mustards, 88, **206–8**.
—, partition coefficient of, 22.
Nitrous oxide, 17, **23**.
— — and procaine, 53.
— —, partition coefficient of, 22.
Noradrenaline, 9, **78** et seq, 81–5, **87–8**.
— and circulation, 103.
— — cocaine, 52.
— — guanethidine, 90.
— — hypotensive drugs, 104.
— — imipramine, 41.
— — prostaglandins, 99.
— — reserpine, 31, 105.
— release, drugs affecting, 90.
—, structure, 80, 86.
— uptake, inhibitors of, 90.
Noradrenergic nerves, 82.
Nordefrin, *see* α-methylnoradrenaline.
Norethandrolone, 167.
—, structure, 166.
Norethindrone, 164.
— acetate, 164.
Norethisterone, 162.
Norethynodrel, 162, 164.
—, structure, 163.
Norinyl, 164.
Norlestrin, 164.
Normal curve, 213, 214.
— equivalent deviation, 221.
— frequency curve, 221.
Normetanephrine, 81, 82.
19-norsteroids, 164.
Nortriptyline, 90.
Novobiocin, 192.

Nuclear magnetic resonance, 19.
Nucleic acid, 130, 180, 197, 208.
—— synthesis, 206.
—— — and proguanil, 196–7.
Nystatin, 182, 185, **192**.

OD 50, 221.
Octopamine, 81, 87.
—, structure, **81**, 86.
Oestradiol, **159**, 160, 162.
Oestriol, **159**, 160, 162.
Oestrogens, 142, **158–60**, 164, 224.
— and adrenal cortex, 153.
—— thyroid, 147.
—, structures, 161.
—, therapeutic use of, 160.
Oestrone, 159, 160.
Oleandomycin, 192.
Opium, 35–6, 225.
— as anaesthetic, 17.
Opsin, 132.
Organic arsenicals, **177**, 226.
— mercurials, 169–70.
Organophosphorus compounds, 61, **72**.
— anticholinesterases, 225.
Orinase, *see* Tolbutamide.
Ornithine cycle, 175.
Ortho-Novum, 164.
Osmotic diuresis, 173.
— gradient, 168.
Osteomalacia, 133.
Osteoporosis and androgens, 167.
—— corticosteroids, 158.
Ouabain, 107.
—, structure, 109.
Ovary and androgens, 165.
—— menstrual cycle, 164.
Ovomucoid, 92.
Ovulation and gonadotrophins, 144.
—— progesterone, 162.
Oxacillin, 187.
—, structure, 186.
Oxamycin, 182.
Oxazole ring, 231.
Oxidation of drugs in body, 13.
Oximes, 62.
Oxotremorine, 4, 7, **14**.
Oxtriphylline, 100.
11-oxycorticoids, *see* Glucocorticoids.
Oxygen consumption and thyroid, 147.
Oxyntic acid, 117.
Oxytetracycline, 188.
Oxythiamine, 128.
Oxytocin, **97**, 143, 145.
Oxyuris, 203.

P-2-AM, *see* Pralidoxime.
PABA, *see* 4-aminobenzoic acid.
PAM, *see* Pralidoxime.
PAS, *see* p-aminosalicylic acid.
PTP, *see* Post-tetanic potentiation.
Pancreas. **149** et seq.
Pancytopenia and hydralazine, 105.
Pantothenic acid, 126, **129**.
— —, structure, 127.
Papaver somniferum. 35.
Papaveretum for premedication, 21.
Papaverine. 35.
Para-aminobenzoic acid, *see also* p-aminobenzoic acid, 51, 53, 127, 130.
—, structure, 179.
Paracetamol, 113, 114, 115, **116**.
—, structure, 114.
Paraffin, liquid, 121.
Parallel quantitative tests, 224.
Paralysis agitans, treatment of, 94.
Paramethasone, 157.
— acetate, 156.
Parathormone, 86.
Parathyroid, 133, **148–9**.
'Park peptide', 182.
Parkinsonism, 9, 94.
Paromomycin, 191, **199**.
Partition coefficients, 22.
Pellagra, 126, **129**.
Pempidine, 65, **73**.
—, as hypotensive, 104.
—, structure, 74.
Penicillenyl derivatives, 187.
Penicillin, 174, 184. **185–7**, 189.
— and cell walls, 205.
—, discovery of, 178, **225**.
—, excretion of, 13.
—, resistance to, 185.
—, structure, 186.
—, toxicity, 227.
— G, 185.
— V, 187.
Penicillinase, 184, 187.
Penicillium, 193.
Penicilloic acid, **185**.
Penicilloyl, 187.
Pentaerythritol tetranitrate, 106, 107.
Pentamethonium, 65, **73**.
—, structure, 74.
Pentamidine, **200–1**.
Pentobarbital, 26.
Pentobarbitone, 26, **27**.
Pentolinium, 65, 73.
—, structure, 74.
Pentothal, 26.
Pentyl trimethylammonium, 4.
Pentylenetetrazol, *see* Leptazol.

Pepsin, 117, 118.
Peptic ulcers, 117–18.
Peptides, vasoactive, 96, **183**.
Peptidyl transferase, 183.
Perchlorate, 145.
— and thyroid, 148.
Peripheral neuritis and isoniazid, 191.
Peristalsis, 121.
Permeability of cell membranes, 66, 78, 85.
Pernicious anaemia, 126, 137.
— — and liver extracts, 130.
Peruvian bark, 177.
Pethidine, 36–7, 38.
— for premedication, 21.
Petit mal, 29.
Phaeochromocytoma, 88.
— and β-blockers, 90.
Phanodorm, *see* Cyclobarbitone.
Pharmacological analysis, quantitative, **223–4**.
Phenacemide, 30.
Phenacetin, 113, 115, **116**.
—, structure, 114.
Phenanthridine, 201.
Phenazocine, 37.
Phenazone. 113, **116**.
—, structure. 114.
Phenelzine, **40**, 81.
Phenethicillin, 187.
—, structure, 186.
Phenformin, 152.
Phenindamine, 93.
Phenindione, 141.
—, structure, 140.
Pheniprazine, 40.
Phenobarbital, *see* Phenobarbitone.
Phenobarbitone, 27, **29**.
— and folic acid, 137.
—, duration of action of, 26.
—, metabolism, 14.
—, structure, 30.
Phenol red. 174.
Phenolphthalein, 122.
Phenols, polyhydric, 145.
Phenothiazine, 41.
— derivatives, **31–2**.
— — and temperature. 113.
— for premedication, 21.
— ring, 232.
—, structure, 31.
— tranquillizers, 41, 225.
Phenoxyacetic acid, 187.
Phenoxybenzamine, 85, **88**.
— and noradrenaline, 82, 90.
— — serotonin, 96.
—, aziridine of, 89.
—, structure, 89.

Phenoxyethylpenicillin, 187.
Phenoxymethyl isoquinolines, 192.
Phenoxymethylpenicillin, 187.
—, structure, 186.
Phentolamine, 85, **88.**
—, structure, 89.
Phenylacetic acid, 185, 187.
Phenylbiguanide, 193.
Phenylbutazone, 115, **116,** 174.
—, structure, 114, 175.
Phenylethanolamine-N-methyl transferase, 79.
Phenylethylamine, 86.
Phenytoin, **29–30,** 110.
— and folic acid, 137.
— — thyroid, 146.
—, structure, 30.
Phloroglucinol, 203.
Pholcodine, 37.
Phosphagen, 113.
Phosphatase, alkaline, 144.
Phosphates, 86, **121.**
— and liquid paraffin, 121.
— — vitamin D, 133.
Phosphatidylethanolamine, 132.
Phosphodiesterase, 42, 86, 100.
Phosholine, 72.
—, structure, 73.
Phospholipase A, 99.
Phospholipids, 99.
Phosphorus and androgens, 167.
—, radioactive, 138, **209.**
Phosphorus[32], see Radioactive phosphorus.
Phosphorylase, 86.
Phthalide-isoquinoline, 45.
Phthalylsulphathiazole, 189.
Physostigmine, **62,** 72.
—, structure, 73.
Phytate, 135.
Picrotoxin, **45,** 46.
—, structure, 43.
Picrotoxinin, 45.
Pilocarpine, **65–6.**
—, muscarinic action, **75.**
—, structure, 76.
Pinworms, 202–3.
Piperazine, 202–3.
— ring, 231.
Piperidine ring, 231.
Piperocaine, 51.
Piperoxan, 88.
—, structure, 89.
Pitressin, see Antidiuretic hormone.
Pituitary gland, **143** et seq.
— — and chlorotrianisene, 160.
— — — clomiphene, 162.
— — — contraceptives, 164.
— — — corticosteroids, 152.

— —, anterior lobe, **143–5.**
— —, — — and menstrual cycle, 159.
— —, posterior lobe, 97, 143, **145.**
— —, — —, assay of, 212, 216, 223–4.
— hormones and insulin, 150.
Placebo, 227.
Placenta and oestrogens, 159.
— — oxytocin, 97.
— — progesterone, 162.
Plasma level, 10.
Plasmodium sp., **195** et seq.
Platyhelminthes, 202–4.
Pleural effusion and radioactive gold, 210.
Pollen, 94.
Polycythaemia vera, **138,** 209.
Polyethylene glycol, 123.
Polyhydric phenols, 145.
Polynitrate reductase, 106.
Polyvinylpyrrolidone, 92.
Porphyrins, 137.
Postsynaptic inhibition, 45.
— inhibitory transmitters, **44.**
— membrane, 56.
Post-tetanic potentiation, 29.
Postural hypotension, 65.
Potassium, 108, 169, 172, 224.
— and ACTH, 144.
— — androgens, 165.
— — corticosteroids, **155.**
— — digitalis, 109, 110.
— ions and kidney, 168.
— salts and posterior pituitary extract, 212.
Practolol, **89,** 110.
—, structure, 91.
Pralidoxime, 62.
—, discovery of, 225.
—, structure, 73.
Prednisolone, 156.
—, structure, 157.
Prednisone, 156.
—, structure, 157.
Pre-erythrocytic stage of malaria parasite, **195–6,** 198.
Prefrontal lobotomy, 36.
Pregnancy and oestrogens, 159.
— — tetracyclines, 188.
— — thyroid, 146–7.
Pregnenolone, 154.
Premedication, **21,** 66.
Presynaptic inhibition, **44.**
— membrane, 57.
Prilocaine, 52.
—, structure, 51.
Primaquine, 196, **198.**
—, structure, 197.
Pro-Banthine, see Propantheline.

Probability scale, **221.**
Probenecid, 174.
—, structure, 175.
Probit, 221–2.
Procainamide, 110.
Procaine, 49–51, **52–3,** 110.
— benzylpenicillin, 11.
— penicillin, 186.
—, structure, 51.
Progesterone, 154, 158–9, **162–4.**
— and adrenal cortex, 153.
— as anti-oestrogen, 160.
—, structure, 163.
Proguanil, 195–7.
Prolactin, 143, **144.**
Promazine, 31, **32,** 41.
Promethazine, 37.
— for motion sickness, **120.**
Pronethalol, 89.
—, structure, 91.
Prontosil, **178,** 189.
Propanediol derivatives, 31, **32.**
Propantheline, 67, **77.**
—, structure, 76.
Prophylaxis, causal in malaria, **195** et seq.
Propionyl choline, 1, 2, 3, 4.
— — and striated muscle, **7.**
—, structure, 3.
Propranolol, 85, **89–90.**
— and digitalis, 110.
— — hypotension, 104, 107.
— as antiarrhythmic, 110.
—, discovery of, 225.
—, structure, 91.
Propylene glycol, 123.
Propylthiouracil, 146.
Prostaglandins, **98–9.**
— and contraceptives, 164.
Prostate, cancer of, and radioactive gold, 210.
— — — — sex hormones, 160, 205.
Prostenoic acid, 98.
Prostigmin, see Neostigmine.
Protamine and heparin, 139.
— insulin injection, 151.
Protease, 146.
Protectives, 123–4.
Protein anabolism and testosterone, 167.
Prothrombin, 138, 140.
— and vitamin K, 134.
Provest, 164.
Pseudocholinesterase, 53, 60, 70, 75.
Psychomotor epilepsy, 29.
Psychoses and corticosteroids, 158.
Pteridine, 180.
—, structure, 127.

2NH$_2$-4-OH-pteridine, 130.
Pteroic synthetase, 184.
Pteroylmonoglutamic acid, *see* Folic acid.
Pulmonary oedema and frusemide, 171.
Pulse and anaesthesia, 20.
— rate and thyroid, 148.
Pupils and anticholinesterases, 75.
— — general anaesthesia, 20–1.
— — morphine, 36.
— — physostigmine, 75.
Purgatives, **120** et seq.
— and antihelminthics, 202, 203.
—, anthracene, **122–3**.
—, bulk, 121.
—, 'contact', 122.
—, irritant, 121.
—, lubricant, 121.
—, saline, 121.
Puri-nethol, *see* Mercaptopurine.
Purine analogues, 208.
— metabolism, 173.
— nucleotides, 107.
— ring, 232.
Purines, 136, 206.
— and folic acid, 130.
Puromycin, 142, 147, 183.
'Purple Hearts', *see* Drinamyl.
Pyrazinamide, 192.
Pyrazine ring, 231.
Pyrazole ring, 231.
Pyridine, 129.
— ring, 231.
Pyridoxal, 127, 129.
— kinase, 129.
— phosphate, 129.
Pyridoxamine, 129.
— phosphate, 129.
—, structure, 127.
Pyridoxine, *see* Vitamin B$_6$.
Pyrilamine, *see* Mepyramine.
Pyrimethamine, 195–7.
Pyrimidine analogues, 208.
— ring, 128, **231**.
Pyrimidines, 136, 195, 198, 206.
Pyrithiamine, *see* Neopyrithiamine.
Pyrogallol, 81.
Pyrogen-free water, 113.
Pyrogens, 113.
Pyrrole ring, 231.
Pyrrolidine ring, 231.
Pyruvic acid, 128.

Quinacrine (Mepacrine), 198, 204.
Quinalbarbitone, 27.
—, duration of action of, 26.
Quinidine, 90, **110**.
—, structure, 109.

Quinine, 110, **198**.
—, structure, 197.
Quinoline ring, 232.
Quinone coenzymes, 140.

RNA, 183, 184, 191, 206.
— and hormones, 142.
Radioactive gold, 209.
— iodine, 148, **209**.
— isotopes, **209–10**.
— phosphorus, 138, **209**.
Rashes, *see also* Skin.
— and actinomycin D, 209.
— — antimony, 204.
— — hydralazine, 105.
— — penicillin, 186.
— — phenindione, 141.
— — phenytoin, 30.
— — sulphonamindes, 189.
— — sulphonylureas, 152.
— — thiouracil, 146.
— — troxidone, 30.
Rat poison, 141.
Rauwolfia derivatives, 31.
— serpentina, 31.
Reagin, 94.
Receptor sites, mixed, 68–70.
Receptors, muscarinic, 54, **65–7**.
—, nicotinic, 54, **56** et seq.
α-receptors, **85** et seq, 103.
β-receptors, **85** et seq, 103.
β$_1$ and β$_2$ receptors, 87, 89.
Reflexes and anaesthetics, 18, 20.
— — strychnine, 44.
—, effects of drugs on, 15.
Renal colic and atropine, 67.
Renin, 155.
— and aldosterone, 172.
Renshaw cells, 54, 68.
Reserpine, **31**, 39, 88, 94, 96.
— and noradrenaline release, 82, 83, 90.
— as hypotensive, 105.
— — tranquillizer, 31.
— group, 78.
—, structure, 28.
Resistance and trypanosomes, 200.
— to antimalarials, 198.
— — chemotherapeutic drugs, **184–5**.
— — streptomycin, 189.
—, transferable, 185.
Resistant strains of bacteria, 184.
Resorcinol, 145.
—, structure, 146.
Respiration and anaesthesia, 20.
— — caffeine, 42.
— — ethamivan, 46.
— — filix mas, 204.
— — nalorphine, 38.

— — nicotine, 64.
— — nikethamide, 45.
— — picrotoxin, 45.
— — salicylates, 116.
Respiratory centre and morphine, 36.
— distress of newborn, 46.
Reticular formation and anaesthesia, 19.
Reticulocytopenia, 208.
Reticulosarcoma, 206.
Retinene, 132.
Retinopathy, chloroquine, 197.
Rhamnose, 109.
Rhodopsin, 132.
Rhubarb, 122–3.
Riboflavine, *see* Vitamin B$_2$.
— phosphate, 128.
Ribonucleoside, 208.
Ribonucleotide, 208.
Ribose, 128.
Ribosomes, 183–4, 192.
Ricinoleic acid, 122.
Rickets, 133.
Rickettsiae and chloramphenicol, 189.
— — tetracyclines, 187.
Rifampicin, 191–2.
— structure, 190.
Rifampin, *see* Rifampicin.
Ringer's solution, 230.
Rings, chemical, index of, 231–2.
Ringworm, 192.
Ristocetin, 182, 184.
Roughage, 121.
Roundworms, 202–3.
Rutin, *see* Vitamin P.
Rutinose, 127.

SRS, *see* Slow reacting substance.
SRS-A, *see* Slow reacting substance.
St. Anthony's fire, 98.
Salbutamol, 87.
—, structure, 86.
Salicin, 114.
Salicylate poisoning, 173.
Salicylates, **114–16**.
—, absorption of, 12.
— and uric acid, 174.
— — urine pH, 175.
Salicylazosulphapyridine, 189.
Salicylglycine, 115.
Salicylic acid, 113.
— —, structure, 175.
Salicyluric acid, 115.
Saline purgatives and anthelminthics, 203.
Salix alba, 114.
Sampling, errors of, 213.

Sarin, 72.
—, structure, 73.
Schistosomiasis, 204.
Schizonts, 195–6, 198.
Schizophrenia and hallucinogens, 47.
— — tranquillizing drugs, 31.
Scopolamine, see Hyoscine.
Screening, 3.
Scurvy, 125–6.
Sea water, 230.
Seborrhoeic dermatitis and vitamin B_2, 128–9.
Secobarbital, 26.
Seconal, 26.
Secretin, 120.
Secretions and atropine, 67.
Sedation and prostaglandins, 99.
Sedatives, **25** et seq.
—, non-barbiturate, 27–9.
Selective action, 1.
— antagonists, 7, 8.
— chemotherapy, 178.
Semilente insulin, 11.
Senna, 122–3.
Senses, special and strychnine, 45.
Septrin, 188.
Sera, assay of, 211.
Serotonin, 90, **94–7**.
— and Bezold receptors, 105.
— — histamine, 92.
— — LSD, 47.
—, antagonists, 96.
—, structure, 95.
Sex hormones, **158** et seq.
Sexual changes and corticosteroids, 158.
Side actions of drugs, **1**.
Sigmoid curve, 220–3.
Silicic acid, 118.
Silver nitrate, 123, 177.
Simmonds' disease, 143.
Site of action of drugs, 4–9.
Skeleton, blood flow in, 10.
Skin, see also Rashes.
— and vitamin A, 133.
—, blood flow in, 10.
— effects in toxicity tests, 226.
Sleep, 25.
Sleeping sickness, 200.
Slow reacting substance, 92, 94, **99**.
Smallpox and methisazone, 193.
Snake venom, 84.
Sodium, 108, 169, 172.
— and ACTH, 144.
— — androgens, 165.
— — corticosteroids, 152, 155, 158.
— ions and kidney, 168.
— permeability, 85, 86.

— — and catecholamines, 85.
— — — veratrine alkaloids, 105.
Sodium antimony dimercaptosuccinate, 204.
— — —, structure, 202.
— benzylpenicillin, 11.
— bicarbonate, 118.
— — and urine pH, 175.
— citrate and urine pH, 175.
— hypochlorite, 193.
— iodide (I^{131}), 148.
— nitrite, 106.
— phosphate, 209.
— salicylate, 115.
— stibogluconate, 200.
— sulphate as diuretic, 173.
— — — purgative, 121.
— tauroglycocholate, 120.
— thiopental, see Thiopentone sodium.
Soluble insulin injection, 151.
Solutions, aqueous, 230.
Soneryl, 26.
Sotalol, 89.
—, structure, 91.
Spermatogenesis, 165.
Sphincter of Oddi, 37.
Spinal anaesthesia, 51.
— cord, **68–9**.
— — and convulsants, 44.
— — — strychnine, 44.
Spiramycin, 192.
Spirochaetes and antibiotics, 181.
Spironolactone, 155, **172–3**.
—, structure, 173.
Sporozoites, 195–8.
Sprue, 126, 137.
S-shaped curve, 2, 220–3.
Standard deviation, **214**, 215, 221.
— error, 214.
— preparations, 212.
Staphylococcus and penicillin, 185.
Starch, 123.
Statolon, 193.
Steroid ring system, 232.
Steroids, structures, 154.
—, synthetic, structures, **157**.
Stibamine, 200–1.
Stibocaptate, 204.
Stibophen, 204.
—, structure, 202.
Stilbamidine and histamine release, 92.
Stilboestrol, 162.
—, structure, 161.
Stimulants of central nervous system, **39** et seq.
Stokes–Adams syndrome, 87, 103.
Straub's method, 70.
Streptidine, 189.

Streptococci and sulphonamides, 188.
Streptomyces sp., 136–7.
Streptomycin, 181, 184–5, **189–91**, 225.
—, excretion, 13.
—, resistance to, 184.
—, structure, 190.
Streptose, 189.
Stress, 155.
Stroke output, 101.
— — curve, 102.
Strophanthin G, see Ouabain.
Strophanthus, 107.
— gratus, 109.
Strychnine, **44–5**, 46.
— poisoning, 45.
—, structure, 43.
Substance P, 223.
Substrate competition, 83.
— control, 6.
Succinylcholine, see Suxamethonium.
Succinylsulphathiazole, 189.
Sugar metabolism and insulin, 150.
Suicidal tendencies and reserpine, 31.
Sulfisoxazole, 188.
—, structure, 189.
Sulphadiazine, 182.
Sulphafurazole, 188.
Sulphamerazine, 189.
Sulphamethizole, 188.
Sulphamethoxazole and trimethoprim, 188.
Sulphamethoxypyridazine, 188.
Sulphanilamide, **178**, 180.
—, structure, 179.
Sulphaphenazole, 188.
Sulphasalazine, 189.
Sulphated polysaccharides, 139.
O,N,sulphato-glycosamino-glucuronate, 139.
Sulphinpyrazone, 174.
—, structure, 175.
Sulphonamides, 181, **188–9**.
— and procaine, 53.
— — resistance, 185.
— — trimethoprim, 184.
—, antithyroid action, 145.
—, as antibacterials, 178, 180.
—, — carbonic anhydrase inhibitors, 170–1.
—, discovery of, 178.
—, excretion, 13.
—, structures, 146, 189.
Sulphonates, alkyl, 208.
Sulphonyl ureas, **151–2**.
Sulphuric acid and thyroxine, 147.
Sulphydryl groups, 171.

Index

Suppressive treatment of malaria, 197.
Suramin, 200, **201**.
Suxamethonium, **60–1**, 70.
— and halothane, 22.
— — neuromuscular transmission, 70.
— structure, 71.
Sympathetic block, 104–5.
— nerve stimulation, effects of, 84 et seq.
— — — and circulation, 101.
— — — — peristalsis, 121.
Sympathomimetic substances, 83, 86 et seq.
— — and antihistamines, 94.
— —, structures, 86.
Synephrine, *see* Octopamine.

T.E.A., *see* Tetraethylammonium.
T.E.C., *see* Triethylcholine.
T.E.P.P., *see* Tetraethylpyrophosphate.
TFA, *see* Tetrahydrofolic acid.
TM10, *see* Xylocholine.
T.M.A., *see* Tetramethylammonium.
TSH, *see* Thyrotrophin.
Tachycardia and iron, 136.
Tachyphylaxis, 82.
Taenia saginata, 204.
Tannic acid, 123.
Tannin, 123.
Tapazole, *see* Methimazole.
Tapeworms, 203–4.
Tartrates, 121.
Teichoic acid, 182.
Teeth and tetracyclines, 187.
Tensilon, *see* Edrophonium.
Testes and oestrogen, 159.
Testosterone, 142, **165–7**, 224.
— cypionate injection, 167.
— —, structure, 166.
—, degradation of, 165.
— enanthate, 167.
— implants, 167.
— propionate injection, 167.
— —, structure, 166.
Tetanus and tubocurarine, 61.
Tetany and calcium deficiency, 133.
— — parathyroid, 149.
Tetracaine, *see* Amethocaine.
Tetracyclines, 181, 184, **187–8**.
— and resistance, 185.
—, excretion, 13.
—, structures, 188.
Tetraethylammonium, **65**, 68.
—, structure, 74.
Tetraethylpyrophosphate, 72.

Tetraethylthiuram disulphide, 34.
Tetrahydrocannabinol, 47.
Tetrahydrofolate, 130, 135.
Tetrahydrofolic acid, **137**, 138, 180, 208.
— —, structure, 179.
β-tetrahydronaphthylamine and temperature, 113.
Tetramethylammonium, 3, 4, 63, **64–5**.
—, structure, 74.
Thalidomide, 226.
Thebane, 35.
Theobromine, 41–2.
— and smooth muscle, 100.
Theophylline, **41–2**, 86.
— and smooth muscle, 100.
Thermodynamic activity, 19.
Thiacetazone, 192.
Thialbarbitone, 26.
Thiamine, *see* Vitamin B_1.
— pyrophosphate, 128.
Thiazides, 171.
Thiazole ring, 128, **231**.
Thimecil, *see* Methylthiouracil.
Thioamides, 145.
Thiobarbiturates, 25.
Thiobarbituric acid, **25**.
Thiocyanate, 145.
— and thyroid, 148.
Thiol compounds, 200.
Thiomersal, 193.
Thiopentol, 26.
Thiopentone, 10.
— and methoxyflurane, 23.
— sodium, 24.
— —, duration of action of, 26.
Thiophene ring, 231.
Thiouracil, 146.
Thiourea, 145.
—, structure, 146.
Threadworms, 202–3.
Threshold dose, 215.
Thrombin, 138–9.
Thrombocytopenia, 208.
— and vinblastine, 209.
Thromboplastin, 138–40.
Thrombosis and contraceptives, 165.
Thymidine, 130.
Thyrocalcitonin, 133, **149**.
Thyroglobulin, 145–6.
Thyroid 145 et seq., 209.
— and TSH, 143.
— binding proteins, 146.
— deficiency, 147.
— hormones, structures, 145.
— hyperactivity, 147–8.
— inhibitors, 148.
— stimulator, long-acting, 143.

Thyrotoxic goitre and radioactive isotopes, 209.
Thyrotrophin, 99, **143**, 147.
Thyroxine, 142–3, **145–8**.
— and TSH, 143.
— — temperature, 113.
Tobacco, 63–4.
Tocopherols, *see also* Vitamin E, 134.
Tolazoline, 88.
—, structure, 89.
Tolbutamide, 151–2.
Tolerance to barbiturates, 27.
— — cocaine, 52.
— — morphine, 36.
— — nitrites, 106.
Tolnaftate, 192.
Toluidine blue, 138, 139.
Toxicity tests, 220, **226–7**.
Toxins, assay of, 211.
Tragacanth, 123.
Tranquillizing drugs, **31** et seq.
Transferrin, 135.
Transmitter release, 18.
Trans-retinene, 132.
Trans-vitamin A, 132.
Tranylcypromine, 41.
—, structure, 40.
Trasylol and bradykinin, 97.
Trematodes, 202, **204**.
Trial, clinical, 226–7.
Triamcinolone, 156.
Triamterene, 172.
—, structure, 171.
Triazole ring, 231.
Trichinella, 202.
Trichlorethylalcohol, 27.
Trichlorethylene and procaine, 53.
—, partition coefficient of, 22.
Trichuris trichiura, 203.
Tricyclic group, *see also* Dibenzazepine derivatives.
— — and noradrenaline, 90.
Triethanolamine nitrate, 106, 107.
Triethylcholine, **58**, 63.
Triethylenemelamine, 208.
Trifluoperazine, 32.
Triflupromazine, 31.
—, structure, 32.
3,4,6-trihydroxyphenylethylamine, 82.
Triiodothyronine, 145–7.
Trimethadione, *see* Troxidone.
Trimethoprim, 180, 184, 188.
— and sulphadiazine, 182.
— — sulphamethoxazole, 188.
—, structure, 181.
Trimethyl xanthines, 100.
Triphosphopyridine nucleotide, 129.

Index

Triple response, 92–3.
Tritium, 79, 81.
Trolnitrate, see Triethanolamine.
Trophozoites, 195–6.
Tropolone, 81.
Troxidone, 30.
Trypan blue, 177.
— red, 177.
Trypanosomes, 177, **200–1.**
Trypanosomiasis, 177.
—, structures of drugs used for, 201.
Tryparsamide, 177, **200.**
—, structure, 201.
Tryptophan, 94.
Tryptophan-5-hydroxylase, 94.
Tuberculosis and streptomycin, 191.
— — tetracycline, 187.
—, chemotherapy of, **191–2.**
Tubocurarine, 7, 55, **61,** 68, 72.
— and histamine release, 92.
—, excretion, 13.
—, structure, 71.
Tumours, chemotherapy of, 205 et seq.
Twin cross-over test, 220.
Typhoid and ampicillin, 187.
— — chloramphenicol, 189.
Tyramine, 81, 83, **87.**
— and monoamine oxidase inhibitors, 41.
— — noradrenaline, 82.
—, metabolism of, 13.
—, structure, **81,** 86.
Tyrode solution, 230.
Tyrosine, 7, **78–9,** 117.
— hydroxylase, 78.
—, structure, 80.
Tyrothricin, 183.

UDP, see Uridine diphosphate.
Ubiquinones, 140.
Ultralente insulin, 11.
Ultra-violet irradiation and vitamin D, 133.
Unit, definition of, 211.
Urea stibamine, 200.
Urethane, 209.
Uric acid and ACTH, 144.
— — — xanthines, 42.
— — excretion, 173–4.
— — and thiazides, **171.**
— —, structure, 174.
Uricase, 173.
Uricosuric drugs, 173–4.
—, structures, 175.
Uridine diphosphate, 182.
Urinary infections and sulphonamides, 188.

Urine pH alterants, 174–**5.**
Urochloralic acid, 27.
Urticaria, 94.
Uterus and ergometrine, 98.
— — menstrual cycle, 159.
— — oxytocin, 97, 145.
— — prostaglandins, 99.
— — serotonin, 95.
— — vasopressin, 97.

Vagus, 120.
— and atropine, 67.
— — cardiac glycosides, 108.
— — gastric secretion, 117.
— — peristalsis, 120.
'Vagus stuff', 224.
Valerylcholine, 3, 4, 6.
Vancomycin, 182.
Vanillic acid, 46.
Variance, 214.
Vasoconstriction and cocaine, 52.
— — ergot alkaloids, 98.
— — nicotine, 64.
Vasoconstrictor drugs and kidney, 168.
Vasodilatation and bradykinin, 96.
— — local anaesthetics, 50.
— — nicotinic acid, 129.
— — procaine, 53.
Vasomotor centres and xanthines, 42.
Vasopressin, see also Antidiuretic hormone, **97,** 145.
Venous return curve, 102.
Ventricular fibrillation, 110.
— — and cocaine, 52.
Veratridine, 105.
Veratrin alkaloids, 105, 119.
Vermifuges, **201** et seq.
Veronal, 26.
Vinblastine, 208–9.
—, structure, 207.
Vinca alkaloids, 208–9.
Vincristine, 208–9.
—, structure, 207.
Viomycin, 192.
Vision, see also Eye.
— and quinine, 198.
— — strychnine, 45.
— — vitamin A, 132–3.
Vitamin A, **132–3.**
— —, structure, 131.
— B$_1$, 126, **128.**
— —, structure, 127.
— B$_2$, 126, **128–9.**
— —, structure, 127.
— B$_6$, 126, 128, **129.**
— —, structure, 127.
— B$_{12}$, 126, 128, **130.**

— —, structure, 136.
— B$_c$, 130.
— B complex, **128** et seq.
— C, **125–6.**
— —, assay of, 212.
— —, structure, 127.
— D, **133.**
— — and liquid paraffin, 121.
— — — tetany, 149.
— —, deficiency, 133.
— D$_2$, 131, **133.**
— —, structure, 131.
— D$_3$, see 7-dehydrocholesterol, 133, 224.
— —, structure, 131.
— E, **134.**
— —, structure, 131.
— H, 126, 128, **130.**
— —, structure, 127.
— K, **134.**
— — and dicoumarol, 140–1.
— — — liquid paraffin, 121.
— K$_1$ and K$_2$, 134.
— — —, structures, 131.
— M, 130.
— P, **126,** 128.
— —, structure, 127.
Vitamins, assay of, 211, 216.
—, fat soluble, **132** et seq.
—, — —, structures, 131.
—, water soluble, **125** et seq.
—, — —, structures, 127.
Volatile and gaseous anaesthetics, **21–4.**
Volume, units of, 229.
Vomiting, 119.
— and actinomycin D, 209.
— — aminophylline, 100.
— — anthelminthics, 203.
— — antimony, 204.
— — arsenicals, 200.
— — chlorambucil, 207.
— — digitalis, 109.
— — ergot alkaloids, 98.
— — filix mas, 204.
— — iron, 136.
— — mercaptopurine, 208.
— — morphine, 35.
— — nicotine, 64.
— — nitrogen mustards, 206.
— — oestrogens, 160.
— — quinine, 198.
— — streptomycin, 191.
— — tetracyclines, 187.
— — urethane, 209.
— — veratrin alkaloids, 105.

Warfarin, 140–1.
Weight gain and corticosteroids, 158.

Weights, units of, 229.
Whipworm, 202–3.
Willow bark, 114.
Withdrawal symptoms of morphine, 36.
Withering, William, 107.
Work and xanthines, 42.
Worms, **201** et seq.
—, classification, 202.
Wuchereria bancrofti, 203.

Xanthine derivatives, **41–2**, 86, 100.
— — and gout, 174.
Xenon, 6.
Xylenol, 193.
Xylocholine, 83.

Yeasts, 192.
— and antibiotics, 182.
— — nystatin, 185.

Yohimbine, 88.
—, structure, 89.

Zinc oxide, 123.
— salts of insulin, 11.
— — as astringents, 123.
— sulphate as emetic, 119.
— suspension insulin injections, 151.
'Zone of inexcitability', 61.